Practice Management Consultant

A Compendium of Articles From Practice Management Online

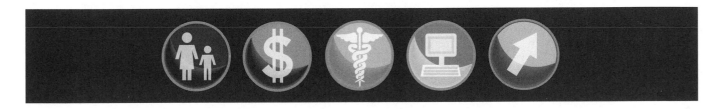

American Academy of Pediatrics

DEDICATED TO THE HEALTH OF ALL CHILDREN™

Library of Congress Control Number: 2009910006
ISBN: 978-1-58110-374-8
MA0534

Table of Contents

Introduction

In many ways, pediatric practices are in a state of economic crisis in a rapidly changing health care environment. From vaccine payment and supply issues to competition from large-scale retail-based clinics, pediatric practices both large and small are facing many business issues and constraints. In order to provide high-quality care and to survive in today's health care environment, pediatricians and their office staff must

- Stay abreast of important business and practice management aspects of a pediatric medical practice in the same way they stay current on medical/clinical information.
- Ensure the stability and potential for growth of pediatric practice through rapidly changing times—mergers and acquisitions of hospitals and clinics, consumer-driven health plans, performance-based payment, increased regulations, and increasing overhead and shrinking margins.
- Have a system in place to quickly integrate new practice concepts and knowledge into the standard processes of the practice.
- Have practical, easily accessible business and practice management information available when it is needed.

Historically there has been little or no preparation in residency programs for the business aspects of practice. With that in mind, the American Academy of Pediatrics (AAP), an organization of 60,000 pediatricians, has developed an extensive collection of pediatric-specific practice management resources to assist pediatricians with managing a practice that provides high-quality care and is financially viable.

This compendium, *Practice Management Consultant*, is a collection of key articles from the *Practice Management Online* (PMO) Web site (http://practice.aap.org), a comprehensive and continually updated online practice resource for AAP members. Many of the articles in this compendium have never before appeared in print!

The compendium covers a wide variety of practice management topics that are pertinent to both new practices just being set up and mature, "well-oiled" practices—and everyone in-between. The articles are organized by general categories.

- Getting Started/Practice Basics
- Office Operations
- Business Considerations and Contracts
- Employment/Personnel
- Finance and Payment
- Medical Liability and Risk Management
- Patient Management
- Quality Improvement
- Medical Home
- Physician Health/Wellness
- Career Transitions

There is also a helpful appendix that includes many sample office forms and letters that can be used to inspire your own office documents (and be sure to visit PMO for even more samples). As you will see, *Practice Management Consultant* is destined to become an integral part of your successful practice, and will be valued by both physicians and office staff.

I'd like to thank several people who have been involved in the evolution of PMO from the beginning—bringing that terrific resource from an idea to reality and thus inspiring this print compendium. These include a small group of AAP members from the Section on Administration and Practice Management and the Committee on Practice and Ambulatory Medicine—Anne Francis, MD; Norman "Chip" Harbaugh, MD; Robert Walker, MD; and Jerald Zarin, MD—and AAP staff members Heather Fitzpatrick, Sunnah Kim, Jeff Mahony, Robert Sebring (retired), Mark Grimes, Maureen DeRosa, and Ed Zimmerman. Eventually a larger PMO Editorial Advisory Board was formed (see current listing in this compendium's front matter) that has helped guide the continuing enhancements to the site and its valuable content. And I'd like to thank Trisha Calabrese, an AAP staffer who now is dedicated full time to PMO, who has been indispensible in keeping the site the most essential resource for the business needs of pediatricians.

Jerald L. Zarin, MD, MBA, FAAP
Chair, Practice Management Online Editorial Advisory Board

Section 1

Getting Started/Practice Basics

Residency Training in General Pediatrics (Medical Students)

Excerpt from Pediatrics 101

Pediatric residency training consists of a 3-year program of core pediatric experiences and elective rotations that follows successful completion of medical school. Individuals are eligible to sit for the certification examination administered by the American Board of Pediatrics only after completion of a residency program accredited by the Residency Review Committee (RRC) for Pediatrics of the Accreditation Council for Graduate Medical Education (ACGME). It is the Pediatric RRC that sets the requirements for accredited programs.

Residency education is primarily centered in university, children's, community, and military hospitals. As changes in the health care system result in more care being provided in the ambulatory and community environment, clinical experiences during residency in these settings are also becoming more commonplace.

Although individual residency programs may vary in setting, size, patient population, and resident number, their common goal is to provide educational experiences that prepare graduates to be competent general pediatricians. It is expected that graduates of these programs will be able to provide comprehensive, coordinated care to a broad range of children from birth through adolescence and young adulthood. To accomplish this goal, all programs must provide experience in the following areas*:

- Inpatient pediatric care including children with general and subspecialty problems acute and chronic in nature
- Emergency and acute illness care in emergency department and ambulatory clinic settings
- Continuity care, during which residents take care of a group of pediatric patients longitudinally over the course of their residency, usually in a weekly clinic

- Normal/term newborn care, including longitudinal follow-up of infants discharged from the nursery
- Subspecialty care, including required rotations in neonatal and pediatric intensive care. Required months devoted to adolescent medicine and developmental/behavioral pediatrics complement a minimum of 6 months of other subspecialty elective rotations chosen from a list provided by the Pediatric RRC.

TIP: **The American Board of Pediatrics offers 2 special routes for pediatrician scientists who are qualified to shorten pediatric training by 1 year or combine research with their residency training. More information on these opportunities—the Accelerated Research Pathway, the Integrated Research Pathway, and the Special Alternative Pathway—is available from the American Board of Pediatrics.**

Throughout their 3 years of training, residents participate in regularly scheduled teaching/attending rounds and conferences, where issues including medical ethics, quality assessment and improvement, medical informatics, and health care financing are covered in addition to the clinical aspects of care. Pediatric residency programs also provide training in the procedural skills necessary to provide routine and critical/resuscitative care to children. And to further enhance their academic skills, residents are also required to participate in scholarly experiences such as journal club, academic conferences, and clinical and/or basic research activities.

There are 203 accredited pediatric residency programs to choose from in the United States. In some larger programs, there may exist different tracks, for example, one that may place greater emphasis on primary

---

* Accreditation Council for Graduate Medical Education. Program requirements for residency education in pediatrics. ACGME Web site. Available at: www.acgme.org/req/320pr701.asp.

care training or another that may focus on preparation for a career in academic medicine or research. Information on programs and their educational resources is available online from the Fellowship and Residency Interactive Database (FREIDA) sponsored by the American Medical Association as well as the ACGME Web site. In addition, the American Board of Pediatrics (ABP) offers 3 special routes for pediatrician scientists who may be qualified to shorten their training by 1 year or combine research with their residency training. More information on these opportunities—Accelerated Research Pathway, Integrated Research Pathway, and Special Alternative Pathway—is available from the ABP. And lastly, for those who wish to be eligible to sit for both the ABP Certifying Examination and the American Board of Internal Medicine Certifying Examination, there are 4-year programs designated as medicine-pediatrics residency programs that fulfill the requirements of both boards. Information about medicine-pediatrics programs accredited by the ACGME can also be found on the ACGME Web site.

Regardless of the particular program, pediatric residency training is designed to confer the knowledge, skills, and attitudes required for comprehensive, longitudinal, and child-centered health care. Pediatric residents learn to consider behavioral, psychosocial, environmental, and family-unit correlates of disease. They learn to care for children who are chronically ill and manage acute events, as well as promote wellness and prevention. Because pediatric residents work with so many other members of the health care team in the management of children, they learn to be collaborative in their approach to care. Although pediatric residency training can be physically, intellectually, and emotionally challenging, it is this common devotion to the care and well-being of children that makes pediatricians among the most professionally satisfied of all physicians.

Licensure and Board Certification (Residents)

Excerpt from Pediatrics 101

The National Board of Medical Examiners® (NBME®) and the Federation of State Medical Boards (FSMB) sponsor the United States Medical Licensing Examination™ (USMLE™).

Students and graduates of medical schools in the United States and Canada that are accredited by the Liaison Committee on Medical Education or the American Osteopathic Association Bureau of Professional Education register for the USMLE with the NBME.

Students and graduates of medical schools outside the United States and Canada register for the USMLE with the Educational Commission for Foreign Medical Graduates.

Medical students take the 3-part examination during medical school and residency. After passing all 3 parts, they are eligible to apply for their medical license.

According to the USMLE, most medical students take Step 1 of the in-training examination after the second year of medical school, Step 2 during the fourth year of medical school, and Step 3 during the first or second year of residency.

Medical licenses are granted by state boards of medical examiners. Medical students who plan to practice in another state are advised to apply for a medical license with that state's licensing board as early as possible (generally early in the third year of residency). Links to individual state boards are on the American Medical Association (AMA) Web site (www.ama-assn.org/ama/pub/category/2543.html).

This is also the time to apply for a federal Drug Enforcement Administration number, which permits physicians to prescribe controlled substances.

Certification by the American Board of Pediatrics (ABP)

In 2003 the 78% certification rate for pediatricians exceeded the national average (72%) as well as the rate of certification among internal medicine physicians (74%).

According to the ABP, physicians must complete the following steps to sit for the board certification examination:

1. Graduate from an accredited medical school in the United States or Canada or a foreign medical school recognized by the World Health Organization.
2. Complete 3 years of training in pediatrics in an accredited residency program.
3. Verify satisfactory completion of residency training.
4. Acquire a valid, unrestricted state license to practice medicine.
5. Pass the 2-day written examination for certification.

Board certification in pediatrics may be renewed every 7 years by successfully completing the program for maintenance of certification in pediatrics, which includes passing a recertification examination.

Online Resources

From the American Academy of Pediatrics
- PREP: Pediatrics Review and Education Program contact information: www.aap.org/profed/prep.htm
- *Career Planning: How to Prepare for the Boards,* dates for scheduled board review courses, information about audio courses and books: www.aap.org/sections/resident/prepareboards.htm

From the AMA
- *Getting a License—The Basics,* an article by the FSMB that sketches out considerations for those applying for a medical license; related links provide information about guides to state licensure requirements and links to national organizations: www.ama-assn.org/ama/pub/category/2644.html

From the USMLE
Review steps 1, 2, and 3 of the examination
- Web site: www.usmle.org/

From the ABP
- General examination admission requirements: www.abp.org/
- A description of the ABP and the subspecialty certificates it awards: www.abp.org/
- A description of subspecialty certificates awarded in conjunction with other certifying boards, with contact information: www.abp.org/

Introduction to AAP Sections and Councils

Sections

More than half of the American Academy of Pediatrics (AAP) membership belong to one or more sections. Sections were developed within the AAP for members who share a pediatric subspecialty, surgical specialty, special area of interest, or stage of life. Sections cultivate ideas and develop programs within their subspecialty or special interest that improve the care of infants, children, adolescents, and young adults. Although their primary goal may be education of colleagues, sections are also involved in policy development, public education, and advocacy for children. As a section member, you will have the opportunity to share ideas with and learn from colleagues who share your specific interests and/or subspecialty background.

Councils

Councils represent one of the newer opportunities within the AAP. They represent the evolution of sections and committees working in the same field into a new, integrated structure. Each council is the primary source of expertise in a given field within the AAP. An executive committee of elected leaders governs each council. Although councils fulfill the functions traditionally held separately by national committees and sections, their scope, as a single entity, is expanded to encompass a broader vision and a wider array of activities. Councils generate policy, create educational programming and resources, develop and promote advocacy initiatives, support translation of policy and education into practice, and integrate and evaluate these efforts to maximize impact. The council structure is designed to give members a strong voice in policy development and in other council activities.

For more information about the development of councils, see the council fact sheet (http://www.aap.org/sections/councilfactsheet2005.pdf) and an article (http://aapnews.aappublications.org/cgi/content/full/26/6/7) published in the June 2005 issue of *AAP News.*

Both sections and councils have an executive committee and subcommittees, so leadership opportunities are bountiful. Members are eligible to join multiple sections and councils that are of interest to them based on their member type and the membership criteria established by the section and/or council.

For information on specific sections and councils, visit their home pages (http://www.aap.org/sections/shome.htm). To apply online, visit www.aap.org/moc/memberservices/sectionform.cfm.

For information on membership, contact the AAP Division of Member Services at 800/433-9016 or membership@aap.org.

American Academy of Pediatrics Chapter Pediatric Councils

Chapter pediatric councils are forums whereby pediatricians meet with health plan medical directors to discuss carrier policies and administrative practices affecting access to, quality of, coverage of, and payment for pediatric services. Chapters with established pediatric councils report that they have been instrumental in bringing pediatric issues to the attention of health plans and affecting change. Pediatric councils have the potential to facilitate better working relationships between pediatricians and health insurance plans and improve quality of care for children. Ideally, changes may lead to more appropriate coverage for pediatric services, as well as smoothly and efficiently run pediatric practices and health plan claims adjudication. A pediatric council is not a forum for joint contract negotiation, individual contract discussion, or other fee-related concerns. Visit www.aap.org/moc/reimburse/pedcouncil/default.htm for chapter-specific resources on developing and maintaining pediatric councils.

Resources for Chapters

The American Academy of Pediatrics (AAP) encourages chapter development of pediatric councils and has made available resources to assist chapters in developing and maintaining pediatric councils.

- Pediatric Council Start-up Kit: http://www.aap.org/securemoc/reimburse/PedCou1.pdf
- Letter to health plans about pediatric councils: http://www.aap.org/securemoc/reimburse/pediatriccouncils.pdf
- Pediatric Council Webinar on Vaccine Financing: http://www.aap.org/securemoc/reimburse/webinarvaccinearchive.doc
- Pediatric Council Immunization Toolkit: http://www.aap.org/securemoc/reimburse/pcit/pcit.htm
- Pediatric council e-mail distribution list
- Monthly Updates on Private Payer Advocacy: http://www.aap.org/securemoc/reimburse/PSAUpdates.htm
- Online Hassle Factor Form to report and prioritize payer issues: http://www.aap.org/securemoc/reimburse/hasslefactor/

For information on AAP private payer advocacy, contact the Division of Health Care Finance and Quality Improvement at dhcfqi@aap.org.

Chapters With Pediatric Councils by District (and Year Started) as of November 2007									
I	II	III	IV	V	VI	VII	VIII	IX	X
CT (2005) MA (1996) RI (2006)	NY 1 (2006) NY 2 (2002) NY 3 (2007)	MD (2004) NJ (2000) PA (2001) WV (2006)	KY (2006) NC (2002) SC (2002) TN (2004) VA (2002)	MI (2005) OH (2005)	IA (2006) IL (2007) KA (2005) WI (2004)	AK (2007) MS (2007) TX (2005)	AZ (2007) CO (2007) HI (2004) MT (2007) NM (2006) UT (2004)	CA (2007) (All 4 California chapters formed a district-wide council.)	FL (2002) PR (2007)

Opening a Practice: A Pediatrician's Perspective

"I love walking into my office in the morning and realizing it really is mine."

Stan Sack, MD, FAAP
Member of the American Academy of Pediatrics
Section on Administration and Practice Management

Stan Sack, MD, FAAP, always desired an opportunity to reside and practice pediatrics in Florida. Unexpectedly, he received information from a hospital that was recruiting a pediatrician to start a practice in Key West, FL. In return, the pediatrician would be provided with start-up expenses and an income guarantee. The location made this opportunity very desirable to Dr Sack, so he applied. As he went through the interview process, it became apparent that there was a clear need for his services, which made the opportunity even more attractive.

Soon after he accepted the offer, he spent his first several months in the practice of his employer/predecessor. This provided him with an opportunity to meet future patients and families and for them to get to know him as well. It also gave him insight into how to manage a solo practice. After his employer/predecessor left the practice, Dr Sack remained in the same office and kept the same patients. In addition, he retained the staff—an office manager/biller, a registered nurse, and a part-time receptionist. As part of his arrangement with the hospital, Dr Sack used the services of the public relations department to market his newfound practice. He continuously advertised his practice in the local newspaper and provided presentations on the local cable station. Moreover, because his office is located on the major route through town, he displayed a prominent sign advertising his practice. Finally, Dr Sack reserved a phone number with the word PEDS in it.

As Dr Sack began to build a practice of his own, his state medical society provided him with a practice management consultant. Because Dr Sack is a member of his medical society, he received this benefit at no charge. In addition, Dr Sack paid the consultant a small stipend to review his business plan.

As he established his own practice, Dr Sack set his fees based on those that were established by his predecessor. Going forward, he feels that it will be important to learn more about negotiating effectively.

Dr Sack admits that the biggest challenge in opening a practice was figuring out what needed to be done and in what order.

He states that his most valuable lessons learned were

- Start as early as you can.
- Try your best to prioritize and learn what takes the longest.
- Use other local physicians as resources. Physicians in your specialty are also very helpful. He believes that had he consulted with them earlier, he probably could have saved quite a bit of money on several fronts.
- "If you really want to do it, don't be afraid—it remains to be seen if I will be financially flush, but if someone as non-entrepreneurial by nature as [me] can get this far, anyone can!"

Dr Sack advises anyone considering opening a practice to weigh everything and question yourself. In the end, for the right opportunity and location, he believes that it's worth it. He admits that opening a practice takes a lot of hard work and planning; however, if you surround yourself with the right people, it makes the job much easier. While there are many concessions, sacrifices, and vagaries (eg, where is health insurance going to come from when the Consolidated Omnibus Budget Reconciliation Act [COBRA] runs out), there are many unexpected benefits too.

If you are interested in starting your own practice and have questions, you can e-mail Dr Sack directly at stnsck@aol.com.

Practice Types

Excerpt from Launching Your Career in Pediatrics Handbook: Getting Started

There are a variety of practice options and structures available to pediatricians. Following is an overview of the various structures.

Solo Practice

Solo practices are for pediatricians who want to own and manage their own practice. This physician is responsible for all aspects of the practice, including establishing policies and guidelines, staffing, office hours, finances, and legal.

Expense Sharing

This type of practice may be as simple as 2 pediatricians sharing office space and staff but operating as

Solo Versus Group Practice

Solo Practice	Group Practice	Hospital Owned	Federally Qualified Health Center	Academic Health Center
More individual freedom	Less individual practice freedom	Not as much physician autonomy	Not as much physician autonomy	Not as much physician autonomy
Longer work hours—clinical and business	Shorter work hours	Work on a schedule	Work on a schedule	Work on a schedule
Complete responsibility for the business	Less need to be involved in business aspects	Subject to employee constraints	Subject to employee constraints	Subject to employee constraints
High public/patient visibility	Less personal visibility with public and patients	Marketing department	Marketing department	Marketing department
Extremes of financial return	Built-in on-call coverage	Centralized patient record keeping	Centralized patient record keeping	Centralized patient record keeping
Business risk	Lower medicolegal/business risk	Low to no legal/business risk	Low to no legal/business risk	Low to no legal/business risk
Less opportunity for informal professional consultations	More opportunity for informal professional consultations	Required referral patterns	Required referral patterns	Required referral patterns
More limited working capital	Access to larger amounts of working capital	Cost allocation to physicians	Limitations due to federal funding regulations	Access to larger amounts of working capital

Possible administrative limitations |
Total involvement in business concerns	Less opportunity for involvement in business concerns	System-determined decisions	System-determined decisions	System-determined decisions
High-tech practice will depend on expenses	Greater chances to be involved in high-tech practice	Better access to equipment and better equipment	Better access to equipment and better equipment	Better access to equipment and better equipment
Set growth pattern	More limits on rapid income growth	Steady flow of income	Steady flow of income	Steady flow of income
Determine benefit structure	Established benefit structure	Established benefit structure	Established benefit structure	Established benefit structure

Source: American Academy of Pediatrics Committee on Practice and Ambulatory Medicine. *Management of Pediatric Practice.* 2nd ed. Elk Grove Village, IL: American Academy of Pediatrics; 1991 and American Academy of Pediatrics. *A Guide to Starting a Medical Office.* Elk Grove Village, IL: American Academy of Pediatrics; 1997.

independent practices. This provides some relief from the financial burden of overhead and office operations and provides some relief from finding night-call coverage. Patients should be made well aware that the 2 physicians have separate practices. If there is no written agreement and patients assume that the physicians are partners, both physicians may be implicated in malpractice litigation.

Partnership

A partnership is an association of 2 or more persons for the purpose of carrying on as co-owners of a business for profit. The partners in this arrangement invest together to make a profit. In this structure, each partner has equal rights and management and also shares the risks and responsibilities. New partners are usually brought in after acquiring the consent of all existing partners. Like marriages, there needs to be compatibility in medical practice and management philosophies among partners. Partners can also expect to receive a formal accounting of all partnership affairs. On the other hand, all partners may be liable for each individual partner's wrong acts or acts of commission or omission assumed by the partnership as a whole, inviting individual liability for any legal action against the partnership. Also, in much the same way partnership gains are shared equally, so may losses be expected to be shared.

Multi-specialty (Large and Small)

Single-specialty groups pool the resources of several pediatricians. The legal arrangement becomes important and is essential to define the roles and responsibilities of the partners. Multi-specialty groups provide a pool of other medical and management skills, but with significantly less personal autonomy.

Corporate Practice

Working for a large corporate health care provider is another option. Corporate practice reduces the personal and financial risk to the individual physician, while also providing opportunities to shelter income through a qualified retirement program. A large health maintenance organization (HMO) office allows pediatricians to practice without business or administrative concerns. This provides a great deal of security in terms of salary and benefits and eliminates the need to be concerned about administrative and business aspects of practice. Government and federal health care facilities provide another practice outlet.

Academic practices provide many of the same benefits. Lastly, niche practices such as emergency department or delivery room coverage, working with specific disease entities like obesity, or substance abuse centers provide yet another practice outlet. Advantages include limited liability to the individual practitioner, centralized management, continuity of life beyond the career trajectories of existing physicians, pension and profit-sharing plans that may be superior to solo practice or partnerships, tax incentives, and presence of other benefits that are more cost-efficient because of scale (eg, health benefit, life insurance, disability, malpractice discount). Disadvantages include need for an extensive organization to manage personnel, legal paperwork, tax, and accounting; need for higher start-up costs; and potential tax consequences (eg, corporate vs income tax). Corporate practices may exist in several forms—HMO groups, government or federal health care centers, hospital-based practices (eg, academic groups, hospitalist groups, emergency department physicians), and boutique practices (eg, substance abuse, surgical centers). These may all be structured very differently depending on local standards, community and state laws, and preferences of organizing groups. Each may have various arrangements for a physician's role and responsibility within the group, including profit sharing, vesting time, amount of call, and academic partnerships.

Academic and Hospital-Based Practices

With the growing demands of outpatient practices, hospital-based practices are growing in almost every community. They may develop as an initiative of local physicians, or hospitals may choose to contract with them. They may offer around-the-clock care that primary physicians find difficult to provide. Having hospitalists has been shown to improve quality measures—including length of stay, mortality, and 30-day readmission rate—in several common inpatient diagnoses. Evidence also shows that hospitalists reduce costs and length of stay while achieving the same or better patient outcomes achieved by non-hospitalists. Hospitalists often practice in group-type structures; they may be simple informal arrangements among a group of physicians within a community who share hospital calls with or without teaching responsibilities, or they may be more elaborate corporate organizations that employ individual physicians. Some may even be organized on a national scale, with local "franchises" that operate within a community but are answerable to corporate headquarters. They may cover one or multiple hospitals depending on the demand and the particular relationships that exist between the group and hospital administration. In much the same way corporations offer benefits of scale in terms of sharing expenses, employee benefits, and tax advantage, groups that are more organized offer the advantage of monitoring the quality of care provided by their physicians. These groups may have methods in place to assess outcomes, lengths of stay, patient satisfaction, and reimbursement values.

Physicians who practice within such a setting report the following advantages:

- Satisfaction of working within a team
- Satisfaction of contributing to the improvement of inpatient care or hospital processes
- Flexibility of work hours (ie, not necessarily 9:00 am–5:00 pm)
- Opportunities for various educational interactions (eg, with other specialists, residents, medical students)
- Opportunity to have nonmedical responsibilities (eg, administration, quality assurance) as much or as little as one wants
- Large variety of clinical cases, which are often acute and whose successful outcomes provide enormous satisfaction
- Being kept on one's toes

Most physicians who work in this setting will report difficulty and even boredom with the daily grind of an office practice, which often seems to involve the same medical problems over and over. These physicians also perceive the business side of keeping a practice afloat not to their liking. They express a high comfort level with a hospital setting and the pace that such work involves. On the other hand, depending on the level of specialty required, length of training time, and challenge of working in a high-pressure field that may be dominated by males, some women may not find this to be a suitable practice alternative. Furthermore, practice turnover may turn the work hours from an advantage to a disadvantage, since regardless of the number of covering physicians, the group will still be committed to providing 24/7 care.

Physicians in practice transitioning to or new graduates contemplating a hospitalist position should ask themselves a number of questions.

- What is the nature of the organization? Is it a corporation, a partnership among physicians, or a hospital-based group? Will a physician be an employee of the corporation or of the hospital? What is the basis of the corporation's relationship to the hospital?
- What is the organizational structure? Who will serve as my direct supervisor(s) and what are his or her responsibilities?
- What is the group's composition? Are they all general pediatricians? Are there family or nurse practitioners? Who are the actual physicians participating in the call rotation? What are the responsibilities of each physician who takes calls? What is the call rotation schedule?
- Are there outpatient responsibilities or emergency department coverage apart from inpatient calls? Where will these be conducted?
- Which hospitals does the group cover? If more than one, are there different responsibilities or expectations with each hospital setting? Are the patient load and population different with each hospital? If one is relocating, what is the approximate distance between each hospital and one's residence? Is there a central office location for the group?
- What are other physician responsibilities apart from direct patient care? Are there administrative duties or teaching responsibilities? Are these expected, required, or optional? If one were to supervise or teach, does this involve nurse practitioners, physician assistants, other nursing personnel, residents, or medical students?
- Does the group have subspecialty or surgical support? If so, who and where? Does it require transferring patients from a primary hospital to a tertiary one?
- What is the rate of physician reimbursement? What is the basis of this scale (eg, seniority, productivity, patient load, call load)? How is one's productivity calculated and what factors go into this calculation? How does one's productivity affect compensation and future raises?
- What benefits are offered to physicians? Do these include health coverage, malpractice liability, other insurance coverage, and retirement funds? If transferring from another practice, will the group offer tail coverage?

- What constitutes terms of separation, termination, and contractual breach? Are there any restrictive covenants (eg, geographic practice restrictions)?
- What are the laws of the state governing all of this and what are the responsibilities and liabilities if one assumes this position? You may need to consult your state medical board or a local lawyer.

Retail-Based Clinics (RBCs)

While the AAP does not support the RBC model of care for children, families are using these types of clinics. Located in retail settings (eg, pharmacies, supermarkets), these clinics provide families with a convenient location and the ability to multitask. While this may seem like a benefit to the family, the care provided at an RBC is very limited and only fragments the medical home. Practices must educate their patients on the importance of the medical home, but also provide a practice setting that meets the needs of busy families today. Practices must acknowledge the changing health care market and respond to remain competitive. Providing a medical home for patients can be challenging financially and administratively, but it is the best model of care for children.

More resources on RBCs can be found on *Practice Management Online* at http://practice.aap.org/content.aspx?aID=1511.

Credentialing

Excerpt from Launching Your Career in Pediatrics Handbook: Opening a New Practice

The process of becoming credentialed to open a medical practice is time consuming and laborious, and involves lag time in terms of completion. When beginning, be aware of which processes take the longest and which are more rapid and straightforward, and prioritize accordingly. Although universal applications exist for some issues, they are rare, and there is little way around the busywork to be done. However, many applications ask for the same information, and keeping essential data handy and organized can save time. Be prepared to budget at least a few thousand dollars for the process. Some entities do not charge a fee; others do. Additionally, unanticipated expenses may be incurred, such as getting duplicates of appropriately sized diplomas. At times you may have to depend on organizations and individuals to send the necessary information. Check with your state medical society for state-specific information.

American Board of Pediatrics

The American Board of Pediatrics (ABP) offers certification in general pediatrics as well as pediatric specialties. This information will be needed when going through the credentialing process. The ABP also maintains Maintenance of Certification. Visit http://www.abp.org for more information.

Obtaining Hospital Privileges

Hospital credentialing committees meet periodically, usually monthly. It can take several months to be approved, so start early. Fortunately, many hospitals accept that privileges are applied for and do not require the process to be complete before processing applications. Also, many hospitals will grant temporary privileges, if needed, before the credentialing process is complete.

Credentialing With Health Insurers

Most large insurers and all managed care organizations (MCOs) will require credentialing for participation as a provider in their plans. It is necessary to start this credentialing process as soon as you have enough of the required information to do so; many insurers take 3 to 6 months and, at times, a preapplication step is required as well. Some hospitals offer credentialing services for a fee, which may save considerable time. These services often are able to negotiate contracts with insurers. For information on universal credentialing, visit http://practice.aap.org/content.aspx?aid=2196. Another solution is to access Council on Affordable Quality Healthcare online at www.CAQH.org, which provides a single application for many payers.

Occupational Safety and Health Administration

All practices must be in compliance with Occupational Safety and Health Administration standards. These encompass a large number of requirements including employee dress, waste disposal, and universal precautions. While meeting some of these requirements is straightforward and intuitive, some may entail a process that takes several weeks. Biohazard removal, for example, may require a scheduled educational session before the office can be set up to handle biomedical waste. Thus it is worthwhile to address this at least several weeks before anticipated opening. For additional information, visit www.osha.gov.

Employer Identification Number

All businesses require an employer identification number, also known as a federal tax identification number. Your practice attorney or accountant can obtain one for you. It is also possible to obtain one online. Plan on a few weeks for this process.

State Tax Identification Number

Check with your state to see if a separate state tax identification number is required. A link to state agencies, as well as information on obtaining a federal tax identification number, can be found at www.irs.gov.

State Medical License

Whether you are starting your own practice or entering private practice as a physician employee, it is extremely important to start your license application early. States differ in their approach, but it is not unheard of for a license to take a year or more to obtain.

It is not unreasonable to begin the license application process before deciding on an ultimate location.

Begin to gather information from all colleges and universities, as well as your medical school, residency, and places of employment on the forwarding of all of your records. Most will want copies of diplomas, residency certificates, and board certification. Be prepared to explain any breaks in the educational process and don't forget courses taken elsewhere. When in doubt, it is best to be thorough, honest, and complete with any explanations.

Some states have extra requirements, such as a special examination or letters of recommendation. Read the application early so none of these requirements are missed; notification from state boards on missing material is often slow and can waste valuable time. Most states have an online information system that informs you of the process, needed materials, and contact information specific to that state.

Drug Enforcement Administration

An application should be filed with the Drug Enforcement Administration (DEA) for a DEA number, which is required to prescribe any medication. This is usually a fairly rapid process. Individuals who already have a DEA number should keep the agency informed of any address changes. For more information, visit www.deadiversion.usdoj.gov.

State Narcotics License

Check with the state medical board to see if a separate state-controlled substance license or permit is required. It is usually less involved to obtain this than the medical license itself.

National Physician Identifier

In 2008 a requirement was initiated for all physicians to have a unique National Physician Identifier (NPI) number. Among other uses, it is the number recognized by most insurance payers and is necessary for payment for services. This is usually a fairly straightforward process. Apply at www.cms.hhs.gov/NationalProvidentstand.

Business License

In addition to federal and state licensing, be sure to check with your city and county about the possible need for obtaining a business license. If needed, this is usually an inexpensive, routine process and in most cases can be done after some of the more involved tasks are completed. Be aware of specific requirements—most will want a copy of your medical license, and many will want information about your location, including access and trash removal.

Laboratory License

Decide if you would like to have an in-house laboratory and, if so, what tests you will be performing. Any testing at all—even a rapid test for blood in the stool—requires an application with Clinical Laboratory Improvement Amendments (CLIA) (http://wwwn.cdc.gov/clia). This is a process that may take several months and is worth starting earlier rather than later. Some states charge additional fees and have an additional application process for in-house laboratories. A CLIA license is not required if all testing is to be sent out.

Assessing the Community

Excerpt from Launching Your Career in Pediatrics Handbook: Getting Started

Whether you are considering opening a practice, joining a practice, or relocating, there are a number of things to consider before making the final decision. In real estate, the 3 most important considerations when buying a house are location, location, and location! The same is true of a pediatric practice. Many of the decisions about practices and lifestyles will be determined by your preferences about where you would like to live and work.

Following are some tips on selecting a community in which to practice:

- The most basic approach to assess the requirements for pediatricians is to determine the employment opportunities and competition for patients.
- Consider trends in the local obstetrician demographics.
- Contact the local chamber of commerce to find migration trends and the opening of schools, homes, and hospitals. This is often a good predictor of whether the location will be viable.
- It is important to know if the community in which you plan to practice is a younger community with new families emerging or an aging retirement community.
- Identify where patients live. The rule of thumb is that patients will drive 20 minutes to see a doctor. Any farther, patients will look for a doctor closer to where they live. However, this rule may not apply to rural physicians.
- Consider the number of retail-based clinics (RBCs) in your area. If there are no RBCs, this is a good time to establish your pediatric office in a central location near a major retail location to get ahead of the competition in the future. If RBCs do exist, make sure the practice you are starting or joining is providing competitive hours and values customer service. Families are using RBCs mainly out of convenience. If your practice can compete by providing the same or better level of convenience, your expertise as a pediatrician will far outweigh the services provided at an RBC. It's a win-win situation for you and your patients. More resources

on RBCs can be found on the AAP Practice Management Online Web site at http://practice.aap.org/content.aspx?aID=1511.
- Consider the number of pediatric care professionals in the area.

Urban Versus Rural Locations

There are many differences between practicing in a rural versus an urban location. Those who choose to practice in a rural area usually prefer to do so in an effort to use all skills learned during residency. It is common for practicing pediatricians in rural areas to perform resuscitations, intubations, and lumbar punctures. It is often their responsibility to stabilize and care for children who are chronically ill. See Table 1 (http://pediatrics.aappublications.org/cgi/content/full/107/2/e18/T1) in "Trends in the Rural-Urban Distribution of General Pediatricians" *(Pediatrics.* 2001;107:e18) for more information.

Practicing in an Urban or Rural Population	
Urban	**Rural**
More technology	Less technology
More networking opportunities	Independent practitioner with fewer networking opportunities
Fewer on-call and weekend hours	Need to be available more (on call, after hours, and weekends)
More commuting time	Larger salaries
More physicians = more competition	Greater need = less competition
Access to subspecialists and children's hospitals	Often will need to contract with subspecialists

Where Children and Their Families Go for Health Care

The American Academy of Pediatrics partnered with Dartmouth Medical School, Center for the Evaluative Clinical Sciences, to develop Mapping Health Care Delivery for America's Children (http://www.aap.org/mapping/). This Web site provides the status of current available national, state, and city data on the following:

- Children younger than 18 years per clinically active pediatrician
- Percentage of clinically active pediatricians who are female
- Median household income
- Percentage of Hispanic children younger than 18 years
- Percentage of children 5 to 17 years old in linguistically isolated households

It is important to note that while some areas in the United States seem to have a large number of pediatricians, these pediatricians are still employed and working.

Marketing Your Pediatric Practice

There are 2 important considerations when marketing your practice. First, if you are looking to acquire new patients, you will want to develop a marketing strategy aimed at attracting new patients. Some tips are provided in this article. Next, it is important to ensure that your existing patients are satisfied with the care that you provide. Happy patients will refer their friends and family!

There are a variety of ways to market your practice.

- **Get involved in the community and make your name and practice known.** Consider sponsoring events or newsletters in the community, get involved at local child care centers, speak to parent groups, meet local obstetricians and gynecologists, become familiar to the nurses in the maternity ward at the local hospital, and publish health articles in the local newspaper.
- **Advertise.** Provide brochures or flyers throughout your community. Be sure to include pharmacies, schools, child care centers, newspapers, cable stations, local obstetricians' and gynecologists' offices, and yellow pages. Consider writing a column for the local newspaper or do a radio show, if possible.
- **Web site.** Create a Web site for your practice. The Web site should include your office hours, staff and providers, and overall policies of the practice. Be sure to tell the potential patient why he or she should visit your practice.

Most importantly, provide excellent care to your current patients.

Tips to Increase Patient Satisfaction

- Consider doing a follow-up phone call on all sick visits.
- Provide patients with monthly or quarterly newsletters via e-mail. Compiling an e-mail list can be done by contracting with outside vendors or maintaining a current list of your patients' e-mails. This is a great way to address common questions or remind patients of influenza season.
- Consider extending office hours (eg, 7 days a week, evening hours). This is especially important if you are competing with retail-based clinics.
- When educating patients and families, be sure that they understand your instructions. Be sure that when creating educational materials, you consider the readability level (should be at the eighth-grade level). For additional information on health literacy, visit www.aap.org/commpeds/resources/health_literacy.html.
- Be sure that your office staff are friendly, patient, and empathetic. If patients have a bad experience with office staff, they are likely to change providers.
- Limit the amount of time that patients are to wait in rooms to be seen.
- Be up front with your patient policies and ask patients to sign a copy of the policy.
- Be sensitive when handling patient complaints. Visit http://practice.aap.org/content.aspx?aid=1258 for tips.
- Conduct a patient survey to find out what your patients think. A sample can be found at http://practice.aap.org/content.aspx?aID=2374.

See the Section on Administration and Practice Management e-mail list conversation summary titled "Marketing Your Pediatric Practice" at http://practice.aap.org/content.aspx?aID=2227 for additional tips.

For additional tips on Web site design, see "Using Web Sites to Market Your Pediatric Practice" at http://practice.aap.org/content.aspx?aID=2335.

Number of Patients Per Pediatrician

The number of patients that a pediatrician sees in 1 week and in 1 year varies by preference. Following are information and resources that provide an overview of some general guidelines. It is important to note that there is a difference between the estimates of the number of visits and the number of patients.

Patients Seen Per Year

Pediatric Research in Office Settings, the national practice-based network of the American Academy of Pediatrics (AAP), conducted a study called "Size and Age-Sex Distribution of Pediatric Practice: A Study From Pediatric Research in Office Settings." This study (published in 1999, using data collected in 1991 and 1992) showed that each practitioner cared for an average of 1,546 patients. The number of patients per practitioner was significantly higher in less populated areas (1,915) and in solo practices (2,097). The average number of patients per practitioner derived from these private practice data is in line with health maintenance organization–based estimates. A summary of this study can be found at www.aap.org/pros/agrpubl.htm.

The article titled "How Many Pediatricians Does It Take to Change a Practice?" (http://archpedi.ama-assn.org/cgi/content/full/159/5/500) states that 1 practice of 7 pediatricians and 3 nurse practitioners sees approximately 35,000 patients a year. It is important to note that a pediatrician may have 3,000 visits from approximately 1,500 patients each year.

Patients Seen Per Week

According to AAP Periodic Survey #43 (http://www.aap.org/research/periodicsurvey/ps43soci.htm), conducted in 2000, the average number of patients that a pediatrician sees in 1 week is 93.6. This survey also provides data on the reasons for patient visits, average length of a typical preventive care visit, and the percentage of patients per week by age group.

Mapping Health Care Delivery for America's Children (http://www.aap.org/mapping/) provides national and state-specific data on pediatric health care delivery in each primary care service area, the newest and best units of primary health care utilization. It provides an accurate picture of where children and their families go for health care and, consequently, zoom in on local health care markets.

Finally, the Key Measures link on the AAP Open Access Scheduling Web site (http://www.aap.org/visit/openaccess.htm) provides things to consider when determining the patient load necessary for a practice.

Visit http://practice.aap.org/content.aspx?aid=1690&nodeID=1102 to learn more about the "Profile of Pediatric Visits."

For more information, contact AAP staff in the Division of Pediatric Practice at dopp@aap.org or call 800/433-9016, ext 4784.

See also a Section on Administration and Practice Management discussion on Managing Patient Load (http://practice.aap.org/content.aspx?aID=1970).

How Can Pediatric Practices Respond to Retail-Based Clinics?

It is important for pediatricians to understand what makes retail-based clinics (RBCs) attractive to families and consider incorporating changes to the practice that acknowledge and meet those needs.

Respond Through Changing Office Operations

- Consider evening and weekend hours to avoid having patients miss school or work.
- Set up immunization clinics at various times.
- Incorporate open access scheduling into the practice.
- Develop linkages for referrals and follow up with RBCs.
- Pediatricians should contact their malpractice carriers to determine the extent of any shared liability and whether such clinics may be codefendants in any potential litigation.
- Because pediatric practices will now be competing with RBCs for third-party payment, practices should identify ways to streamline billing and collections, such as electronic connectivity with carriers for claims submissions and payment as well as negotiate for favorable or priority payment over RBCs. Be aware that some insurance carriers are waiving copayments for RBCs.

Communicate With Families

- Families should be notified by the pediatrician that referrals, prescriptions, letters, etc, cannot be provided by the pediatrician based on care provided at RBCs, unless the pediatrician has an opportunity to examine the child and review clinic reports.
- Discuss with families and RBCs what information can be shared and under what circumstances.
- Educate families about RBCs.
- A template letter is available at http://practice.aap. org/content.aspx?aID=1943 to inform patients when an RBC will be opening in the area. This letter can also be modified, so it is appropriate to send to patients who have already been seen at an RBC.
- A sample fact sheet is available at http://practice. aap.org/content.aspx?aID=1945 to provide families with a discussion of the myths and facts of RBCs.

- The American Academy of Pediatrics Ohio Chapter developed a fact sheet for pediatricians to share with families (http://practice.aap.org/public/ Primary%20Care%20Physicians%20vs%20 Retail%20Health%20Clinics.pdf).

Take a Leadership Role in the Community

Several chapters, medical groups, and others have been involved with RBCs within their hospitals and communities.

- The Arkansas Chapter has written a letter to Wal-Mart stating their concerns (http://practice. aap.org/public/AR%20chap%20ltr%20to%20Wal-Mart%20Aug%202006.pdf).
- The Virginia Chapter newsletter contained an article regarding RBCs, written by AAP Board Member Dave Tayloe, MD, FAAP (http://practice. aap.org/public/Virginia%20Chapter%20article-Summer06.pdf).
- Pediatricians in St Louis organized when they learned that Take Care Health Systems^{SM} had contracted with their Children's Hospital. Press releases can be viewed at http://practice.aap.org/ public/pmo_book086_document005A_en.doc and http://practice.aap.org/public/pmo_book086_document005B_en.pdf.
- Talking points were developed to provide pediatricians the information they need to appropriately respond to their patients and the public when asked about RBCs (http://practice.aap.org/content. aspx?aID=1947).

More resources are available on *Practice Management Online* at http://practice.aap.org/topicBrowse.aspx?no deID=1000.1072.1082.1108.1109.

Section 2

Office Operations

Designing an Efficient Office

When pediatricians open a practice, they often wonder how to appropriately design their office. Following are some key considerations when beginning to structure the office design:

- Will you own or rent?
- How will you finance the property?
- What are the building codes?
- How will you design the office setting so that the flow pattern is logical?
- What is the staffing structure? Are staff shared between pediatricians or are they assigned to a particular pediatrician?
- How prepared will your office be for an emergency?
- How many examination rooms do you need, and what will be the sizes of these rooms?

Once these questions are addressed, the following guidelines can assist you in designing a workable office that allows you to provide high-quality, efficient care to your patients.

Research and Plan

- Talk with others about how they designed their offices. Inquire about what worked and what did not.
- Visit other practices of similar size to learn about the practical aspects of office design.
- Consider contracting with consultants (eg, architect, office design expert, building contractor, financial advisor, banker, attorney).
- Include staff in your discussions and consider their suggestions when designing the office.

Space Requirements

- A solo practice may require a building with a minimum of 1,000 sq ft. For offices with 3 pediatricians, 2,500 sq ft or more may be more practical. The number of physicians will influence the number of examination rooms, private offices, and administrative space.

- Provide ample space for ancillary services and staff.
- Consider the potential increase in patients and staff and allocate a reasonable amount of space for potential growth.

Reception Area

- This area should be easily accessible from the sign-in area.
- The reception area should be well marked and resemble a "living room" in the pediatrician's professional home.
- To estimate the number of chairs needed, follow this formula—the maximum number of patients + 50% of that number for relatives and friends x 20 sq ft. The minimum size of a reception area is 144 sq ft. If patients are moved to examination rooms quickly, a smaller reception area may be appropriate.
- Separate seating is preferred over couches.
- All chairs should be stable.
- Provide coat hangers, toys, and books (the toys and books should be accessible to children).
- Light colors and decorations are preferable.
- Display patients' artwork on a bulletin board.
- If space allows, provide separate rooms for sick- and well-child visits. Parents often appreciate this. One way to separate the rooms is with a partition in the reception area. One side should clearly be designated as the area for those children who are sick and the other for those who are well. For more information on infection control in office reception areas, see the American Academy of Pediatrics policy statement, "Infection Prevention and Control in Pediatric Ambulatory Settings" (*Pediatrics.* 2007;120:650–665, http://aappolicy.aappublications.org/cgi/content/full/pediatrics;120/3/650).

Examination Rooms

- Allow 3 to 4 rooms per pediatrician. This promotes efficient patient flow.

- The size of the examination rooms should be large enough to hold the examination table, medical equipment, chairs, and those who will be in the room. Usually 8' x 10' is ideal for infants and young children, and 12' x 12' is good for adolescents.
- A scale and sink do not have to be in every room. A centralized weight station and sink may be used.
- Each examination room should have a cabinet and place to dispose of hazardous materials.
- Mirrors in examination rooms can be a great source of entertainment for infants and young children.
- Rooms should have doors and soundproof walls to ensure patient confidentiality.
- Place a sign on the inside of examination room doors alerting parents to keep toddlers and young children away from the door.
- A number, color, or object should mark the hallway leading to the examination rooms so that children can see them.

Incorporating Electronic Health Records Into Examination Rooms

- Allocate ample space for the system.
- Place the system so that you can face the patient and your back is never to the patient.
- Consider dictation pods.

Nurse's Station

- One to 2 assistants need a workspace of approximately 70' x 100'. An additional 20 sq ft should be allocated for each additional assistant.
- This area should have storage for medical supplies and equipment and a refrigerator to store medications, immunizations, and hyposensitization materials.
- This space should have enough room for a computer or workstation. Nurses who are providing telephone care or obtaining laboratory results or radiology reports can also use this area.

Laboratory Space

- If extensive laboratory procedures and testing are done in the office, a separate laboratory is needed. Otherwise, this can be combined with the nurse's station.
- Cabinets, freestanding work space, and a storage room should be included.

- Electrical outlets and a sink are also necessary.
- Multiple electrical outlets are necessary.

Other Considerations and Tips When Designing a Practice

- Chair rails can help avoid damage to walls.
- Be conscious of placement. Things that are placed in low areas can and will be accessed by children. If there are things you do not want children to get, keep them high and away from children.
- Keep patient and parent education materials available in easy-access locations (eg, examination rooms, reception area).
- Lighting should be adequate.

Tips on Designing a Parking Lot

- Check with your zoning board to be sure that you are in compliance with the city regulations.
- An architect can assist with the design of the parking lot.

This information was extracted from the American Academy of Pediatrics Committee on Practice and Ambulatory Medicine *Management of Pediatric Practice.* 2nd ed. Elk Grove Village, IL: American Academy of Pediatrics; 1991:27–31.

Additional Resources

- "Office Design That Works," *Medical Economics,* July 6, 2007. This article provides a sample floor plan and pictures of a physician's office.
- "Starting a Practice 5–6 Months Out: Office Design and Supplies," *Medical Economics,* June 18, 2004. This article provides information on renting or purchasing office furniture, supplies, and other important information to consider when opening a practice.

For more information, contact AAP staff in the Division of Pediatric Practice at dopp@aap.org or call 800/433-9016, ext 4784.

Setting Up a Computer System

Excerpt from Launching Your Career in Pediatrics Handbook: Opening a New Practice

As you set up your practice, an integral part of your business operations may involve purchasing and implementing a computer system. Even if you are not very comfortable with computer systems, many are easy enough to use with adequate training. Consider that more and more practices are adopting electronic health records (EHRs) and with more regulations such as Health Insurance Portability and Accountability Act (HIPAA) and electronic prescribing, a computer system may be inevitable in the future of health care.

There are several levels of how a computer system can be integrated into your practice. The cost is determined by what level of involvement you desire. If you are just setting up your practice, it may be easier to start with an EHR rather than trying to convert your practice at a later time. However, it is significantly more expensive and time consuming to implement an EHR system as you start your practice. Some hospital systems are helping practices by offsetting expenses with a system that is compatible with the hospital's system. This would be worth investigating if it is true in your area.

Steps for Choosing a Computer System

1. Determine to what extent you would like to use a computer in your practice.
2. Perform a financial analysis to see what is affordable and what your return on investment (ROI) would be. Investigate options such as hospital system financial support. Contact banks or lenders in your area if financing will be needed.
3. Research vendors and systems.
4. Meet with several vendors for product demonstrations. If possible, visit pediatric practices that are currently using the system.
5. Contact the American Academy of Pediatrics (AAP) Section on Administration and Practice Management (SOAPM) (http://www.aap.org/sections/soapm/soapm_home.cfm) and the AAP Council on Clinical Information Technology (COCIT) (http://www.aapcocit.org), and review the publications and advisories on *Practice Management Online* (PMO) and the COCIT review of available systems (additional information follows).

6. As you refine your search, make sure you understand the initial costs of acquisition and implementation, as well as any ongoing maintenance costs.
7. Once a decision is made, define an implementation and a transition strategy. Information is available through SOAPM, COCIT, and PMO to help you plan these processes (additional information follows).
8. Schedule installation of required wiring, networks, telephony, hardware, and software. This is especially important if you are constructing a new office and can install the necessary wiring during the building process.
9. Plan and carry out implementation of products with all necessary training and customization.

How Will the System Be Used?

When looking to purchase a computer system for your practice, the first question that you must answer is, "For what will I be using the system?" The answer will determine the type of system you need, the investment that will be required, and the timeline for installation.

The simplest use of computers in an office is like what you would do at home—word processing, spreadsheets, simple accounting, and possibly Internet access.

The next step would be to use a computer system to run practice management software (PMS). This software typically would allow you to use a computer for appointment scheduling, billing, and storing patient demographics.

The final step for using a computer in a pediatric office is for EHRs. This is essentially patient charting completely on the computer.

The cost of and time for installation increases as you proceed from stand-alone computer to full-scale PMS and EHR. Sample costs are listed in the Table.

Electronic Cost Comparison			
	Single-User Computer	**PMS**	**PMS and EHR**
Software cost	$500–$1,000	$1,000–$5,000/FTE	$1,000–$50,000/FTE
Hardware cost	$2,000 desktop	$1,000–$2,500 per desktop/laptop/tablet $2,000–$4,000 per server Additional for printers, scanners, modems, networking equipment	
Implementation cost	$75–$150 per hour of training/implementation (usually some hours included in purchase price) Average 35 h for implementation for EHR		
Time frame	2 wk–1 mo	3 mo	3–6 mo
Implementation difficulty	Simple	Moderate	Complex
Maintenance/support (yearly)	None–$100	$500–$1,000/FTE	$1,000–$4,000/FTE

Abbreviations: PMS, practice management software; EHR, electronic health record; FTE, full-time equivalent.

Financial Analysis

Depending on which system you buy, there is usually a significant up-front expense. However, it is extremely important to investigate what the recurrent expenses include. Hardware and software maintenance can be very costly and are a necessary burden to keep your business running. Additionally, hidden expenses for upgrades, support, and additional training should be outlined before you sign any contracts.

Benefits of an Electronic Health Record

Why go electronic if it costs so much? There are many benefits to being on a computer system. You gain accuracy, efficiency of charge capture and billing, legibility, and accessibility. Improvement of coding is more easily achievable with electronic capture. Increased legibility and better documentation result in improved patient care and decreased medical liability. Depending on your practice, you may see improved work flow. Locating and pulling charts are no longer an issue with EHRs. This results in more rapid processing of refills and forms. There are no longer concerns about lost charts. If you do internal billing, you can take advantage of electronic filing and posting, which can significantly reduce your accounts receivable. These are some of the most tangible benefits to being electronic. While not helpful for most pediatricians, there are also significant savings of transcription costs. With these benefits, it generally takes 2 to 3 years to get an ROI. The other important point is that it is far easier and less costly to start a practice with information technology (IT) in place than to implement at a later date.

The AAP SOAPM e-mail list provides pros and cons from various members. Visit http://practice.aap.org/content.aspx?aID=1971 to view comments. Also see the article titled "Electronic Health Records: Should I Convert My Office to Paperless?" (http://practice.aap.org/content.aspx?aid=1969). There are many resources to help you to calculate your ROI available from *Physicians Practice* (http://www.physicianspractice.com) and the Medical Group Management Association (http://www.mgma.com). Because you are just starting in practice, you may need to talk to other practitioners to get a better feel for work flow, time costs, and expenses.

Evaluating Software

Once you've determined the computer needs of your practice, the next step is to evaluate vendors of PMS and EHR software. One of the best ways to evaluate software is to ask around in your local community or the AAP to see what other pediatric practices are using. The Certification Commission for Healthcare Information Technology (http://www.cchit.org) is an organization that certifies health care software that meets certain standards. The AAP COCIT Web site (http://www.aapcocit.org) also has many valuable resources.

The AAP offers answers to some frequently asked questions as well as reviews from fellow AAP members.

- "Electronic Medical Record FAQ": http://www.aapcocit.org/EHRfaqs.pdf
- EHR reviews: http://www.aapcocit.org/EHR/readreviews.php

- "Implementing an Electronic Health Record": http://www.practice.aap.org/ehr.aspx

There are some features of the PMS and EHR that you should investigate that are unique to pediatrics.

Practice Management Software

- Is it capable of family billing using head of household?
- How are siblings linked in the system? If you update one child's address, will all the siblings be updated?
- Can you put alerts on the account for special situations (eg, child with special needs requires extra time for appointments)?
- Can you design appointment templates that can specify different types of appointments (eg, well-child appointments vs sick-child appointments)?
- Can you easily move appointments from one physician's schedule to another?
- Is it capable of running queries so that you can do studies or single out patients within certain demographics (eg, to determine your payer mix or how you are being paid for certain procedure codes)?

Electronic Health Records

- Does it have growth charts? Does it have specialized growth charts (eg, preemie charts, Down syndrome charts)?
- Can you create forms (eg, school)?
- How well does it handle immunization records? Can you add new ones (as vaccines are developed)? How does it handle reminders if a child is due for vaccines? Can it communicate with statewide immunization registries?
- How do you enter notes? Via templates? Can you type free text also? Can you customize the templates?
- How does it handle documenting a sick visit in addition to a well check?
- Does it have coding assistance?
- Does it offer electronic prescribing? Does it have a weight-based prescribing system for calculating pediatric dosing?
- Does it have laboratory report integration and ordering? Can you set pediatric norms for laboratories? Can you interface with local hospital laboratories and major laboratories? For how much?
- Can you use images or photos (eg, drawing of lesions)?
- Can you capture signatures (eg, for waivers)?
- Is there an online interface available where parents can request refills, schedule appointments, or preregister online?
- Are there pediatric-specific educational handouts?
- Can you integrate a spirometer, electrocardiogram machine, or vitals machine?
- Is it capable of sending charges electronically?
- Will it support patient self–check-in?

General

- What is your support turnaround (including after hours and weekends)?
- How frequently do you have upgrades? Who does those upgrades?
- Are upgrades included in the maintenance cost?
- Who performs support for your system? Is there someone local who will come on-site? Or is it done remotely?
- Is there a resource for users of the same specialty to network and share ideas for using the system?
- How long has the company been in business? What is the company's business plan? Does it give you a feeling of confidence in that it will be there for the duration of your practice?
- How do you store backups for patient data? Is it done locally? Is there off-site storage?
- What are the security features? HIPAA compliance features?

Once you have chosen several vendors, schedule demonstrations. Make sure that the vendors demonstrate a pediatric scenario for you. For such an expensive capital purchase, it is wise to meet with at least 3 different vendors. When you have decided which ones you like the most, visit practices that are using these systems in real life. These practices can give you a much better feel for how the system works in everyday pediatric practice. It is also a good idea to get information about obstacles they encountered, how they would do things differently if they could, and whether they would purchase the system again knowing what they do now. The implementation of an EHR in an existing practice can be a very painful process. Depending on what stage they are at in the implementation process, you could take their advice accordingly. In general, once you are 2 to 3 years into a system, you will find that the EHR was a good choice and that you wouldn't go back. However, those first years can be very strenuous as you make the transition!

Technical Support

There are many ways to implement a computer system. The larger your practice and the more features you make electronic, the more likely you are to need technical support. This may take the form of a staff member who is technically savvy and a local engineer from your vendor. It may be a local computer support business or your local "geek squad." If your system is large enough, you may need to hire an IT specialist. Regardless of the system, you are likely to encounter needs for upgrades and maintenance (eg, backups), as well as troubleshooting problems. The problems will range from simple (eg, the mouse doesn't work) to complex (the network is down for your satellite office). In general, it is wise to have someone you can call for help when these issues arise.

Data Storage, Backups, Power Outages, and Disaster Plan

Lastly, it is important to consider how you will protect your data. There are frequently news reports of patient data being stolen by employees. Once you are electronic this issue should be examined carefully. It is much more difficult to steal 1,000 paper charts than to steal a computer containing that same information. Investigate your vendor's capacity for security and virus protection. EHRs must be compliant with specific HIPAA rules. Backup for your data can be done many ways depending on your system. Investigate options with your vendor. If your system is on-site, certain precautions should be taken to have some form of off-site storage for your data.

You should also have a disaster plan in place. This will be important in case of extreme disaster to your practice (eg, fire, water damage), but also in other cases when something as simple as the power goes out to your building. For power outage or when the system is down for some reason, a common plan is to go onto paper. The data are scanned into the computer when power is restored. Design a plan that works for you and your practice.

For information on implementing an EHR, visit http://practice.aap.org/ehr.aspx.

For additional information on PMO about EHRs, visit http://practice.aap.org/content.aspx?aid=2496. This section of PMO also provides articles provided by those practices who switched to EHRs.

Practice Work Flow and Policies

Excerpt from Launching Your Career in Pediatrics Handbook: Opening a New Practice

There are many things to consider when designing the infrastructure of your pediatric practice. This section will provide tips on the following:

- Selecting an Office Location and Space
- Setting Office Hours
- Making the Best Use of Your Office Hours
- Creating Customized Schedules
- Using Patient Flow Patterns
- Creating Office Policies
- The Employee Handbook
- Health Insurance Portability and Accountability Act Policies and Procedures
- Red Flag Rules
- Occupational Safety and Health Administration
- Other Policies
- Purchasing Techniques: Controlling Purchase Costs of Supplies and Vaccines
- Vaccines
- Telephone Triage
- After-hours Phone Care
- Coverage and Referrals

Selecting an Office Location and Space

For information and tips on designing an efficient office, visit http://practice.aap.org/content.aspx?aid=1982&nodeID=1077.

Additional Resource
"Do I Need Separate Waiting Rooms for Sick and Well Children? A Practice Management FAQ" is available at http://practice.aap.org/content.aspx?aid=2226&nodeID=1077.

Setting Office Hours

If you are joining an established practice, your hours are set for you by the practice, based on your negotiations at the time of contracting. If you are taking over an established practice, the community will likely expect you to continue the prior practice's hours or to expand them—reducing them from the outset would likely have a negative marketing effect.

Most pediatricians go into practice with the idea of balancing work and family time. Ideally speaking, the decision of office hours should be part of your market analysis, done as the first step in assessing and selecting the community and location in which you wish to practice, not after you have made the selection, picked space, ordered supplies, and made commitments. Your care, your demeanor, and your availability are the major determinants of the practice's success.

Here are some things to consider.

1. The style of practice you want, and if you have a family, what your family can accept. It is critical that the family unit have appropriate expectations, a full understanding of what is being undertaken, and a realistic estimate of the effort needed to succeed.
2. The practice competitiveness of an area or community. If you are the only pediatrician in town, you can tilt the balance toward your own needs. On the other hand, if you select a highly competitive area, you will need to find ways to attract patients. That might mean expanded hours or night, evening, and weekend hours, which would require more work time.
3. The coverage you might be able to expect, and what responsibilities as well as benefits accrue through any coverage arrangement.
4. What are the community resources? Are there local retail-based clinics, urgent care centers, or after-hours centers? If so, this could enhance your practice if you achieve a cooperative working agreement. However, they can also be competitive facilities drawing patients away.
5. Understand the community needs—socioeconomic, prior health care availability, customs, and traditions.

Options to consider for making your hours more effective include

1. *Early bird hours* (eg, walk-in, first-come first-served, minor problems, and quick fixes designed to get children into school and parents off to work). You might be able to see 5 to 10 patients quickly, relieving the crowding in the morning and afternoon schedules. Parents look positively on the quick-in-and-quick-out as a benefit, and enjoy the consideration shown by not making them take a

half day off from work or have the child miss school. Early bird hours could begin at 7:30 or 8:00 am, depending on when school starts in your community. *Caveat:* For early bird hours beginning at 8:00 am, set the walk-in registration time from 7:45 to 8:15 am. Do not set the early bird time from 8:00 to 9:00 am. If you do, you might find 5 to 10 people walking in at 8:55 am, expecting to be seen by 9:00 am.

2. *Teen time* (ie, evening hours for adolescents). They appreciate it when they come into a true adolescent practice and not to see a "baby doctor." Office décor is also important!

3. *Talk time* (ie, certain hours set aside in advance for parents who need extended talk time for chronic diseases, educational issues such as learning disorders or attention-deficit/hyperactivity disorder, or behavioral issues). By having a specific period set aside, you meet the needs of the parents and patient and avoid having the staff schedule a standard appointment time that is not adequate, causing you to inevitably run late and disconcerting all the following scheduled appointments.

4. *Specialty time* (ie, focus on your individual interest in practice). This can be done one patient at a time or in groups, depending on the subspecialty.

5. *Group baby care.* Some practices set aside an hour and schedule 5 to 6 similar-aged infants for the same time. The nurses begin the visit by obtaining a history of each infant. The physician examines the infants in sequence, expanding on history issues. Next, all of the families sit down as a group with the physician for question-and-answer time and anticipatory guidance time. Many parents ask the same questions; many forget what to ask but hear another parent ask it for them. This format also allows for group support as the parents develop social relationships with other parents with similar-aged children. Consider this option as an elective solution—parents can opt in or out at any time; however, it is common for many groups to continue this format into the early school years.

These solutions are attempts to take patient needs into account, which is difficult if you have set 10- or 15-minute, or modified wave, appointments. They compartmentalize your chosen hours. Remember—marketing quality of service is just as important to a practice's success as quality of care.

Sample Office Schedule		
Solutions	**Days of Week**	**Hours**
Early bird time	Monday–Friday	8:00 am (parents to arrive no later than 8:15 am)
Regular appointments	Monday, Wednesday, Friday	9:00 am–4:30 pm
Regular appointments	Tuesday, Thursday	1:00–4:00 pm
Talk time	Tuesday	9:00 am–12:00 pm
Teen time	Tuesday	4:00–7:00 pm
Baby groups	Thursday	9:00–11:00 am
Toddler groups	Thursday	11:00 am–12:00 noon

In this sample schedule, your hours would essentially be Monday through Friday from 8:00 am until 5:00 pm (last appointment, 4:30 pm). As the practice develops, you can modify the schedule. As you potentially add on partners, nurse practitioners, or physician assistants (PAs), you can continue to modify your schedule.

Making the Best Use of Your Office Hours

The most common scheduling methodologies are fixed appointments and wave or modified wave scheduling. These formats apply to the timing of appointment scheduling. There are also open access and modified open access—these apply to the style of scheduling.

1. *Fixed* (ie, the time and length are preformatted). For example, appointments are offered every 10, 15, or 20 minutes. When you first start in practice, it would be better to allow more time as you get to know patients and they get to know you. Then, as you get used to your routine and patients become familiar through repeated visits, you can change the time slots.

2. *Wave* (ie, schedule all the patients for a given segment, usually a half hour or an hour). In this scheduling method, instead of scheduling 4 patients 15 minutes apart, all 4 are set for on-the-hour, and the physician sees each one in sequence of arrival. The first gets seen immediately; the fourth gets seen after the first 3. The advantage is that some patients arrive on time and some are late. The wave takes this into account. The disadvantage is if they all arrive on time, and the fourth

has to wait 45 minutes or more to be seen. *Caveat:* You must also be very careful to select the type of patients your staff schedules. If they schedule 4 adolescent well-care visits, you might have difficulty completing the work.

3. *Modified wave* (ie, same 4 patients, same hour; however, the first 2 are told to be there on the hour, and the second 2 are told to be there in a "second wave," 15, 20, or 30 minutes after the first 2). This method gains (for the most part) the benefits of wave, but lessens the disadvantages of long waits for later appointments. For additional information on wave scheduling, see "Wave Scheduling" (http://practice.aap.org/content.aspx?aid=1920).

4. *Open access* (ie, offering same-day scheduling for all visits, preventive or illness/injury). While it does not rule out parent-choice, in-the-future appointments, the goal is to take care of today's work today and minimize future appointments, so as not to have a full schedule before you open the doors. Most practices can estimate the daily patient flow and schedule providers' work times to accommodate the need. For established practices, there might be a conversion time because they may already have appointments well in advance. For new practices, starting with a clean slate, it is much easier to implement. Logic says you will do a certain number of preventive care and interval visits over the span of a month—whether you do it in a standard prebooking "first available appointment" or open access "any available appointment today," you will likely see the same number of patients of both types over a month. The one disadvantage is that parents may not always be available, primarily for preventive care visits, at the time you have open that day. For additional information on open access scheduling, visit http://practice.aap.org/ content.aspx?aid=384&nodeID=3014 and http://practice.aap.org/content.aspx?aid=1108&nodeID=3027.

5. *Modified open access* (ie, booking preventive care and long consultations at the convenience of the parent with the traditional "first, or later, available appointment basis" but using typical open access style for illness/injury or interval visits). This is the style the vast majority of small practices use because it takes care of today's work today, especially for those issues parents feel are urgent (ie, illness/injury), yet allows the parent to select a preventive care appointment that is convenient

for themselves and their child. It also allows the practice to set aside additional time if it is apparent that the child has multiple or in-depth problems the parent expects to discuss.

Final Considerations in Setting Hours

Setting hours is critically important because parents consider availability and accessibility just as important as care quality and health care insurance participation. It needs to be part of your marketing plan to build your practice. Decide which you wish to do *before* you select where you will open a practice. The greatest mistake is to pick a location without understanding what will be needed to be successful in that location.

One lesson learned after many years of practice is that if you take care of your community, it will take care of you. If you are considerate of your community, it will be considerate of you, and it is your greatest support in practice.

The other lesson is to make use of *Practice Management Online* (PMO) as your major referral for suggestions and information, built on the experiences of thousands of pediatricians who have already gone through the same processes you are about to encounter.

PMO has additional resources for reducing no-shows.
- Cost-effective Ways to Reduce No-shows: http://practice.aap.org/content.aspx?aid=2098)
- "Missed Appointment Policy": http://practice.aap.org/content.aspx?aid=2024
- Sample missed appointment letters: First and second letters, http://practice.aap.org/content.aspx?aid= 2093; third (and final) letter, http://practice.aap.org/content.aspx?aid=2095&nodeID=3017

Creating Customized Schedules

The most highly efficient practices use this labor-intensive method. It is unlikely that a new practice will have the experience and data to implement it fully, but some basic techniques can be used and more complex management developed as the practice matures. The base template is the modified open-access system described previously. One person in the practice, preferably a physician with business skills, takes responsibility for maximizing the number of visits that can be handled by the practice. This can only be done if the scheduling doctor has several attributes.

1. An understanding of the practice's seasonal variations in demand for certain types of visits. For example, each schedule should be customized with more slots assigned to well visits in the summer season and more acute care visits assigned in the winter season.
2. An understanding of how each provider works. There are clear differences in provider styles and they cannot all have the same schedule. Some work very quickly, some less so. Some take on more complex specialized patients and need a schedule that reflects this. If there are multiple locations, they may have different characteristics. All of this must be meshed with your productivity schema so that everyone has the opportunity to be rewarded for their own productivity.
3. The time and compensation to monitor how the practice is booking on a daily basis and to make requisite modifications to the system on an ongoing basis. There must be an extra salary for this person over and above their patient productivity compensation.
4. The authority to totally control the schedule of the providers. No one but the scheduling doctor has the authority to alter the schedule. If other providers need to make changes, they must be authorized by the scheduling physician prior to being implemented. This goes for vacations, days off, and other commitments. If schedules need to be changed, even with short notice, providers must cooperate with these changes as much as possible.
5. The data systems needed to figure all of this out and the ability to try to get patients to move their well visits to low-demand periods such as April and May to even out the summer crunch of such visits. This may require active calls to patients to solicit such visit times.
6. The ability to customize the schedule with certain types of visits at certain times, with rules about changing such job stream templates for appointment staff to follow. These job streams may vary by season, office, and individual provider.

As is obvious, this type of system is not for everyone. However, if fully implemented, this type of schedule can earn a practice far more revenue than nearly any other single management technique of handling patient care.

Using Patient Flow Patterns

Employers and families are looking at their health care costs closely. The pediatric services that your practice provides are increasingly being rated for value and quality by insurance companies and your patients.

Pediatricians, as primary care providers and pediatric specialists, are dealing with fixed insurance payments that do not allow them to routinely pass on increased costs to payers. Perception of patient flow through the practice provides the base to adapt and manage patient visits to the advantage of the providers and patients. Here are some tips to ensure patient flow.

1. Assess how a patient encounter progresses from the patient's point of view. This can be done by shadowing a patient through the visit, using a kitchen timer attached to a clipboard or notepad where the staff notes encounter times.
2. Start from the initial scheduling, the chart pull, or electronic medical record (EMR) review. Identify the points of care where your staff engage with the patient and prep for the visit. You can then review as a team (providers and front desk, clinical, and billing staff) to identify areas that catch patients in time delays.
3. Gridlock in patient flow can be found during the check-in process, provider appointment times, interruptions in providers' work flow, documentation practices, examination room setups, clinical processes, scheduling, and checkout.
4. Prioritize changes based on staff, provider, and patient survey information. Initiate one change per area at a time; ensure that adaptation and evaluation are complete before going on to the next one. A sample patient survey can be found on PMO at http://practice.aap.org/content.aspx?aID=2374.

Goals of change should be to increase provider, patient, and staff satisfaction while increasing revenue and cutting expenses.

Identifying the flow of patients may also have an immediate effect on revenue. The location of the checkout or collections desk can have a significant effect on co-payment collection. As the patient checks out after the visit, a properly placed desk can improve contact with the patient and increase chances for collection. Co-payments are often given less attention in the world of collections because of the small amounts, but these dollars can quickly add up. By making sure that all patients pass by the checkout desk before leaving the office, optimizing patient flow can provide another opportunity to collect the co-payment as the patient schedules the next appointment.

Creating Office Policies

Because of the multiple regulatory agencies that monitor the health care industry, physician offices must have policies and procedures established in addition to those required by employment and labor laws. When first beginning this process, the alphabet soup of regulatory bodies can be overwhelming. However, there are key policies and procedures that every physician's office should have, and PMO has many examples to get you started. Some labor law policies are required only if you have a certain number of employees and may not apply to a practice that is just starting up. It is especially important to review your policies with legal counsel because the wording of your policies may have significant legal ramifications.

The Employee Handbook

The bulk of office policies are included in the employee handbook. This handbook is given to every employee on hire. You should keep documentation that each employee has received, understood, and agreed to its terms.

Employee handbooks are often called policy and procedure manuals. The purpose of the handbook is to provide a written statement of the policies of the business and how the business is to be conducted. The company employee handbook is one of the most important communication tools between your company and your employees. It presents your expectations for your employees, and it also describes what they can expect from the business. It needs to be as clear and unambiguous as possible. Misunderstandings or misstatements can create legal liabilities for your business. In legal disputes courts have considered an employee handbook to be a contractual obligation, so word it carefully and with professional legal assistance. The handbook provides an objective reference for you and your employee in the case of disputes over behavior or performance.

This handbook should contain enough detail to avoid confusion, but not so much as to overwhelm—for instance, there may be other documents (eg, group insurance, retirement plan) that more appropriately provide details. In the handbook, you are providing a clear summary and stating the most important points of each issue addressed. It is important to be familiar with the myriad of laws and regulations for employment. Your local medical society may be a good source of information about human resource laws and requirements. Additionally, it is a good idea to consult with your business attorney about any laws on which you are unclear.

The following is a list of potential sections for your employee handbook:

- Introduction
- Mission Statement
- Equal Employment Opportunity Statement
- Accommodating Disabled Workers (Americans with Disabilities Act)
- General Policies
  - Personal Information
  - Attendance
  - Use of Company Property
  - Dress Code
  - Safety and Accident Rules
  - Fire Prevention
  - Smoking
  - Illegal Drug and Alcohol Use and Abuse
  - Sexual Harassment
  - Employee Conduct Guidelines
  - Conflict of Interest
  - Performance Reviews
  - Personal Telephone Use
  - Inclement Weather
  - Employment Referrals
  - Employment of Relatives
  - Personnel Record
- Compensation and Benefits
  - Payroll
  - Work Hours and Reporting and Attendance Policy
  - New Employee Orientation Period
  - Holidays
  - Vacation
  - Sick Leave
  - Family and Medical Leave
  - Maternity Leave
  - Funeral Leave
  - Jury Duty
  - Military Service
  - Leave Without Pay
  - Overtime
  - Break Periods
  - Group Insurance Benefits

- Short-term Disability
- Continuation of Medical/Consolidated Omnibus Budget Reconciliation Act
- Worker Compensation
- Retirement Plans
- Tuition Assistance
- Employee Assistance Program
- Medical Services Provided to Employees and Their Immediate Families
- Employment Separation/Termination
- Closing Statement
  - This states that the most recent version of the handbook supersedes all previous versions of the handbook.
- Employee Acknowledgment Form
  - To be signed by each employee. When you create new policies and update your employee handbook, you should get new acknowledgment forms signed.

For more details on each of the policies, there are several Web sites and books that can assist you. For employee handbooks for medical practices, check with Medical Group Management Association (MGMA).

PMO has a sample employee handbook available at http://practice.aap.org/content.aspx?aID=2091.

Health Insurance Portability and Accountability Act Policies and Procedures

The Health Insurance Portability and Accountability Act of 1996 (HIPAA) was created to ensure that patient privacy was protected. It required that businesses who deal with protected health information follow certain policies to protect patient privacy. In addition, it required that procedures were in place to deal with violations of these policies. If an investigation by the Department of Health and Human Services determines that a person or entity has violated these policies, significant civil and criminal penalties can be incurred.

There are 3 major sections of HIPAA and all covered entities were required to be compliant with all of these standards after 2005. The 3 sections are the Privacy Standards, the Transactions and Code Set Standards, and the Security Standards.

The HIPAA Privacy Standards require physicians to protect the privacy of patients' medical information. Physicians are required to regulate the ways in which they use and disclose patients' protected health information. Physicians are required to offer patients

certain rights with respect to their information, such as the right to access and copy, the right to request amendments, and the right to request an accounting. Lastly, physicians must have certain administrative protections in place (eg, a privacy officer, staff training, implementation of appropriate policies and procedures, disciplinary actions, and recourse) to further protect the privacy of patients' information.

The HIPAA Transactions and Code Set Standards govern the format for electronic transactions between physicians and health plans and other entities. For example, the claims that physicians submit to payers must be in a specific format.

The HIPAA Security Standards further require physicians to protect the security of patients' electronic medical information through the use of procedures and mechanisms that protect the confidentiality, integrity, and availability of information. Physicians must have in place administrative, physical, and technical safeguards that will protect electronic health information that the physician collects, maintains, uses, and transmits. The standards cover all electronic forms of patient medical information, including faxes, e-mail, and EMR/electronic health records.

The full HIPAA law is complex and arduous to read. The US Department of Health and Human Services provides a comprehensive guide to covered entities (eg, doctor's offices) at www.hhs.gov/ocr/privacy/hipaa/understanding/coveredentities/index.html.

The American Academy of Pediatrics (AAP) has *HIPAA Online: A "How-To" Guide for Your Medical Practice* available at http://practice.aap.org/hipaa.aspx.

You may also find additional assistance in creating policies from the American Medical Association and Medical Group Management Association.

Red Flag Rules

Starting in 2009, medical practices are considered creditors and must abide by the red flag rules as set forth by the Federal Trade Commission. These rules protect against identity theft. Because nearly all medical practices file insurance claims and wait to bill patients the remainder of the fee, or have some patients on some type of payment plan, they are "lending" money to patients and are therefore considered creditors.

If a provider is considered a creditor, the covered account is a consumer account designed to permit multiple payments or transactions, or any other account for which there is a reasonably foreseeable risk of identity theft. For a medical practice, this would be patient billing records.

Medical practices would be required to develop an identity theft program that contains reasonable policies and procedures to
• Identify relevant patterns, practices, and specific forms of activity that are red flags, signaling possible identify theft.
• Detect these patterns or red flags.
• Respond to those detected to prevent and mitigate identity theft.
• Ensure the program is updated periodically to reflect changes in risks.

In administering such a program, a creditor would need to
• Obtain approval of the program from its board or board committee.
• Involve the board or senior management designee(s).
• Train staff.
• Exercise oversight of service provider arrangements.

For additional information about the red flag rules and for a sample policy, see http://practice.aap.org/content.aspx?aid=2687.

Additional information is available at http://www.ftc.gov/bcp/edu/pubs/articles/art11.shtm and http://www.aha.org/aha/advocacy/compliance/redflags.html.

Occupational Safety and Health Administration

Occupational Safety and Health Administration (OSHA) regulations were created to provide a safe and healthful workplace to employees. All medical offices are required to be in compliance with OSHA standards.

There are several key hazards that need to be addressed in a medical office. However, please see the OSHA official Web site for the complete list of regulations.

The following information comes from the OSHA publication, *Medical & Dental Offices: A Guide to Compliance with OSHA Standards*. These are the most common standards that apply to medical offices.

Blood-borne Pathogens Standard (29 CFR §1910.1030)

This is the most frequently requested and referenced OSHA standard affecting medical and dental offices. Some basic requirements of the OSHA blood-borne pathogens standard include

• A written exposure control plan, to be updated annually
• Use of universal precautions
• Consideration, implementation, and use of safer, engineered needles and sharps
• Use of engineering and work practice controls and appropriate personal protective equipment (gloves, face and eye protection, gowns)
• Hepatitis B vaccine provided to exposed employees at no cost
• Medical follow-up in the event of an exposure incident
• Use of labels or color-coding for items such as sharp disposal boxes and containers for regulated waste, contaminated laundry, and certain specimens
• Employee training
• Proper containment of all regulated waste

Hazard Communication (29 CFR §1910.1200)

The hazard communication standard is sometimes called the "employee right-to-know" standard. It requires employee access to hazard information. The basic requirements include
• A written hazard communication program
• A list of hazardous chemicals (eg, alcohol, disinfectants, anesthetic agents, sterilants, mercury) used or stored in the office
• A copy of the material safety data sheet for each chemical (obtained from the manufacturer) used or stored in the office
• Employee training

Ionizing Radiation (29 CFR §1910.1096)

This standard applies to facilities that have an x-ray machine and requires the following:
• A survey of the types of radiation used in the facility, including x-rays.
• Restricted areas to limit employee exposures.
• Employees working in restricted areas must wear personal radiation monitors such as film badges or pocket dosimeters.
• Rooms and equipment may need to be labeled and equipped with caution signs.

Exit Routes (29 CFR Subpart E §1910.35, §1910.36, §1910.37, §1910.38, and §1910.39)

These standards include the requirements for providing safe and accessible building exits in case of fire or other emergency. It is important to become familiar with the full text of these standards because they provide details about signage and other issues. OSHA consultation services can help, or your insurance company or local fire and police service may be able to assist you. The basic responsibilities include

- Exit routes sufficient for the number of employees in any occupied space
- A diagram of evacuation routes posted in a visible location

Electrical (Subpart S-Electrical 29 CFR §1010.301 to 29 CFR §1910.399)

These standards address electrical safety requirements to safeguard employees. OSHA electrical standards apply to electrical equipment and wiring in hazardous locations. If you use flammable gases, you may need special wiring and equipment installation. In addition to reading the full text of the OSHA standard, you should check with your insurance company or local fire department, or request an OSHA consultation for help.

Poster

Every workplace must display the OSHA poster (OSHA publication 3165) or the state plan equivalent. The poster explains worker rights to a safe workplace and how to file a complaint. The poster must be placed where employees will see it. You can download a copy or order one free copy at www.osha.gov or by calling 800/321-OSHA (321-6742).

Reporting Occupational Injuries and Illnesses (29 CFR §1904)

Medical and dental offices are currently exempt from maintaining an official log of reportable injuries and illnesses (OSHA form 300) under the federal OSHA record-keeping rule, although they may be required to maintain records in some state plans. If you are in a state plan, contact your state plan directly for more information. All employers, including medical and dental offices, must report any work-related fatality or the hospitalization of 3 or more employees in a single incident to the nearest OSHA office. Call 800/321-OSHA or your state plan for assistance.

Resources

- Medical & Dental Offices: A Guide to Compliance with OSHA Standards: www.osha.gov/Publications/OSHA3187/osha3187.html
- Compliance assistance resources: www.osha.gov/dcsp/compliance_assistance/index.html#Resources

Other Policies

Clinical Laboratory Improvement Amendments/COLA Accreditation

The Centers for Medicare & Medicaid Services regulates all laboratory testing performed on humans in the United States through the Clinical Laboratory Improvement Amendments (CLIA). If you plan on having an in-office laboratory that performs CLIA tests that are not waived, then you must be in compliance with CLIA. COLA is an organization that provides accreditation to CLIA-compliant laboratories.

Resources

- www.cms.hhs.gov/clia
- www.cola.org

Medical Assistants

Many states allow medical assistants (MAs) to administer vaccinations or medications under the supervision of a physician. However, most require some sort of training. It is a good idea to have formal written policies and procedures addressing the type of training program that you will use and how the MAs will be supervised. In several states, MAs are not allowed to give injectables, so be sure to check to see what laws apply to you. Your state board of medicine or equivalent should be able to assist you.

Reconstituting Medications

If you plan to give injectable medications that require reconstitution, such as ceftriaxone, you may have to develop policies and procedures for this process. Some states require practices that reconstitute medications to follow US Pharmacopeia guidelines for sterile mixing techniques. Some states only allow registered nurses (RNs), physician assistants, or physicians to do the mixing. Check with your state board of medicine for rules for your state.

Dispensing Medications

As a convenience to your patients, you may choose to dispense some commonly used medications (eg, amoxicillin, albuterol) for patients to purchase. This can be done in a variety of ways, including using prepackaged medications through commercial services. However, each state will have its own legal requirements for the dispensing of medications in a non-pharmacy. Again, check with your local agency for legal requirements.

Preparing Your Office for a Disaster

For information about how to prepare your office for an emergency or disaster, visit Preparation for Emergencies in the Offices of Pediatricians and Pediatric Primary Care Providers (http://practice.aap.org/content.aspx?aid=2057&nodeID=1105).

Additional Resources on Policies

PMO has several sample policies available. Visit http://practice.aap.org/topicBrowse.aspx?nodeID=4000.4033 for additional information.

Purchasing Techniques: Controlling Purchase Costs of Supplies and Vaccines

Medical supplies and vaccines account for a large percentage of pediatric practice overhead. Vaccine costs in nonuniversal states can be 20% to 25% of your expenditures. Controlling purchasing costs allows you to manage one element of overhead expenses in your business.

Group Purchasing Organizations

A group purchasing organization (GPO) helps physician practices minimize costs of medical supplies and vaccines by collectively joining practices with other physicians in volume purchasing. Large-volume purchasing power gives a group of physicians the clout to bargain for price reductions on medical supplies and vaccines. You can belong to multiple GPOs for individual supplies and use the price lists to build the best purchasing plan for your practice.

Develop a spreadsheet with the supply item listed in the first column, and in subsequent columns enter the price taken from each GPO price list. This makes it easy to compare your cost for an item when ordering. You can go the additional step of developing your own shopping list for each GPO, but don't forget to compare prices with the original spreadsheet at least quarterly. Generally, GPOs only provide price lists to those interested in becoming members.

Another cost assurance responsibility is to compare the invoice with your contracted price. Delegate this to a staff member in billing who is used to dealing with the dollars and has the time to do the comparison.

PMO has a list of GPOs available at http://practice.aap.org/content.aspx?aid=2381. If your area is not serviced, consider joining together with other practices to negotiate a buying contract with manufacturers. AAP chapters and pediatric councils are a great place to look for partners.

Discounts and Rebates

Always inquire about rebates and discount ordering. Be alert to the end of the financial quarters when the companies are trying to improve their numbers. Advantage should be taken of online ordering discounts (about 2%), prompt pay discounts, and manufacturer's promotions (most often 2%–3%). These promotions frequently are combined with 90-day invoice dating. This gives the practice a few months to provide the vaccine and obtain payment.

Payments

Practice payments made with a credit card can provide a financial advantage to the practice in 2 ways. A credit card payment can be scheduled for payment just prior to the date of the prompt pay cutoff date. This adds the credit card billing cycle time to the time between purchase and payment. Choose a credit card that offers additional perks, such as frequent flyer miles, that can be used for attending conferences or continuing medical education (CME) meetings, reducing other expense line items.

Inventory

Inventory is a cost-saving measure that is often overlooked in a practice. Knowing what you own and when it expires can save you money by preventing duplication of items, loss of product by expiration dates being overlooked, and performance of procedures more tediously when you had purchased a clever product that was going to make your job easier! A sample list of supplies needed to start a practice can be viewed at http://practice.aap.org/content.aspx?aid=2395.

Delegate

Staff members need to be accountable for the supplies and usage in their area. Lists and computer prompts are helpful tools to give them to make it easier to remain compliant.

Remember that your goal is to provide the best pediatric care for the least cost.

Vaccines

The following information about administering vaccines in the office is available on PMO.

Cost of Giving Vaccines in Your Office

To calculate your total vaccine costs, enter your information into all 3 calculators at http://practice.aap.org/vaccinecalculator.aspx and click the Calculate Total Cost button at the bottom of the page. You can also use the individual calculators to calculate partial vaccine costs. These calculators give the practice cost of administering 1 dose of vaccine over a 3-month time frame.

Liability Insurance

- "Improve Vaccine Liability Protection": http://practice.aap.org/content.aspx?aid=1602
- "Reducing Vaccine Liability: Strategies for Pediatricians": http://practice.aap.org/content.aspx?aid=545
- "Insurance Coverage for Vaccine Loss": http://practice.aap.org/content.aspx?aid=2228

Storage and Handling

- "Safe Storage of Vaccines": http://practice.aap.org/content.aspx?aid=2205
- "Lessons Learned From Hurricane Katrina: Ensuring Proper Vaccine Management Handling and Administration During a Disaster": http://practice.aap.org/content.aspx?aid=1979

Coding for Vaccines

- "Coding for Pediatric Preventive Care": http://practice.aap.org/content.aspx?aid=2052
- "When Is It Appropriate to Report 99211 During Immunization Administration?": http://practice.aap.org/content.aspx?aid=2119
- "Vaccine Coding Table": http://practice.aap.org/content.aspx?aid=2334

Managing Vaccine Refusal

- Parental Refusal to Vaccinate Form: http://practice.aap.org/content.aspx?aid=1605
- "Responding to 7 Common Parental Concerns About Vaccines & Vaccine Safety": http://practice.aap.org/content.aspx?aid=106

Purchasing Vaccines

- "Vaccine Purchasing Groups": http://practice.aap.org/content.aspx?aid=2381

Reminder/Recall

- "Vaccine Reminder Recall Systems: A Practical Guide for Pediatric Practices": http://practice.aap.org/content.aspx?aid=2674

Telephone Triage

An essential function of a pediatrician is to provide advice and guidance to parents. However, not every issue requires a doctor's appointment. Therefore, a pediatric practice will need someone to provide advice to parents over the telephone. This serves to help the families, as well as to triage patients to determine when and if a child needs to be seen in the office.

During the workday, most offices will have an experienced pediatric nurse (usually an RN) provide advice as determined by the physicians of the practice. Many will use nationally recognized pediatric telephone advice protocols such as those created by Barton D. Schmitt, MD, FAAP.

The number of advice nurses to staff depends very much on the volume of phone calls handled. When you are first starting your practice, the volume may not be enough to warrant a full advice nurse full-time equivalent (FTE). You may have a cross-trained nurse who helps in the clinical area and with handling phone calls between patients. As the practice grows, additional staff may be needed. A fully established practice will usually require one full advice nurse FTE for every 4 providers.

In the past, most pediatric offices provided phone call triage and advice services at no additional cost. However, recently there has been a great deal of interest in charging parents for telephone care, particularly after office hours. There are very specific guidelines for billing insurance for telephone care, and payment varies greatly based on insurance companies and your individual contracts. The AAP has guidelines for pediatricians on charging for telephone care at http://practice.aap.org/telecarepmt.aspx.

Additional Resources

- *Developing a Telephone Triage and Advice System for a Pediatric Office Practice:* http://eweb.aap.org/pub39209
- *Pediatric Telephone Protocols: Office Version,* 12th Edition, binder: http://eweb.aap.org/pub56118

After-hours Phone Care

After-hours phone calls can be handled by the physician on call. However, many practices use after-hours triage services to provide frontline phone care. There are many after-hours triage services across the country and it is important to select one that is experienced in handling pediatric phone calls. Some practices use their own advice nurses to take after-hours calls. For additional guidance, see "Weigh Costs and Benefits When Selecting After-hours Triage Service" at http://aapnews.aappublications.org/cgi/content/full/25/4/182.

Additional information can be found at
- "After Hours Calls: Evaluating Options": http://practice.aap.org/content.aspx?aid=386
- "Finding an After Hours Call Center": http://practice.aap.org/content.aspx?aid=390

Coverage and Referrals

Tips on Finding Coverage From Other Pediatricians

- Join the local AAP and attend meetings.
- Join your local hospital's medical staff and attend meetings.
- Be willing to be in hospital or organization committees; they force you to go out and talk to your peers.
- As few and far between as they are now, attend sponsored dinners and socialize.
- Advertise in the local AAP magazine or bulletin.
- Be willing to provide coverage to others as well.
- Check with your community hospital or emergency department to see if it has coverage pools.
- Attend newborn deliveries and form a relationship with local obstetricians-gynecologists; they can point you to other providers in the area.

Tips on Finding Referrals

- Attend CME seminars or conferences provided by your closest tertiary or children's hospital.
- Ask other providers in your area who they refer to.
- When you get a referral from a specialist, call and ask about the practice.
- Ask neonatologists at your community nursery for leads.

Wave Scheduling

Elizabeth Woodcock, MBA, FACMPE, CPC

If work ebbs and flows throughout the day or no-shows plague your pediatric practice, you may want to try wave scheduling. Wave scheduling differs from the familiar practice of dividing the hour into neat time slots for each patient appointment and trying to fill each one. Wave scheduling means appointing patients in waves. This scheduling methodology comes in different forms. It could mean that your practice schedules all of each hour's patients at the top of the hour, or schedules most of them at the top of the hour and only a few during the hour. To illustrate, following are different forms of wave scheduling.

Full Wave Scheduling

Eight patients are scheduled at 8:00 am, 8 at 9:00 am, 8 at 10:00 am, etc. For pediatric practices with significant no-shows and late arrivers, schedule the entire hour's worth of patients at the top of the hour. Decide how many patients to schedule based on (1) the number of no-shows expected and (2) the average duration of appointments. If patients are seen every 10 minutes, but you expect 20% of them to be no-shows, then schedule 8 patients for the 6 slots to be filled that hour. The advantage of this method is that, even if 6 patients scheduled during that hour don't show up, you'll be on to the next hour's wave by 50 minutes after the hour. You can expect that at least one in the next wave of 8 patients will come in early. In any case, see patients based on their order of arrival. (Explain this to patients when they schedule appointments to avoid frustration at arrival. Pediatric practices that are open about the wave scheduling and the reason behind it discover that most patients embrace it.) If you're scheduling every 10 minutes, patients who arrive on time often have to wait a long time and rarely get seen on time. In the wave model, parents who are conscientious will have their children seen first. Even if the patient doesn't arrive first for the "wave," the average wait is 20 to 30 minutes and the maximum wait is 45 to 50 minutes, if the hour is scheduled appropriately. This contrasts to practices plagued by no-shows and late arrivals, where average waits are often more than an hour, and maximum waits routinely stretch to several hours.

Modified Wave Scheduling

Four patients are scheduled at 8:00 am, 2 patients are scheduled at 8:15 am, and 2 patients are scheduled at 8:30 am. During the next hour, 4 patients are scheduled at 9:00 am, 2 at 9:15 am, 2 at 9:30 am, etc. Pediatric practices that deal with a small but disruptive problem with no-shows and late arrivals should try modifying the wave further so that more patients are scheduled toward the top of the hour, but some are still scheduled during the hour. For a practice that expects 20% of patients to be no-shows and others to arrive late, this modified model still means that you're likely to have 2 patients who are ready to be seen at all times. If 2 of the top-of-the-hour patients don't show up, you can see the 2 who do and be ready for the one 8:15 am patient who arrives on time. If the other 8:15 am patient is late, you can see him at 8:25 am, and the 8:30 am wave will be ready.

The beauty of the wave methodology is that it allows you to account for multiple appointment types (eg, acute visits and well-child checks). Schedule the longer appointments at the top of the hour regardless of the methodology you choose because it will give staff adequate time to perform intake duties and allow some wiggle room if patients arrive late.

The rationale of wave scheduling is to strike a balance between optimizing your time—the greatest asset of a pediatric practice is the providers' time—and respecting the parents' and patients' time. A traditional schedule, where patients are expected to show up and be right on time, just does not work for all patient populations. Wave scheduling is an option for those pediatric practices where parents and patients aren't always as compliant as we'd wish them to be.

Wave scheduling isn't a perfect scheduling methodology. But that's just the point. It accommodates parents' and patients' imperfections with showing up on time, or showing up at all, and optimizes your providers' time, but does not punish those parents who are compliant with the appointment times you've provided.

Author Elizabeth Woodcock, MBA, FACMPE, CPC, is an Atlanta-based practice management speaker. Contact her at elizabeth@elizabethwoodcock.com.

Open-Access Scheduling

Open access, sometimes called "advanced access" or "same-day" scheduling, allows pediatric practices to not only provide timelier health care, but also more patient-centered and efficient care for children. Open access involves redesigning scheduling systems to allow practices to offer same-day appointments to all patients, regardless of the nature of their problems, whether routine or urgent. The guiding principle is, "do today's work today."

This seemingly impossible feat is accomplished by gradually eliminating the preexisting backlog of patients from practice schedules and carefully matching the daily supply of clinicians to the daily demand for visits. The underlying theory is that demand is predictable. Thus practices can match their appointment supply to demand on an ongoing basis.

Would Open Access Improve My Lifestyle as a Pediatrician?

Yes! Implementing open access scheduling can result in fewer patient calls after hours, fewer emergency department (ED) visits and hospitalizations, and a more predictable schedule. When patients are able to see you the same day they want to be seen, they are less likely to call you after hours. Also, if patients are seen promptly on the day they call, they are less likely to go to the ED during normal office hours. A patient seen by an unfamiliar doctor in the ED is more likely to be admitted. Finally, one of the most frustrating aspects of being a physician is not being able to leave the office at 5 pm on time when the office closes. With open access, it is rare to have several "add-ons" or "walk-ins" to see at the end of the day. Patients who call for same-day appointments are placed in appointment slots during the regular scheduled day.

Will My Staff Benefit From Open Access?

Staff morale is high in practices where schedulers and receptionists can offer patients appointments the same day. Why? Because patient satisfaction is generally higher and staff do not have to deal with angry parents who want their sick child seen when the schedule is full.

Will My Patients Like Having Open Access?

Most patients are pleasantly surprised when they are offered same-day appointments. Some still prefer to book appointments into the future. However, you are putting the patient in the driver's seat. They decide when it is convenient for them to see you as opposed to the traditional model. Also, by having fewer "add-ons" or "walk-ins" without a scheduled time, you reduce waiting for the other patients, therefore, making your office more efficient.

My Phones Are Already Very Busy. Will Open Access Make Them Even Worse?

Just the opposite happens. The phone system is usually a symptom of poor access. People call to make an appointment, but because the schedule is full, they are kept on the phone longer while they are being triaged. This causes a backlog and increases congestion on the phones. Very frequently it is the same people that call day after day to try to get in to see you. This adds to the volume of phone calls and ties up your phones. In most open access practices, the phones improve as access improves. The phones actually get better with open access.

Can Open Access Improve My Bottom Line?

Open access affects different practices in different ways. In capitated plans, there are a few benefits. By having more availability in your schedule every day, you are able to increase your panel size and thereby increase monthly revenues. Also, by encouraging continuity of care and having same-day appointments, ED visits and hospitalizations are decreased, making you eligible for utilization bonuses.

There are also several benefits for fee-for-service plans. One of the principles of open access is to maximize each visit. If a child is brought in for a diaper rash but needs a 4-month-old well-child check, the preventive care is conducted and the diaper rash is assessed during the same visit. This increases the total relative value units per visit, thereby increasing your revenues.

Open access can save you money by

- Decreasing turnover with staff because of improved morale
- Improving utilization of nursing staff by eliminating most nurse triage
- Reducing no shows and cancellations dramatically
- Improving patient satisfaction, which translates into more new patients and increased revenue for the practice

Do All Appointments Have to Be Scheduled the Same Day?

Patients can still book appointments in advance. When the patient calls, your receptionist should always offer a same-day appointment. However, if the patient prefers to book the visit in the future for their convenience, it should be up to the patient. If you need a follow-up visit, you can book that appointment because you know that patient is going to need to be seen in the near future.

Keep in mind that the amount of appointments booked into the future varies with the time of the year. In the summer, before school begins, the majority of visits are going to be well-child checks and sports physicals. These can be booked in advance. Thus, in the summer, your percentage of prebooked appointments might be less. The opposite is true in the winter. Most of your visits are going to be sick visits. Your same-day appointments will probably comprise more of your schedule.

Can We Still Schedule Well-Child Checks in Advance?

Yes, but just how far in advance is something your practice needs to decide on as a group. In our experience, most pediatric practices find that booking further than 4 to 6 months in advance is not necessary if patients are assured that when they do call, they can get an appointment right away.

What If the Patient Calls at 4:30 pm and Wants to Be Seen the Same Day?

Your practice needs to have a plan for this occurrence. In some practices, the patient is seen the same day regardless of the time they call. In other practices, anybody that calls after 4:30 pm or 5:00 pm is offered an appointment first thing the following morning. When doing "today's work today," your practice will need to decide when "today" officially ends.

I Like This System, but There Is No Way I Can Convince the Rest of the Practice to Do It. What Can I Do?

If you are convinced, start a small pilot study with just your patients. Explain open access to the rest of the group and measure outcomes before and after. After you have small successes with your pilot, it will be easier to spread this to the rest of the group.

This Open Access Sounds Great, but It Looks Like a Lot of Work to Set It Up, and I'm Very Busy Already.

It does take some initial effort, but with 1 or 2 hours a week you can probably implement many components of open access. Start with a small pilot with maybe just one physician, and then spread it to the rest of the group. The benefits will greatly outweigh all the time that you put in initially.

FAQs developed by Xavier Sevilla, MD, FAAP. Dr Sevilla is the 2003 Honorable Mention of the AAP Steering Committee on Quality Improvement and Management Annual Quality of Care Award. Dr Sevilla was recognized for effectively implementing open access scheduling in his migrant office in rural Florida.

If you need help with open access, or if you have any additional questions, we can help you. Contact Junelle Speller for more information or to provide feedback at jspeller@aap.org or 847/434-7650.

After-hours Calls: Call Centers Versus Telephone Answering Services

Choosing an After-hours Call Center

After-hours call centers provide professional representation for the pediatric practice. Therefore, inquiry should be made about the professional level of the individuals answering calls, how they are trained and supervised, if they are certified, and which triage manuals and software are being used. You should also learn the name and degree of participation by the supervising physician. Inquiring about the volume of calls handled by the center, the number of physicians it serves, and its formal affiliations with insurers and hospitals may also be useful.

Both the service itself and its professional employees should be licensed in your state and should carry their own liability insurance.

The malpractice insurer for the pediatric practice and its participating health care plans should agree in writing that use of this outside provider for after-hours calls does not violate contractual agreements. It is strongly recommended that a practice physician should review triage protocols at regular intervals to be certain that they conform to practice recommendations and advice. Discrepancies should be noted and discussed with an appropriate call center representative.

Choosing a Telephone Answering Service

In most cases, telephone answering service personnel have no formal medical training and minimal medical knowledge. Their primary function is to relay messages accurately and in a timely fashion. However, informal triage of calls occurs when the operator must decide whether a physician should be contacted on an urgent basis. It is therefore recommended that the service agree to follow written instructions provided by practice physicians. The list should be short, avoid medical and technical terminology, and allow for over-screening of calls. Except in special circumstances, it is best not to list all of the conditions for which you would like to be called (eg, trouble breathing, high fever, head trauma, etc). The list is too long to be practical and exclusions might create liability. An example of such instructions is given below.

Unless you are otherwise notified, our physician will call in once every 90 minutes for nonurgent calls. However, the physician should be called or paged immediately if

1. The caller believes the call is an emergency. (Best screening question: "Is this call an emergency?" or "Do you feel frightened about the way your child looks or is acting?")
2. The caller believes the problem can't wait until the next call-in time. (Best screening question: "The doctor will be calling in at 9 o'clock, but I can page her if you believe this problem can't wait.")
3. You (the service operator) believe the call is an emergency because of the type of complaint or because the caller seems very nervous.
4. The caller has made multiple calls about the same problem.
5. The patient is an infant younger than 2 months who has a fever or is acting sick.

Preparation for Emergencies in the Offices of Pediatricians and Pediatric Primary Care Providers: A Summary of AAP Policy for Your Practice

Pediatricians and pediatric primary care providers (PPCPs) are essential members of the emergency care system for children. A lack of emergency preparedness can result in increased liability. Pediatricians and PPCPs may be required to provide urgent or emergent care in their offices, at least until emergency medical services (EMS) arrives.

In July 2007 the American Academy of Pediatrics (AAP) published a policy statement, "Preparation for Emergencies in the Offices of Pediatricians and Pediatric Primary Care Providers," drafted by the AAP Committee on Pediatric Emergency Medicine. Following is an overview of the committee's recommendations:

- **Office-based self-assessment:** To be prepared for an office emergency it is important to assess the types of patients that you see, the potential emergencies, and any resources that would benefit the patient in the event of an emergency.
- **Parent and patient education:** Providing effective education and anticipatory guidance to parents can assist with preventing emergencies as well as helping parents determine when children should be directed to an emergency department.
- **Preparing the office and office personnel:** All staff should be able to recognize emergencies (including signs and symptoms) and know how to summon help.
- **Emergency equipment and medications:** Trained staff must have rapid access to appropriate equipment and medications to use at the time of an emergency.
- **Health care professional skills:** In the event of a pediatric emergency, PPCPs must be able to provide basic airway management and initiate treatment of shock.
- **Documentation:** The most effective tool for risk management of office emergencies is documentation of efforts taken to improve office readiness, such as purchase and maintenance of equipment and medications, training provided, and policy and practice for patient education, patient triage, and office flow.

- **Emergency medical services:** Establishing good and close communication with local EMS providers can help inform your office of their unique skill sets and introduce them to the types of emergencies to which they might be called to respond from your office.
- **Advocacy:** PPCPs play a critical role as advocates for high-quality emergency care for their pediatric patients. In partnership with out-of-hospital and hospital-based staff, PPCPs can help ensure the readiness of all components of the emergency care system for children.

Recommended Equipment That Pediatricians Should Have in Their Offices

Airway Management

- Oxygen-delivery system
- Office emergency equipment and supplies
- Bag-valve-mask (450 and 1,000 mL)
- Clear oxygen masks, breather and non-rebreather, with reservoirs (infant, child, adult)
- Suction device, tonsil tip, bulb syringe
- Nebulizer (or metered-dose inhaler with spacer and mask)
- Oropharyngeal airways (sizes 00–5)
- Pulse oximeter
- Nasopharyngeal airways (sizes 12–30F)
- Magill forceps (pediatric, adult)
- Suction catheters (sizes 5–16F) and Yankauer suction tip
- Nasogastric tubes (sizes 6–14F)
- Laryngoscope handle (pediatric, adult) with extra batteries and bulbs
- Laryngoscope blades (0–2 straight and 2–3 curved)
- Endotracheal tubes (uncuffed 2.5–5.5; cuffed 6.0–8.0)
- Stylets (pediatric, adult)
- Esophageal intubation detector or end-tidal carbon dioxide detector

Vascular Access and Fluid Management

- Butterfly needles (19–25 gauge)
- Catheter-over-needle device (14–24 gauge)
- Arm boards, tape, tourniquet
- Intraosseous needles (16 and 18 gauge)
- Intravenous tubing, microdrip

Miscellaneous Equipment and Supplies

- Color-coded tape or preprinted drug doses
- Cardiac arrest board/backboard
- Sphygmomanometer (infant, child, adult, thigh cuffs)
- Splints, sterile dressings
- Automated external defibrillator with pediatric capabilities
- Spot glucose test
- Stiff neck collars (small, large)
- Heating source (overhead warmer, infrared lamp)

Specific Recommended Emergency Medications That Pediatricians Should Have in Their Offices

Drugs

- Oxygen
- Albuterol for inhalation
- Epinephrine (1:1,000)
- Activated charcoal

- Antibiotics
- Anticonvulsant agents (diazepam, lorazepam)
- Corticosteroids (parenteral, oral)
- Dextrose (25%)
- Diphenhydramine (parenteral, 50 mg/mL)
- Epinephrine (1:10,000)
- Atropine sulfate (0.1 mg/mL)
- Naloxone (0.4 mg/mL)
- Sodium bicarbonate (4.2%)

Fluids

- Normal saline solution or lactated Ringer's solution (500-mL bags)
- 5% dextrose, 0.45 normal saline (500-mL bags)

The complete policy statement, recommendations, and various appendices such as a self-assessment tool, reception desk emergency cards, important telephone numbers, and sample scenarios can be found online at http://aappolicy.aappublications.org/cgi/content/full/pediatrics;120/1/200.

Safe Storage of Vaccines

According to *Red Book® Online* Vaccine Handling and Storage (http://aapredbook.aappublications.org/cgi/content/full/2009/1/1.5.2), the American Academy of Pediatrics (AAP) recommends the following:

- Be sure that all vaccines are stored at the recommended temperatures.
- All staff should be trained on the standard procedures for storage conditions and these should be posted on or near each refrigerator or freezer used for vaccine storage.
- Assign a staff member as the vaccine coordinator. This person will be responsible for ensuring that vaccines are handled and stored in a careful, safe, recommended, and documentable manner. A backup person should also be assigned.
- Check refrigerators and freezers to ensure that they are working properly and maintain a refrigerator temperature between 2°C and 8°C (35°F and 46°F) with a target temperature of 40°F, and a freezer temperature of -15°C (5°F) or colder. A certified thermometer should be used and located at the center of the storage compartment.
- Maintain a logbook to document temperature readings. Temperatures should be recorded at the beginning and end of the clinic day. The date, time, and duration of any mechanical malfunctions or power outages should be noted.
- All opened vials of vaccine should be placed in a refrigerator tray. To avoid mishaps, do not store other pharmaceutical products in the same tray.
- Store unopened vials in the original packaging. This facilitates inventory management and rotation of vaccine by expiration date and also protects measles, mumps, and rubella and measles, mumps, rubella, and varicella vaccines from light.
- Indicate on the label of each vaccine vial the date and time the vaccine was reconstituted or first opened.
- Inspect the vaccines weekly for outdated vaccines and remove expired vaccines promptly.
- Store several bottles of chilled water in the refrigerator and several ice trays and ice packs in the freezer to fill empty space. This will also minimize temperature fluctuations during brief electrical or mechanical failures.
- Do not allow staff to store food or drink in refrigerators where vaccines are stored.

- Vaccines should be stored in the central storage area of the refrigerator. Do not store vaccines in the door shelf or peripheral areas.
- Do not store radioactive materials in the refrigerator with vaccines.
- Develop a written emergency plan in the event of a catastrophic occurrence.

The fact sheet "Don't Be Guilty of These Errors in Vaccine Storage and Handling" (http://www.immunize.org/catg.d/p3036.pdf) provides these additional tips: avoid using dorm-style refrigerators and be sure that the refrigerator is closed properly every time.

Finally, consider using a thermometer system that alerts the appropriate party if the refrigerator or freezer temperature is out of range.

Additional Resources and Tools

- CDC Recommendations and Guidelines: Vaccine Storage and Handling: http://www.cdc.gov/vaccines/recs/storage/default.htm
- "Checklist for Safe Vaccine Handling and Storage": http://www.immunize.org/catg.d/p3035.pdf This resource provides a checklist to help safeguard the vaccines.
- "Lessons Learned from Hurricane Katrina: Ensuring Proper Vaccine Management, Handling, and Administration During a Disaster": http://practice.aap.org/content.aspx?aid=1979
- "Notice to Readers: Guidelines for Maintaining and Managing the Vaccine Cold Chain": http://www.cdc.gov/mmwr/preview/mmwrhtml/mm5242a6.htm (*MMWR Weekly,* October 24, 2003)
- "Risk Factors for Improper Vaccine Storage and Handling in Private Provider Offices": http://pediatrics.aappublications.org/cgi/content/full/107/6/e100 (Pediatrics. 2001;107:e100)
- "Standards for Child and Adolescent Immunization Practices": http://pediatrics.aappublications.org/cgi/reprint/112/4/958.pdf
- "Temperature Log for Vaccines (Fahrenheit)": http://www.immunize.org/catg.d/p3039.pdf
- "Vaccine Handling Tips": http://www.immunize.org/catg.d/p3048.pdf

For more information, contact AAP staff at cispimmunize@aap.org; call 800/433-9016, ext 4271.

Lessons Learned From Hurricane Katrina: Ensuring Proper Vaccine Management, Handling, and Administration During a Disaster

Disasters can have a devastating effect on the delivery of health care. The management, handling, and administration of vaccines are aspects of health care that can be successful if proper procedures are in place to prevent any possible challenges. Therefore, it is important for all pediatricians (regardless of location) to be prepared with a comprehensive vaccine management protocol to ensure that vaccines are handled properly before disaster strikes.

What Can Pediatricians Do to Prepare?

- Promote good storage and handling.
  - Regularly monitor refrigerator temperatures.
  - Follow vaccine handling and storage requirements.
  - Check equipment function when placing vaccine orders.
- Develop vaccine management protocols in the event of a power outage. If necessary, move vaccines to a safe storage area.
- Display a vaccine disaster recovery plan.
- Contact distributors to stop bulk vaccines and order deliveries.
- Confirm suspension of Vaccines for Children (VFC) vaccines to the local public health agency.
- Ensure power source backup for vaccine refrigerators.
- Document vaccines determined not viable for later return. Do not discard vaccines that have been subjected to temperature instability. Contact the manufacturer for instructions. In some cases, manufacturers will accept returns after the expiration date for credit. Post a list of manufacturer information lines.
- Be proactive.
  - Back up energy source.
  - Develop protocols for removal of vaccines to a safe storage site if there is a prolonged power outage. Have transfer containers and knowledge of where to get ice or dry ice for transport.
- Protect the vaccine.
  - Maintain the cold chain.
  - Monitor temperatures; don't discard or administer affected vaccines until it has been discussed with public health authorities.
  - Follow proper procedures during a power outage and once power has been restored.

What Can Pediatricians Do During a Disaster?

- Communicate the emergency to provider sites in advance.
- Send additional information (if available) to those practices in the path of danger.
- Communicate with local health departments and officials (stay on message; coordinate activities when possible).

What Can Physicians Do After a Disaster Hits?

- Contact the local health department or the Centers for Disease Control and Prevention for information and guidance.
- Follow interim immunization recommendations and communicate those to your staff.
- Provide recommended vaccines to those living in a crowded setting.
- Notify distributors to resume vaccine deliveries.
- Notify vaccine representatives to resume bulk order shipments.
- Contact the local public health department to determine if VFC vaccine delivery has resumed.
- In the event of a vaccine shortage, work with local public health officials to identify and distribute needed vaccine.

At All Times

- Document all vaccines.
- Provide immunization records within the scope of the practice of the state in which the vaccine is administered.
- Immunization cards should be provided to individuals at the time of vaccination.
- Standard immunization practices should be followed for delivery of all vaccines, including provision of Vaccine Information Statements.

The best thing that a pediatrician can do is to be prepared and have an office protocol and plan in the event of an emergency. Contact your local health department for assistance.

For the full presentation, complete with links to resources, please visit http://practice.aap.org/content.aspx?aid=1979.

Additional Resources

Vaccine Management: Recommendations for Storage and Handling of Selected Biologicals (http://www.cdc.gov/vaccines/pubs/vac-mgt-book.htm)—This resource provides specifics for shipping, condition on arrival, storage requirements, shelf life, instructions for reconstitution of use, shelf life after reconstitution or opening, and special instructions. It also provides vaccine manufacturers' quality control office telephone numbers.

Vaccine Handling Tips (http://www.immunize.org/catg.d/p3048.pdf) —This fact sheet provides details on safe vaccine storage and handling.

For more information on immunization initiatives, contact the American Academy of Pediatrics at cispimmunize@aap.org or 800/433-9016, ext 4271.

Vaccine Reminder Recall Systems: A Practical Guide for Pediatric Practices

What Are Reminder/Recall Systems?

Immunization reminder/recall systems are cost-effective methods whereby children in need of vaccination are identified and contacted to come to the physician's office. Reminder systems track future appointments, whereas recall systems track missed appointments during which immunizations would have been given. Combining reminder and recall systems is a powerful method for ensuring optimal vaccination rates.

Why Are Reminder/Recall Systems Important?

Good immunization practices in private offices are important because of the reliance on office-based pediatricians and family physicians for childhood vaccinations. In general, pediatricians are doing a good job delivering routine vaccines—more than 70% of children receive their vaccines from pediatricians and more than 80% receive vaccines in the private sector. However, more than one-fourth of preschool children lack at least one routine vaccination, and more than two-thirds of adolescents have not received the meningococcal conjugate vaccine or a pertussis booster.

What Are the Benefits of These Systems?

Using reminder/recall systems within a medical home has been shown to improve not only immunization rates but also overall health care. Children who are behind on immunizations are at greater risk of being behind on other preventive services. By using these systems, physicians can increase vaccination rates and promote other important clinical services, such as lead and vision screening.

How Can Reminder/Recall Systems Be Implemented?

To implement a reminder/recall system, consider the following:

- An "immunization information gap" exists. Parents often do not know the vaccination status of their children and pediatricians sometimes perceive coverage among their patients as higher than it really is.
- Pediatricians should ask themselves, "How well am I doing at vaccinating my patients?" To know for

certain, contact the local state health department to request an office assessment of coverage and follow-up.
- Organization is essential. Offices use varied record-keeping systems, such as postcards, telephone calls, or a variety of techniques. The key is to create a system that allows personnel to identify children in need of vaccinations.
- One size does not fit all. Successful recall systems vary from tickler files to community-based immunization registries. These systems are dependent on office personnel's ability to use the system and fine-tune it to meet the specific needs of the practice.

Effective Models and Strategies

The pediatrician's role is to overcome the immunization information gap and ensure that children are vaccinated on time. By adopting the National Vaccine Advisory Committee Standards for Child and Adolescent Immunization Practices and American Academy of Pediatrics (AAP) policy statements on immunization, physicians can enhance their policies and practices and improve the health and welfare of children, adolescents, and their community.

Definitions and Types of Reminder/Recall Systems

The AAP endorses reminder/recall systems through policy statements and reports. The following examples of reminder/recall systems were adapted from the work of the AAP Task Force on Community Preventive Services. Physicians do not have to invest a lot of time or money to develop a successful reminder/recall system. By evaluating their resources and needs, physicians can implement a simple, effective system suited to their practice. For more information about reminder/recall systems, visit the Agency for Healthcare Quality and Research Web site at http://www.ahrq.gov/ppip/postcard.pdf.

1. **Chart Reminders:** Chart reminders can be as simple as a colorful sticker on the chart or can be as comprehensive as a checklist of preventive services including vaccinations. Reminders to physicians should be prominently placed in the chart. Reminders that require some type of acknowledgment, even a simple check mark by the physician, are more effective.

2. **Mail/Telephone Reminders:** Staff, or an automated telephone dial-out system, call the patient or send a postcard/letter reminding the patient that a vaccination is due and offer the opportunity for the patient to schedule an appointment.
   - Typical setting: Private practice and managed care.
   - Advantages: (1) Phone contact can help to ensure that the message is understood and provides the opportunity to schedule an appointment; (2) reaches patients who may otherwise not have scheduled visits; (3) easy to implement, requiring minimal staff time.
   - Disadvantages: (1) Relies on patient to schedule and keep appointments; (2) not useful in practices with high patient turnover or with a population that changes residences frequently; (3) may need bilingual reminders; (4) generating a list of patients who should receive reminders may be difficult in some practices (eg, for those without computerized records); (5) if baseline vaccination rates are high, the incremental increase in vaccination rate attained may not be worth the time and effort invested.
   - Implementation: (1) Determine selection criteria (ie, age and/or diagnosis); (2) generate a list of patients to be reminded (manually or via computerized billing or medical records); (3) review list to remove the names of patients who have died, transferred their care to another provider, entered a long-term care facility, left the practice/area, or received vaccinations; (4) develop reminder; (5) send reminders or place calls (6 calls a day, 5 days a week for 8 weeks = 240 patients contacted); (6) schedule appointments.
   - Resources needed: Staff time, telephone script, or postcards.
3. **Computerized Immunization Reminders:** The computer can print a list of possible reminders that appear on a patient's record. The software can be programmed to determine the dates that certain preventive procedures are due or past due and then print computer-generated reminder messages, usually overnight, for patients with visits scheduled for the next day. Many electronic medical records or immunization information systems (registries) already have this capability built in.
   - Typical setting: Private practice, managed care, hospitals, and long-term care facilities.
   - Advantages: effective, inexpensive once computerized system is in place, efficient.
   - Disadvantages: (1) Only reaches patients with office visits, (2) may be less effective in fee-for-service practices since cost to the patient may be a barrier to vaccination in a fee-for-service practice.
   - Implementation: (1) Design or identify a computerized reminder system to use, (2) train professional staff in the use of the computerized reminders.
   - Resources required: Computer program linked to medical records or billing data to generate reminders, computerized medical records.
4. **Expanding Clinic Hours:** Expanding access can include (1) reducing the distance from the setting to patients; (2) increasing, or making more convenient, the hours during which vaccination services are provided; (3) delivering vaccinations in settings previously not used; and/or (4) reducing administrative barriers to vaccination (eg, "drop-in" clinics or "express lane" vaccination services). This group of strategies has been very effective in increasing immunization rates when combined with other strategies, such as patient reminder/recall, less clearly so when used alone.
   - Typical setting: Private practice, managed care, and hospitals.
   - Advantages: Efficient, may help increase access to care among lower income and other disadvantaged persons.
   - Disadvantages: Increased staff time and expense, new clients may lack records, or recall, of previous immunizations.
   - Implementation: (1) Determine which access barriers are the most important for your setting and your patients; (2) meet with staff to discuss implementation of strategies to improve access; (3) implement strategies, monitor increased vaccination rates in comparison to resources expended.
   - Resources needed: Staff time and potential financial cost (if new clinical setting established to increase access).
5. **Standing Orders:** A standing order is a written order stipulating that all persons meeting certain criteria (ie, age) should be vaccinated, thus eliminating the need for individual physician's orders for each patient.
   - Advantages: Easy to implement using ready-made templates.

- Disadvantages: Only reaches patients already contacting the health care system.
6. **Card file:** A 3x5 card file system can be used to track dates vaccines were given and due dates for future vaccines. Office personnel can review these cards to determine missed appointments and follow up with parents.
7. **Phone lists:** Phone lists can be used to follow up with patients who have future immunizations or have missed appointments. By tracking patients whose immunizations are due soon, physicians show parents they are aware of their children's needs.
8. **Clinical Assessment Software Application (CASA):** The CASA is a database developed by the Centers for Disease Control and Prevention (CDC) to help immunization providers assess immunization rates in their offices. This database can help physicians determine the immunization status of children at critical age markers and antigen-specific levels, as well as the percentage of children who drop out of the vaccination schedule and miss opportunities for immunization. The CASA also produces reports and provides programmatic feedback, and programs are available from the CDC at http://www.cdc.gov/vaccines/programs/cocasa/default.htm.
9. **Immunization Information Systems:** Using a modem to link to the local health department registry allows staff to check or update immunization records daily. This ensures that there are no missed opportunities at any location.
10. **Multiple Systems:** It might be necessary to use several systems. For example, office personnel can ask parents to address reminder postcards. These postcards can be sent prior to the next appointment, and patients who fail to show up can be placed in an "alert" file and called to set up a new appointment.

**For information about other reminder/recall systems, including card files, phone lists, electronic systems, and more, visit the AAP Childhood Immunization Support Program Web site at: www.aap.org/immunization/pediatricians/pdf/ReminderRecall.pdf.

AAP Section on Administration and Practice Management Member Comments About the Use and Implementation of Reminder/Recall Systems

- We mail reminder postcards 1 week in advance of scheduled checkups and call patients the day before their visit.
- We use a computer software package for our recalls. We enter the recall information at the end of each visit and at designated times throughout the month we print our recalls on cards in our office. We hope to have the software electronically manage and process the reminders for later mailing.
- We use postcards as reminders. We fill them out during the physical examination and put them in a "tickler file" to be mailed 1 month prior to next examination.
- In the past, we ran a list from our computer of all patients in a certain age range who had not been in for a routine physical examination during the subsequent 2 years. We then sent a postcard reminder out—we didn't get much of a response!
- We use a telephone-based reminder/recall system. It interfaces with our practice management software and calls all patients who have appointments. We call the night before but it can be set up to call whenever you want.
- In our office, we generate a report from our computer system for reminder of next-day appointments and make the calls from the front desk at the end of the day. We also generate reports based on age in our system to recall patients each month to schedule appointments for well checks for the next month, and our staff make those calls as well.
- Patient reminder phone calls are launched from our appointment system into an electronic message system. This is done 2 days before the scheduled visit to allow parents time to change their appointment, if necessary. If the parent answers the call (as opposed to going to voice message), the parent can confirm the appointment or cancel the appointment. The office receives a summary of all the calls made by the system indicating any actions taken. Patient recalls are used when the patients cannot get an appointment (usually because the next appointment is needed beyond the schedule that has been determined). These patients complete a recall card (address it) and the card goes into a tickler file by month to send the postcard. If

the recall is due to a vaccine shortage (ie, Prevnar) the office keeps a manual recall list.

- We schedule the next well-child visit at the time the patient is in. It is not unusual for our office to schedule 2-, 4-, 6-, 9-, 12-month visits at the baby's 2-week visit. We also send birthday cards so this is how we remind parents to make 1-year, 2-year, etc, well-child visits. We additionally have a kindergarten physical Saturday one time per month from March to August. We have a clown and do nothing but kindergarten physicals and have about 50 kids each of these days. We gather names of kids with a computer inquiry on birth date so that we can send them a letter to schedule the kindergarten physical early. Our computer system will generate letters based on many codes for recall. We do not use this only because our office is set up to pro-actively handle scheduling as mentioned above.

- We are a 10 full-time equivalent practice. We have tried several processes over the years. Our current method is the most successful to date. Our no-show rate is finally at a level we can live with. One of our staff was resigning her position to be a stay-at-home mom. She was one of the clinic aides that placed reminder calls to the following day's scheduled patients. This particular person was very good with the parents and her attempts seemed to have the greatest effect. The trouble was, by placing the calls during the usual 8 to 5 we usually reached answering machines and we found that people didn't listen to their messages. We set up a separate line in the employee's home that reflects our practice name and phone number on caller IDs. The stay-at-home mom begins placing reminder calls in the late afternoon. She resumes after she has fed her family dinner, and tries again while her family does homework, dishes, etc. We find she reaches families in person, because they are home doing the same things that she is doing. If she has not reached a live person by bedtime, she calls these few remaining in the early morning hours while she gets her family up to start the day. She calls into the office with the list of cancels at 7:00 am so those spots are then available to fill with same-day appointments. The time spent averages 2.25 hours per day at entry-level wages plus cost of the phone line in her home. When we compare the effectiveness of our real, live, warm human

reminder call person with the cold, impersonal, mildly effective recording programs, we feel we are getting a bargain.

Reminder/Recall Systems: Useful Web sites

1. AAP Childhood Immunization Support Program: www.aap.org/immunization/about/programfacts. html
2. Centers for Disease Control and Prevention: http://www.cdc.gov/vaccines
3. AAP Council on Clinical Information Technology: http://www.aapcocit.org

Implementation of a Vaccine Reminder/Recall System: A Successful Pilot Project in Pennsylvania

By Kathleen Marker, RN, Practice Manager Consultant

Reminder/recall systems are proven effective in improving vaccination coverage rates, yet it is not realistic for many pediatric practices to obtain outside funding or devote tremendous amounts of staff time to reminder/recall efforts. So, like many programs aimed at helping pediatric practices improve immunization rates, the Pennsylvania Immunization Education Program (IEP) tried hard—and succeeded—in finding practical and efficient ways to help practices implement reminder/recall systems. The IEP reminder/recall project involves reviewing the charts of 19- or 20-month-olds (each practice can choose which age group works best for them) each month, assessing their immunization status, and attempting to bring in those patients who are overdue for immunization. By concentrating on this age group, staff avoid wasting time reaching out to compliant families that are already bringing their children in regularly for care and instead focuses precious staff time on children who are overdue. Focusing on this age group also enables practices to catch-up children by 2.

From December 2003 to June 2004, 14 practices pilot-tested this approach. Two sites dropped out due to influenza season demands on practice resources, but 12 sites found the project doable even during this hectic time. The project included both pediatric and family practices in clinic and private settings. Locating and reviewing the charts took between 1 to 3 hours per site. Between 2 and 60 charts fell into the target age group at each site, each month. The number of overdue patients varied from 2 to 13 children per site per month. Managing the ever-increasing snowball of overdue children that could not be contacted was a challenge. To address this challenge, staff made several attempts to contact each patient but only during the month of their review. All sites elected to do telephone calls for recall. Staff made at least

3 attempts per overdue child. Practice staff were successful in locating most but not all of the overdue children.

Families are more likely to obtain immunization services during the first year of life because drop-off is more common after 12 months of age.

Successfully locating and bringing in the overdue children resulted in approximately half of the overdue children being brought up to date for immunization. Staff found this reminder/recall project simple to understand and do. They were very pleased with the results and all plan to continue this monthly reminder/recall of 19- or 20-month-olds. Numerous additional practices in PA have now started this project. It would be great to build on IEP's reminder/recall effort and do more frequent, more intensive reminder/recall with more ages. But, for practices with limited resources, this project has significant rewards and requires minimal effort utilizing existing staff.

The PA IEP is a collaborative project between the Pennsylvania Chapter of the American Academy of Pediatrics (AAP); Pennsylvania Department of Health; and Pennsylvania Chapter of the American Academy of Family Physicians. Pilot testing of the program has been completed and expansion efforts to develop an easy-to-do reminder/recall system that targets young children are currently underway. The project is the brainchild of IEP Practice Manager Consultant Kathleen Marker, RN, who conceived and pilot tested the effort at her practice and is working with practices that wish to implement it.

For more information, click on "Reminder/recall" at www.paaap.org or e-mail the IEP at: iep@paaap.org.

Implementation of a Computer-Managed Immunization Tracking System: Putnam Valley Pediatrics, Putnam Valley, New York

By William M. Zurhellen, MD, FAAP

Initially, Dr Zurhellen and his staff only tracked immunizations and preventive care; in 1989 the office converted to an electronic medical record (EMR) system, which was built around their original immunization software. The physician or nurse administering the immunization could now enter all immunization information, including the child's preventive care examination information, directly into the system at the time of the visit. Each month the system reviews all medical records and produces a list of children in need of immunizations who do not have a preventive care appointment already scheduled (those children in need who already have an upcoming appointment are not included for obvious reasons); a reminder postcard is generated and mailed to the parent.

The date of the reminder is then recorded in the system so at a later date (the following month, usually) the office can retrospectively review compliance with that specific recall. The system also produces a list of children whose immunization status is up to date but due for a periodic preventive-care examination. These children also get reminder cards. A physician reviews the list to see if there are "slow-responders" who may need a follow-up telephone call. The ultimate goal is to maintain peak immunization rates, as well as peak preventive-care rates, because the same recall system implements both.

Timeline for Implementation

- June 1984 for immunizations
- July 1987 for preventive care
- August 1989 for complete EMR

Key Obstacles

- The office had to write its own software.
- Rule-based logic had to be revised each time the immunization recommendations were changed or when new immunizations were added (about 1–2 hours of programming, done in-house, for each change—note, some are easier, some are harder…).
- Rule-based logic had to be revised each time the practice experienced a vaccine shortage, and then again when the shortage was resolved—because

there is no point in recalling children if no vaccine is available

Key Benefits

- Office keeps peak immunization rates, keeping children healthy and customers (parents/health maintenance organizations) satisfied
- To a certain extent, staff can predict inventory and ordering needs; because the system tracks health insurance information, staff can differentiate between commercial/Vaccines for Children supply needs.
- Staff can maintain even and full scheduling, rather than having "crush demand" periods, by filling empty slots with patients responding to the recall.
- System is cost effective, because 1 or 2 vaccine-administration fees cover the entire cost of the recall (ie, 1 or 2 added encounters generate enough income to cover cost, and any other additional ones provide otherwise-missed incomes).
- By aggressively tracking/reminding preventive care visits, staff significantly reduced the amount of immunization recalls they must perform.

Lessons Learned

- Our office could never have done this with paper-based records, implementing an EMR was the right choice for us.

For more information, write to Dr Zurhellen at Putnam Valley Pediatrics, PO Box 397, Putnam Valley, New York 10579.

Protecting Patient Health Information

C. Morrison Farish, MD, FAAP

"Pay attention to your follow-through; it may be more important than you think."

This sounds like good advice on the golf course or tennis court, but it's also true when it comes to protecting patient health records after you retire or sell your practice.

Your patients have trusted you to respect their privacy, maintain the confidentiality of their health information, and ensure its availability for their continuing care for as long as you've been their doctor. This trust shouldn't end when you relocate or close your practice.

Any career transitions can be dicey, but knowing what to expect and having a clear understanding of your responsibilities about safeguarding patient charts can smooth the way considerably. A clean follow-through is the name of the game.

You have several options for finding a trustworthy custodian to manage your soon-to-be "former" patients' charts. Making a good choice will depend on several considerations (eg, whether you're retiring, the facility is closing, the practice is dissolving, or this transition involves a sale). Your state may have specific laws governing the disposition of medical records and other legal considerations.

In some states, a state archive or health department will store health records from closed facilities. Generally, state regulations recommend records be transferred to another health care provider. If a health care facility or medical practice is sold to another health care provider, patient records may be considered assets and included in the sale of the property.

If a facility closes or a practice dissolves without a sale, records usually can be transferred to another physician who agrees to accept the responsibility. Don't make this a casual agreement. You'll need to be sure that the physician understands what the responsibility entails and agrees to follow through.

If this is not feasible, records may be archived with a reputable commercial storage firm. This is not an inexpensive proposition. The state chapter of American Health Information Technology may be able to advise you of the medical records storage companies in your area if you haven't found a local recommendation from a colleague.

Either way, before the records leave your possession, your patients should be notified and given an opportunity to obtain copies of their health information. Typically patients are notified by mail, e-mail, and by publishing a series of notices in the local newspaper (to reach those for whom you no longer have a current address). State law may specify how much time patients should be given to request their records or how they should be contacted. Only copies of the health records should be given to patients, unless the required retention period has expired.

Liability Issues

Generally, the physician remains liable for accidental or incidental disclosure of health information during or after a facility closes. That's one reason why the physician should take steps to protect the integrity of the records and the confidentiality of the information they contain, while ensuring access for continued patient care.

But there is a much bigger risk here. Let's say that, 5 years after you've closed your practice, one of your former patients decides to file a malpractice claim against you. Should you be unable to produce a medical record, you would have virtually no defense.

State laws and regulations addressing facility or practice closure should be followed. These usually are available from the state department of health. If state laws and regulations are silent on how to proceed, you should consider the following factors:
- Applicable laws/regulations on medical record retention
- Agreements with public and private payers on record retention
- Recommendations from professional organizations
- Legal advice

Retention Requirements

State Laws/Licensure Requirements

A physician is bound by applicable federal and state laws and regulations even after the health care facility has been closed. Many state health departments and licensing authorities govern health care facility closures and specify how and where patient records should be transferred.

To minimize storage and/or transfer costs, you may want to destroy records that are past the required retention period; but be careful. The retention period for health records of minor patients (those who have not yet become legal adults) is often much longer than the retention period for those of adult patients. So, if you see a flat-rate retention period (eg, 5 years, 7 years, or 10 years), chances are it is not referring to records for pediatric patients. Keep looking.

If the state law does not specify the length of time records must be kept, then you need to consider the state's malpractice statute of limitations for minors and make sure that records are maintained until the patient reaches the age of majority (as defined by state law) plus the period of the statute of limitations, unless otherwise provided by state law. A longer retention period is prudent, because the statute of limitations may not begin to run until the potential plaintiff learns of the causal relation between an injury and the care received (discovery) instead of incidence.

You also should contact your professional liability insurance carrier. Because both the insured physician and the carrier must have access to patient records after the closure in the event of a malpractice claim, you'll want to be sure that your plan for keeping records private and available is acceptable with the insurer. Liability insurance risk managers often have sound advice on record retention.

Medicaid Requirements

If you participate in Medicaid, check your provider manual. There should be a specified period in which the records must be kept in their original or legally reproduced form. Your contracts with other payers may have similar requirements.

Other Recommendations

Professional organizations should be contacted for guidelines or recommendations. The American Academy of Pediatrics does not have official recommendations on this topic.

- American Health Information Management Association
- American Medical Association
- Your state medical societies

Legal Advice

Get advice from your legal counsel to determine the appropriate retention period, ensure compliance with state laws and regulatory agencies, and help plan for an orderly closure or transfer.

Following Through

As soon as you anticipate closure or practice breakup, you should begin planning for proper disposition of patient records. Your primary objective is to ensure future access by patients, health care providers, and other legitimate users while protecting the confidentiality of the information contained in the records.

First, make sure all health information documentation is completed before the records are archived or transferred. This includes transcription of dictated reports and interpretation of any diagnostic tests.

Notification

Patients should be given a reasonable amount of time (at least 1 month, unless a longer period is required by state law) to request copies of their records. The notification should include the following:

- Date facility will close.
- A release of information authorization form for patients to complete to receive a copy of their records.
- Specify that only written requests for copies of health information will be honored.
- Underscore any time limits (submission deadlines) on the period during which requests will be accepted.
- Indicate where the records will be stored and how to access them once they have been archived or transferred.
- Provide information on how to seek a new pediatrician.

The custodian of the retained records should retain a copy of the actual letter and/or e-mail sent to patients, along with the mailing list, broadcast e-mail list, post office receipt, all returned (undeliverable) envelopes, and a list of returned or undeliverable e-mails.

Closure With a Sale

If the facility or practice is sold to another physician, patient records may be considered assets and included in the sale of the property. As part of the agreement with the new owners, you, the physician selling the records, should retain the right to access the charts and obtain copies, if needed. In addition, if the new owner considers selling the records to a third party, you should retain the right to reclaim the patient records.

If the facility is sold to a non–health-care entity, patient records should not be included in the assets available for purchase. You should make arrangements either to transfer the records to an archive or another physician who agrees to accept responsibility for maintaining them.

Closure Without a Sale

If the facility closes or a practice dissolves without a sale, arrangement should be made with another pediatrician where patients may seek future care, unless otherwise required by state law. That new pediatrician should agree to maintain the records, permit access by authorized persons, and destroy the records when applicable time periods have expired.

Make sure the pediatrician and his or her staff have a clear understanding of medical record management (record retention, destruction requirement, and confidentiality).

Get it in writing. Prior to transferring records, a written agreement outline in terms and obligations should be executed. The original provider is responsible for ensuring that records are stored safely for an appropriate length of time.

Section 3

Business Considerations and Contracts

Getting a Loan

Excerpt from Launching Your Career in Pediatrics Handbook: Opening a New Practice

How Much?

The biggest factor in determining when you will break even is the amount of money you have to borrow to start up the practice. When determining a loan amount, it is important to consider the cost of equipment, rent, malpractice, and other insurances (eg, workers' compensation, liability). Also, during the first few months, you will be paid on what you borrow or have set aside, as you will have little to no income for 30 to 90 days, depending on how well you did your homework with the local managed care organizations (MCOs).

You will need to borrow or use capital for your income over the first 90 to 180 days; if you borrow more, you will have to pay back more. In addition, check the sample supply and equipment checklist (http://practice.aap.org/content.aspx?aID=2395) to get an idea of how much money you will need to borrow to stock and furnish your practice. For information on obtaining loans, check with various bank Web sites. For additional information, visit the US Small Business Administration (http://www.sba.gov).

Defining a Contract Strategy

Developing a negotiation strategy is an important step in the negotiation process. A pediatrician should have a clear idea of what he or she wants in a contractual relationship. A negotiation strategy is developed on the foundation provided by the medical group's analysis and the managed care organization's (MCO) assessments. Key elements include the following:

- MCO's market position
- Provider group's market position
- Projected role the MCO will play in the practice's market strategy over the next 3 years
- An understanding of the MCO's flexibility and willingness to be creative in contractual arrangements with providers

The negotiation strategy should be written and prepared in advance. This will help the group clarify the issues before engaging in negotiations, which can become heated and drawn out.

An outline should include the following components:

- Contractual Issues—Identification of all problems and the development of realistic business and contractual language alternatives.
- Covered Services—Definition of services to be covered or excluded under the proposed contract.
- Service Area—Determination of whether the contract will be exclusive or semi-exclusive for a defined service area.
- Reimbursement Options—Identification of minimum acceptable reimbursement thresholds for the practice and the definition of reimbursement options to be offered during negotiations.
- Risk Management—Development of stop loss and risk corridor protections based on coverage services and utilization projects.
- Administrative Issues—Specification of claims turnaround, utilization and cost reporting expectations of the MCO.
- Medical Management—Identification of any concerns regarding precertification, concurrent review, and credentialing requirements.
- Other Issues—Projection of potential MCO issues with provider group and definition of volume guarantees in exchange for favorable pricing.
- Cost of Walking Away—Projection of current and future losses should the practice decide not to contract with the MCO.

Although the preparation to this point will be extensive, expressing the strategy in writing will help the practice define and prioritize the issues. Before entering into negotiations, pediatricians should know what issues are deal breakers and which can be traded.

More detailed information is available as PediaLink Module Contract Negotiation With Payers (http://practice.aap.org/content.aspx?aid=1924).

Managed Care Contract Issues

Pediatricians entering into managed care contracts need to take certain steps before signing a contract: assessing their readiness and the readiness of the practice for managed care, assessing the strengths and weaknesses of the managed care plans they are considering, and selecting a professional advisor to assist in the contracting process. Once these steps are completed, pediatricians should carefully review the terms and provisions of managed care contracts. Such contracts should clearly define the responsibilities of the pediatrician and the managed care organization. As in any contracting process, it is important to identify which provisions are negotiable and which are not. Pediatricians need to seek legal review from their own attorney before signing any contract. Working with their professional advisors, pediatricians should attempt to eliminate onerous provisions for the agreement and include language that protects their interests and the interests of their patients.

Depending on the market share of the health plan and the services offered by the pediatrician, the negotiability of the contract will vary. Well-established managed care plans that have a large market share typically use form contracts. Newer managed care plans that have little market share and want broad provider participation will be more willing to negotiate terms. Regardless of the specific entity with which the pediatrician is negotiating, know as much as possible about that managed care plan and that being sensitive to the issues will enhance the pediatrician's opportunities for successful contract negotiations.

Definitions

This section of the contract will contain definitions of key terms. These should be reviewed carefully to ensure that they are not overly strict or vague. *(A Pediatrician's Guide to Managed Care,* 2nd edition [Nelson RP, Minon RE. Elk Grove Village, IL: American Academy of Pediatrics; 2001], page 97)

Medical Necessity Definition

Pediatricians should be wary of working in a contract that gives the managed care plan final authority on certain matters, particularly questions of medical necessity. Such provisions should be reviewed carefully to ensure that they do not impede the pediatrician's ability to exercise his or her best professional judgment in making medical practice decisions. Medical necessity is a mechanism that gives legal authority to a health plan to limit the provision of covered benefits to an enrollee. *(A Pediatrician's Guide to Managed Care,* 2nd edition [Nelson RP, Minon RE. Elk Grove Village, IL: American Academy of Pediatrics; 2001], page 95)

The AAP policy statement "Model Contractual Language for Medical Necessity for Children" provides guidance for payers to adopt more consistent medical necessity definitions that take into account the needs of children. Pediatricians should reference this policy as a guide when negotiating their contracts with health plans.

All Products Clauses

The following suggested contract provision is to make clear that the physician is not required to participate in "all products" offered by the health plan. Rather, the physician is only required to participate in the plan specified in the agreement. Under some arrangements, the parties may contract for multiple plans under the same agreement. Without the protection of this provision, the physician is at risk for participating in other products offered by the health plan that may not be beneficial to the physician's practice.

Subject to the limitations identified herein, Physician agrees to provide or arrange for the provision of [Medically Necessary] Covered Services to all Plan Members on Physician's Patient Panel in accordance with the provisions of this Agreement and Health Plan's applicable rules, regulations, and policies (collectively referred to as "Program Requirements"), a copy of which has been provided to Physician prior to execution of this Agreement and is incorporated by reference herein. Nothing in this Agreement shall be construed to require a Physician to participate in any plan other than the one specified in this Agreement. The list of Covered Services in this Agreement may only be changed by mutual written agreement of the parties. (A Pediatrician's Guide to Managed Care, 2nd edition [Nelson RP, Minon RE. Elk Grove Village, IL: American Academy of Pediatrics; 2001], page 173)

Fee Schedule

Fee schedules are often negotiable, particularly if the pediatrician has a substantial practice or other attractive attributes that give the pediatrician leverage with the health plan. The health plan may try to include a provision stating that the health plan may amend the fee schedule at its sole discretion during the term of the Agreement. Pediatricians should resist such attempts and instead insist on including language that gives the pediatrician the right to approve changes in the fee schedule or to terminate the Agreement if the physician is not willing to accept the health plan changes.

It is also necessary to ensure that the health plan follows *Current Procedural Terminology (CPT®)* conventions, recognizes *CPT* modifiers, and does not bundle or downcode the claims in a way that leads to reduced reimbursement for multiple procedures performed during the same patient visit.

The fee schedule should list the services that the pediatrician commonly performs and the related *CPT* codes and should include a reimbursement rate for each *CPT* code. In addition, the fee schedule should state when services under certain *CPT* codes are performed during the same patient visit, they will be considered separately for reimbursement purposes, assuming they are documented and medically necessary. The fee schedule may also list which procedures will not be considered separate under any circumstances. This approach should avoid future conflicts relating to bundling and downcoding.

Physician shall be entitled to payments by Health Plan for the provision of [Medically Necessary] Covered Services to Plan Members. These payments shall be made in accordance with the Fee Schedule. The Fee Schedule may be amended during the term of this Agreement only by mutual agreement of the parties. The Fee Schedule shall be renegotiated each year on or before the anniversary of the effective Date of this Agreement ("the Anniversary Date"). If renegotiated rates for any year are agreed upon after the Anniversary Date, the new rates shall be applied retroactively to the Anniversary Date. Health Plan agrees to adhere to the most current Current Procedural Terminology (CPT), *including the notes, guidelines, modifiers, and instructions published therein. Health Plan further agrees that any payment policies that deviate from or are not covered by* CPT *notes, guidelines, modifiers,*

or instructions shall be specified in the Fee Schedule. Health Plan agrees not to alter, rebundle, or otherwise edit payment codes unless the edit conforms with the Fee Schedule and CPT. Health Plan agrees that all claims submitted by Physician shall be presumed to be coded correctly unless Health Plan can provide evidence that a claim fails to comply with the Fee Schedule or CPT. If the Fee Schedule is not attached as an Exhibit, or in the event that the Exhibit is not specific enough to put Physician on notice as to Health Plan's payment policies with respect to any Covered Services, Health Plan shall be required to pay the greater of Physician's usual and customary rate or Physician's billed charge for that Covered Service when performed by Physician hereunder. (A Pediatrician's Guide to Managed Care, 2nd edition [Nelson RP, Minon RE. Elk Grove Village, IL: American Academy of Pediatrics; 2001], page 180)

New Vaccines

Pediatricians need to evaluate the immunization benefit and determine how it has been priced. It is strongly recommended that pediatricians negotiate a fee-for-service carve out for immunization. Some managed care organizations pay for immunizations on a separate fee schedule. If immunizations are not covered under an all-inclusive or separate capitation, levels of reimbursement should be identified. Reimbursement should be at least at the level of practice costs (ie, the cost of the vaccine, the cost of associated supplies, and the administrative cost). In situations where immunizations are included in the capitated rate and the price of the vaccine increases, or a new vaccine is introduced and recommended during a contract period, an additional amount should be paid by the health plan to cover this increase during the contract period.

Physician shall be reimbursed by Health Plan in an amount equal to the sum of the cost of the immunizations and injectables (eg, antibiotics, hormones, etc) utilized in the provision of Covered Services to Plan members, including the cost of the drugs and supplies associated with such injections, plus a fee of [$_____] for each immunization or injection administered by Physician.

Note: Physicians should be wary of arrangements pursuant to which the immunization reimbursement amount is based on an average wholesale price as physicians may not be able to obtain such favorable pricing from their suppliers. The language in this provision also states that the physician will receive a separate fee for administration of the immunization or injection. (A Pediatrician's Guide to Managed Care, 2nd edition [Nelson RP, Minon RE. Elk Grove Village, IL: American Academy of Pediatrics; 2001], page 190)

Verification of Eligibility

It is important to clarify how eligibility of health plan coverage will be verified in a timely manner. This should include provisions for the health plan's responsibility for payment when the physician has taken the requisite steps to verify eligibility and the health plan is in error or when services are provided in an emergency situation before eligibility can be verified.

Except in the event that Emergency Services are required or in the event that the Plan Member presents an unexpired identification card evidencing the Plan Member's eligibility for coverage by Health Plan, Physician agrees, as a condition to receiving payment from Health Plan, to contact Health Plan by telephone, facsimile, or other agreed-upon form of communication to verify an individual's eligibility as a Plan Member before providing any Covered Service to treat individual or before referring that Plan Member to another provider for the provision of Covered Services. Health Plan will be bound by its confirmation of eligibility as evidenced by the Health Plan identification card or otherwise given in the manner contemplated by this Agreement, unless Physician has actual knowledge that the Plan Member is not eligible for Covered Services. In the event that a Plan Member loses eligibility during a course of treatment, Health Plan shall be required to pay Physician for all Covered Services to that Plan Member until the date on which Physician has actual knowledge that the Plan Member has lost eligibility under the Plan. In the event of an emergency, Physician shall attempt to verify the individual's eligibility as a Plan Member as soon as reasonably practicable. (A Pediatrician's Guide to Managed Care, 2nd edition [Nelson RP, Minon RE. Elk Grove Village, IL: American Academy of Pediatrics; 2001], page 177)

Practice Overhead

Norman "Chip" Harbaugh, MD, FAAP

Our pediatric practices have been buffeted by the winds of managed care over the last few years. Managing a practice has now become a crash course for an MBA. Recently there has been a lull in the storm as the economy ran without much attention towards medical cost. As the economy slides into a recession, corporations are again looking to trim costs. Medical inflation has returned with a vengeance, and thus is a prime target for corporate cost cutting.

Companies will subsequently be shifting medical costs onto their employees in the form of defined contribution as well as an increase in co-payments. As the co-payments rise to $30.00 to $40.00, the patients' threshold for visiting your office will increase and, thus, decrease revenue. This economic landscape will force us to financially fine-tune our practices.

Overhead is the main variable we can change to increase profit. The median overhead expenses for pediatrics are between 55% to 60%. The possible savings of overhead is as follows (ranked in order):
- Employee cost
- Benefits
- Space
- Malpractice insurance

Employee cost consumes the most practice resources. The median
- Staff salary—22.56%
- Staff benefits—4.68%
- As the unemployment rate increases to 5.7%, the wage inflation pressure will decrease. Look to control these costs over the next 2 years.

Mid-level providers, such as physician assistants and nurse practitioners, are beneficial in not only dispersing patient volume but also in increasing your practice's profitability. See the Mid-level Provider chart below.

The mid-level providers pay for themselves if they see between 10 to 13 sick patients per day. If these visits include well checkups, then the break-even point is around 8 to 10 patients per day.

Pediatricians' salaries have stagnated recently.

Physician Salaries	
	Median
Pediatrics (overall)	$140,690
Pediatrics (1–2 years)	$130,633

Source: US Department of Labor Bureau of Labor Statistics and *Physician Compensation and Production Survey. 2007 Report Based on 2006 Data,* respectively

Studies show that our productivity has increased 2% to 10% per year while our compensation only increased 1% to 6% per year. Our conclusion is that we must maximize our tax-free benefits.

These tax-free **benefits** should include
- Malpractice insurance
- Major medical insurance
- Disability insurance *(though there may be benefits to paying with after-tax dollars.—ed)*
- Life insurance
- Liability (umbrella)
- "Slush" fund (CME, auto insurance, maintenance, gas, cell phone, dues)
- Profit sharing 15% of salary
- Pension trust 6% of salary

Tax-free is extremely important. See the Financial Package table on page 61.

As the table shows, the lower salary of $200,000 with $100,000 tax-free benefits (Example 2) is actually worth $70,000 more than Example 1. This is a 23% increase in profit on the entire package value of $300,000. *(Profit sharing and pension trust will be taxable when the proceeds are used during retirement, but this is much later and may be at a lower tax rate.—ed.) (The author and SOAPM recommend an accountant and/or an attorney knowledgeable in tax to assist in setting up any kind of tax-free benefit program.—ed.)*

Mid-level Provider					
Avg Billed	**75% Collection Rate**	**57% Overhead**	**Collected**	**Avg Pay**	**Profit**
$413,000	$310,000	$176,000	$133,000	$85,000	$48,000

Financial Package		
Example 1 – all taxable salary		**Example 2 – salary and tax-free**
$300,000	Salary (taxed)	$200,000
$0	Tax-free benefits	$100,000
$300,000	**TOTAL**	$300,000
Salary		
	Assuming a 30% tax bracket (which is low but to be conservative)	
$300,000 * .30 = $90,000 tax		$200,000 * .30 = $60,000 tax
	Which results in	
$210,000	**NET INCOME**	$140,000
Benefits		
$ 0	*Value of benefits before tax*	$140,000
$ 0	*less 30% tax*	$ 42,000
$ 0	*Results in a tax free pkg for Example 2 (ie, <$100,000)*	$ 98,000
$ 0	**BENEFIT VALUE**	$140,000
Example 1 – all taxable salary		**Example 2 – salary and tax-free**
$210,000	**NET INCOME**	$140,000
$0	**BENEFIT VALUE**	$140,000
$210,000	**FINAL TOTAL TAKE-HOME VALUE**	**$280,000**

If your present practice is full, then the demand for checkups will be strong. The new doctor's visit profitability threshold will decrease (<10 well-patient visits per day) because the average reimbursement per checkups is greater than sick visits. See the New Doctor chart below.

Employee staff ratio allows practices some reasonable comparison.
- Provider/employees
  - Bad 1/5
  - Good 1/3.5
  - Better/lower 1/3.4 with lab
  - 1/3.2 no lab
  - Low 1/2.8—1/2.3

These ratios should be used as a guide not as hard fact. Be careful in using them.

Hopefully this has been helpful in stimulating desire for productive change. Although we only covered employee cost, change is inevitable and it is the manner in which we embrace or reject it that determines the final outcome.

New Doctor					
Avg Billed	**75% Collect**	**57% Overhead**	**Collected**	**Avg Pay**	**Profit**
$530,000	$397,000	$226,000	$171,000	$112,000	$58,000

Working With Consultants and Advisors

Excerpt from Launching Your Career in Pediatrics Handbook: Opening a New Practice

Why Hire Consultants?

As one can see from this discussion, there are myriad processes the new practice must set up across a broad range of disciplines, including medical, legal, technologic, insurance, business, and management. While many physicians have tried to save money by doing all of this themselves, it may not be the best way to proceed. While doing it alone may be possible depending on the skill set of the physician(s) in the new practice, it is absolutely critical to establish all of these systems correctly the first time out. Given the increasing complexity of these matters and the total lack of physician training and experience with any of them, failure to do so can be very, very expensive to you and your practice in the long run.

Herein lies the dilemma of consultants and advisors. Doctors are notoriously averse to paying others to do tasks that they somehow feel they ought to be able to do for themselves. After all, how hard could it be for the bright individuals who go into medicine? Unfortunately, it is considerably harder than it looks. Choosing the proper help is vital to a new practice. Such help includes a health care lawyer (not a general practitioner), a health care accountant (not only bookkeeper), and a practice management consultant. All of these consultants can entail significant expense in the short run. Doctors are again notorious for viewing such expenses as overpriced and unnecessary. However, when used properly, they will pay for themselves many times over.

Legal Counsel

The most expensive will generally be legal counsel. Some practices choose to have everything set up by their legal advisor. While this may be possible with an experienced health care attorney, their time is the most expensive of all consultants. They may be good at what is legal but may not appreciate the day-to-day dynamics of medical practice management and administration. A good legal mind to advise you on partnership agreements, corporate structure, leases, contract negotiations, and contracts is absolutely vital. Yet many of these tasks can be accomplished just as effectively with lower-cost consultants, with only a final legal review at the end.

Health Care Accountant

A good health care accountant is someone who does more than keep your books. This accountant will help you with budgeting, help you with contacts at local financial institutions, supply you with advice in financing business practices, and provide you with frequent reports based on benchmarking your performance against other practices in the field using national norms and local experience.

Practice Management Consultant

Lastly, hiring an experienced practice management consultant is a good idea. It is important to begin working with a consultant during your third year of residency. Lay and physician consultants are available. Consultants can provide the overview you need to coordinate and get the most out of your other consultants. They can review your practice's processes from a functional end-user point of view and can assist you in assessing whether your plan will work in a real-world setting. Consultants are also available to assist you with coding and physician profit distribution, staffing, salaries, and marketing. Often, they can assist you with drafting documents for later legal review. Consultants are available to help you compare electronic health records and practice management software, negotiate with payers, and construct an office policy manual. Finally, consultants can even help run your practice until you are able to hire your own management team.

Please realize that none of this advice comes cheap, but it is a worthy long-term investment to make sure your new practice is primed for success.

PediaLink Module Contract Negotiation With Payers

Edward N. Zissman, MD, FAAP

Visit http://pedialink.org/cmefinder/videos/Contract_Negotiations_Preview/index.htm for a free preview.

Visit http://www.pedialink.org/cmefinder/search-detail.cfm/key/2f65c7bc-b672-46e9-aa8f-155d5c0e7c87/type/course/grp/2/task/details to take the module.

The American Academy of Pediatrics (AAP) has published its first practice management PediaLink online education module entitled: "Contract Negotiations With Payers." Two years in development, the program was introduced at the AAP Annual Leadership Forum in March 2007. This 5-credit program presents techniques and processes to confidently conduct successful negotiations. Key topics include technical considerations, model contracts, negotiation styles, and a 4-phase negotiation process model.

1. *Preparing and planning* to enter the process of contract negotiation with third-party payers
2. Utilizing proven strategies to successfully *negotiate* the best contract terms
3. Making *decisions* concerning the contract terms
4. *Reviewing* the contract and monitoring compliance with the contract terms

There are 5 overarching elements to consider throughout all phases of negotiation (information, leverage, time, power, and analysis). The program teaches the multiple steps of each phase using an interactive case history and an interactive "negotiations coach."

The module discusses key aspects of communication, including nonverbal communication. It also addresses negotiations concerning vaccines (both the product and the administration services). After discussion of the 5 overreaching elements with definitions and explanations, the module finishes with a very comprehensive checklist of contract issues. This checklist is adapted from: *A Pediatrician's Guide to Managed Care*, 2nd edition (Nelson RP, Minon RE. Elk Grove Village, IL: American Academy of Pediatrics; 2001). All registrants will receive a complimentary copy of this valuable resource. The learners also are taught to access AAP materials, including appeal letter templates and other resources, which can be accessed through the educational activity.

To register for "Contract Negotiations With Payers," go to www.pedialink.org. The center column of this page lists continuing medical education (CME). Click on "view all online CME." This takes you to CME finder. Scroll toward the bottom and click on the Details button of "Contract Negotiations With Payers."

Phase 1: *Prepare and Plan*	
Step 1	Look first at the top 10 Current Procedural Terminology codes for which you bill. Define priority contract issues, including provisions/what services are important to you.
Step 2	Identify your goals, desired outcomes, needs and wants, and reason(s) why you want the outcome.
Step 3	Collect and analyze data about your practice performance. Document the quality of care you offer. Assess the market, different payment models, physician numbers, geography, patient volume, largest area employers, and other areas that relate to your practice.
Step 4	Identify your strengths (niche).
Step 5	Determine who it is that you will be talking to in each step of the negotiation process. Identify the decision-maker who represents the payer on your contract.
Step 6	Research payer interests, needs, and wants, including ascertaining what you perceive to be the payer's interests and desired outcomes.
Step 7	Know federal and state antitrust law, as it applies.
Step 8	Plan your strategy and create your agenda, then prepare to work on it. Plan your strategy and approach to implement your agenda.
Step 9	Rehearse important parts of your agenda and negotiating position.
Step 10	Set your target based on your goals and identify your options, alternatives, and compromise level.

Phase 2: *Negotiate*	
Step 1	Orient yourself toward a successful negotiation. Implement your planned strategy and approach.
Step 2	Establish rapport in phone and face-to-face meetings.
Step 3	Take an active listening stance and skills into every meeting. Focus on understanding, and on being understood.
Step 4	Reassess your predetermined negotiation style based on what you observe and perceive early in the meeting(s). Adapt your style, if necessary.
Step 5	Assert your needs clearly. Align your responses and overall path forward with your expectations, goals, outcomes, needs, and wants.
Step 6	Acknowledge the payer's representative as a person and recognize the payer's point of view.
Step 7	Reframe.
Step 8	Ask problem-solving, open-ended questions to gain deeper understanding and encourage dialogue. Why? Why not? What if?
Step 9	Review and refine options. Brainstorm possibilities and ideas for solutions.
Step 10	Focus on needs, interests, and concerns. Deal effectively with objections and dishonest tactics. Manage impasses with patience and respect. Clarify issues and feelings. Counter offers, using persuasive and bargaining skills.

Phase 3: *Make Decisions*	
Step 1	Identify signals that could indicate that it is time to begin closing the discussion.
Step 2	Restate and evaluate options. Pick a solution (or solutions) from the options, adjust, and work to agree on preliminary outcomes. Build consensus.
Step 3	Decide when to close for agreement, defer/delay, or walk away. If you decided to defer or delay negotiations at this or some other point, evaluate when or if it is reasonable to return to the bargaining table at a later time with new options or explore other payer options.
Step 4	Close for agreement.
Step 5	Recap/summarize to ensure that all parties are clear on agreed-on points.
Step 6	Secure commitment.
Step 7	End the meeting with a mutual commitment to implement determined plans. Build an opportunity to check back with each other to evaluate progress on implementation.

Phase 4: *Review Contract and Monitor Compliance*	
Step 1	Review/evaluate the contract.
Step 2	Conduct a legal review to ensure that the contract is legally binding.
Step 3	Have both parties sign the contract.
Step 4	Evaluate the negotiation process and results.
Step 5	Implement the contract. Ensure that all pediatricians and staff in your practice are fully informed as to all provisions of the new contract.
Step 6	Monitor compliance by the payer and enforce contract provisions.
Step 7	Establish a formal review process to evaluate the overall impact of the contract on your business, patients, practice, and staff.
Step 8	Renew, replace, or terminate the contract. Make your decision based on the payer's performance and the value the relationship brings to your practice.

On successful completion of this online module, you will be able to

1. Identify benefits for you and your practice from improving negotiations with payers.
2. Identify technical considerations and issues for developing a payer strategy, including elements of a model contract.
3. Recognize your negotiation style and its impact on negotiation outcomes.
4. Apply a 4-phase negotiation process (steps and elements) to negotiations with payers.
5. Link to an array of resources related to negotiating with payers.

The primary audience is composed of general pediatricians and general pediatric residents. Secondary audiences include office managers, finance managers, coding specialists, and other employees who are involved in reimbursement for services, employment, or working with vendors.

The registration fee is $100 for AAP members. Five credit hours are earned on completion of this activity.

Learn to Manage Payer Contract Negotiations With Confidence

New from PediaLink! Contract Negotiations With Payers is an online education course that will show you how to use leverage in your negotiations, make informed decisions, and monitor compliance in 4 easy-to-implement steps.

Key Learning Objectives

- Identify negotiation styles and their impact on contract outcomes.
- Identify issues for developing payer strategies.
- Improve negotiation skills.

This activity has been approved for *American Medical Association/Physician's Recognition Award Category 1 Credit.*

Register today and receive *A Pediatrician's Guide to Managed Care* FREE! Visit www.pedialink.org/cmefinder.

Questions Pediatricians Should Ask Before Signing a Managed Care Contract

It is important you read and understand your contract before signing it. Consider having your legal counsel review it. These questions should identify areas in the contract to address during negotiations with the carrier.

1. How important is this contract to your practice?
2. What provisions are most important to you and are they addressed in the contract?
3. What is your payment under this contract?
4. Can the managed care organization (MCO) change payment terms unilaterally?
5. Does the contract give the MCO the right to unilaterally "offset" alleged "overpayments" from amounts otherwise due?
6. What are your rights to appeal a payment decision?
7. Does the MCO have an obligation to pay you promptly?
8. How does the contract define "medically necessary" care?
9. How do you determine whether medically necessary services are covered by a patient's benefit plan?
10. Does the contract (or administrative manual) clearly designate any and all services and procedures subject to prior authorization requirements?
11. How does the MCO verify that a patient is enrolled in a plan?
12. In which products are you required to participate?
13. Does the contract allow the MCO to "rent" you to other entities?
14. Does the contract require compliance with a prescription drug formulary?
15. How can you terminate the contract?
16. Are pediatric medical and surgical subspecialists and children's hospitals members of the panel(s) that contract with the MCO?
17. What mechanism is in place for the MCO to add new procedures, technical advances, and immunizations to their list of covered services in a timely manner?
18. What are the provisions related to collecting co-payments, co-insurance, and deductibles?
19. Does the contract contain a hold harmless clause?
20. Does the contract have an "escape clause" with regard to new patients?
21. What are the claims filing requirements?
22. What are the requirements of physician availability?
23. How can the physician-patient relationship be terminated?
24. Does your contract allow you to write off or discount patient fees?
25. What are the malpractice insurance requirements?
26. What are the provisions for access to medical records?
27. Does the MCO require that physicians use certain practice protocols?
28. How do you plan to monitor compliance by the carrier with the contract?

Consult and compare your contract with the AAP model contract in *A Pediatrician's Guide to Managed Care* available through the AAP Online Bookstore at www.aap.org/bookstore as well as the fourth edition of the AMA *Model Managed Care Contract* at www.ama-assn.org/go/psa.

To assist in your review, use the AAP checklist to assess carrier contracts (posted on the AAP Member Center, private payer advocacy page at www.aap.org/moc/) and compare the contract provisions to the items to consider. Every 6 months or annually, review the contract to ensure carrier compliance with the contract provisions. This review will also identify items to renegotiate at future contract renewals.

The American Medical Association (AMA) is acknowledged for its permission to revise the AMA brochure "15 Questions to Ask Before Signing a Managed Care Contract."

Checklist to Assess Carrier Contracts

It is important you read and understand your contract before signing it. Consider having your legal counsel review it. Consult and compare your contract with the American Academy of Pediatrics (AAP) Model Contract in the *A Pediatrician's Guide to Managed Care* available through the AAP Online Bookstore at www.aap.org/bookstore. To assist in your review, use the checklist below and compare the contract provi-

sions to the items to consider. Record your findings in the Contract Review column and then assess each item to determine the appropriateness of the contract to your business operations. Every six months or annually, review the contract to ensure carrier compliance with the contract provisions. This review will also identify items to renegotiate at future contract renewals

1. How Important Is This Contract to Your Practice?

First you need to objectively determine whether this carrier contract is necessary for your practice and determine at what point you walk away from a bad contract.

Items to Consider	Contract Review	Assessment (keep as is, modify, or negotiate)
• Do you have all the provider manuals and other administrative, utilization management, and quality management procedures in order to accurately evaluate the contract? Although the managed care organization (MCO) may find it burdensome to send out all the necessary documents or manuals to potential participating physicians, it is imperative that you obtain these materials in order to understand your obligations as a participating physician.		
• What does the contract mean in terms of revenue and expenses?		
• How would you replace any patients and/or revenue you might lose?		
• What are your alternatives to this contract?		

2. What Provisions Are Most Important to You and Are They Addressed in the Contract?

Items to Consider	Contract Review	Assessment (keep as is, modify, or negotiate)
• Identify issues that are your bottom line, and ones that you are willing to compromise.		
• Identify issues that you intend to revisit during the next contract renewal.		

3. What Is Your Payment Under This Contract?

If the contract does not compensate you beyond your practice expense, you may lose money on the contract. You can't make up the loss with numbers. A loss is a loss period. So don't be afraid to be the businessperson and ask for more payment. If you think that you are losing money on some of your contracts, it may be a worthwhile investment to retain a practice management consultant to determine why and to reconsider those contracts. This is especially true for immunizations. If you are projected to lose money on the contract, it is not worth your time to consider any of the other factors.

Items to Consider	Contract Review	Assessment (keep as is, modify, or negotiate)
• What are your costs to provide the services required under the contract? While this is not an easy determination, you should have a general idea of the overhead and other expenses associated with running your practice. The Medical Group Management Association has resources for benchmarking your practice expenses including data on rent, salaries, • equipment, etc, for specific specialties in different geographic locations.		
• Does the contract provide enough information for you to determine what you will be paid for the services you provide?		
• Does it include a comprehensive fee schedule? If not, insist that the MCO provide fee schedules for the 20–50 most commonly billed procedures. Also insist that the MCO provide you with detailed information on payment methodology, including recognition of *Current Procedural Terminology (CPT®)* codes and guidelines. MCO reimbursement policies should be transparent so that you can determine your payment under the contract.		
• What is their payment for after-hours and emergency care?		
• Are coding edits transparent? Do they recognize modifiers? Are any services bundled, ie, • 2 or more separately reportable services that are grouped together under one *CPT* code for payment (such as bundling immunization administration with payment for the vaccine)?		
• Are there stipulations in the payment methodology for obesity care and attention-deficit/hyperactivity disorder/mental health? See the Coding Fact Sheets on Obesity at http://www.aap.org/moc/reimburse/codingfactsheet.pdf and Developmental Screening http://www.aap.org/moc/reimburse/.		
• Is the payment based on the Resource-Based Relative Value Scale (RBRVS)? Read the yearly RBRVS brochure from the AAP at http://www.aap.org/visit/rbrvsbrochure.pdf.		
• Many MCOs base their payment methodology on the RBRVS. This is a system designed to value the medical services provided. The value of the services is determined by the relative value units (RVUs) assigned by CMS. These RVUs are determined by totaling the physician work, practice expense (facility or non-facility) and malpractice expense. The total RVUs are then multiplied by a geographic practice cost index (GPCI) designed to reflect the differences in costs of geographic areas. Those values are then multiplied by a conversion factor to determine the dollar amount the service is worth in the Medicare system. Every year the conversion factor changes to maintain budget neutrality. The total dollars spent on health care in the Medicare system are divided by the RVUs performed and the result is the conversion factor. So what does Medicare have to do with pediatrics? Most fee schedules are based on a percentage of Medicare. But instead of negotiating a percentage of Medicare, which fluctuates year to year secondary to the variable conversion factor, negotiate a specific dollar amount conversion factor. You will then have a fixed payment until you renegotiate. The national average conversion factor is $50.		
• Does the contract include provisions for vaccine and immunization administration payments? Insist that there be provisions to address payment for new vaccines, vaccine price increases, and new immunization recommendations in a timely manner. Make sure that all payments are at a level that meets your practice expenses. See The Business Case for Pricing Vaccines and Immunization Administration and the Vaccine Addendum at http://www.aap.org/moc/.		

Items to Consider (cont)	Contract Review	Assessment (keep as is, modify, or negotiate)
• Ask for incentives for immunization registry, electronic medical record, and immunization recall or reminder systems. If your practice is efficient and effective with high immunization rates then the MCO benefits as well with a higher Healthcare Effectiveness Data and Information Set (HEDIS) score. This is a good strategy for negotiation.		
• Does the contract clearly state the method of payment and the time of payment? Consider the financial stability of the third-party payer. Incorporate penalties to the carrier for unnecessarily delayed or late payments. Check with your state's prompt payment laws and incorporate appropriate penalties.		
• Note limitations for collecting payments from patients for non-covered services. Understand what advance beneficiary notices are and use the AAP Use of Waivers in a Pediatric Office (http://www.aap.org/moc/reimburse/Waivers2006.pdf). Are there any requirements or notifications mandated before the non-covered service is performed? If a nonparticipating physician is covering for a participating physician in the plan, how will payment be made?		

4. Can the MCO Change Payment Terms Unilaterally?

Items to Consider	Contract Review	Assessment (keep as is, modify, or negotiate)
• If so, does the contract require the MCO to provide you notice of any reimbursement changes? The third-party payer should not be allowed to unilaterally amend the contract. Both parties should sign amendments to the contract.		
• Is there a mechanism for you to terminate the contract if you object to the changed reimbursement terms? Make sure there is a time frame (30–60 days) for you to terminate the contract due to fee schedule changes.		

5. Does the Contract Give the MCO the Right to Unilaterally "Offset" Alleged "Overpayments" From Amounts Otherwise Due?

Items to Consider	Contract Review	Assessment (keep as is, modify, or negotiate)
• If so, does the contract require the MCO to explain such offsets to the physician? Is there a mechanism for the physician to appeal offsets? Does the contract limit the time frame for these payment offsets? Watch for terms that unilaterally allow the payer to offset the next payment by the amount of a claim the payer thinks was erroneously paid.		
• Many MCOs conduct retrospective audits of physician practices several years after services are rendered and then either demand return of sums allegedly "overpaid" or automatically deduct payment without explanation to physicians. Don't allow these alleged "overpayments" to be refunded for any longer than the timely filing limit.		

6. What Are Your Rights to Appeal a Payment Decision?

Items to Consider	Contract Review	Assessment (keep as is, modify, or negotiate)
• Does the contract provide specific procedures to appeal a reimbursement decision? If the contract refers to administrative policies and procedures, review these procedures specifically to determine your appeal rights.		
• Is the appeals process fair or is it weighted heavily in favor of the MCO? Look out for a provision that states that a physician must abide by the third-party payer's decision in terms of payment for services rendered or whether service will be approved, etc. Never enter into an agreement that automatically waives your rights.		
• Is there any independent review permitted as part of the internal appeals procedure? Make certain a provision exists outlining a process for resolution of disputes such as through arbitration or legal proceedings.		
• Make sure that carrier payments are not withheld during the appeal process. Avoid provisions that allow carriers to withhold payment on non-related claims to offset carrier overpayments.		

7. Does the MCO Have an Obligation to Pay You Promptly?

Items to Consider	Contract Review	Assessment (keep as is, modify, or negotiate)
• Does the contract include a specific payment period, and does the MCO agree to pay interest if it delays payment beyond that period? Many states have laws that require prompt payment of claims.		
• If your state has a prompt pay law or fair business practice act, does the contract comply with the time frames and interest penalties and other claims processing and payment provision? Do you have contacts in the state insurance commissioner's office?		
• To determine whether your state has a prompt payment law, check the Summary of State prompt pay laws at http://www.aap.org/moc/displaytemp/PromptPay7.06.pdf.		

8. How Does the Contract Define "Medically Necessary" Care?

Items to Consider	Contract Review	Assessment (keep as is, modify, or negotiate)
• Does the contract use an objective standard, such as a "prudent physician" standard, or does it give the MCO wide flexibility in determining what is medically necessary?		
• Compare the contract definition of medically necessary care to the AAP statement, "Model Contractual Language for Medical Necessity for Children" at http://aappolicy.aappublications.org/cgi/content/full/pediatrics;116/1/261.		

9. How Do You Determine Whether Medically Necessary Services Are Covered by a Patient's Benefit Plan?

Items to Consider	Contract Review	Assessment (keep as is, modify, or negotiate)
• Does the MCO have a quick and efficient mechanism to determine whether medically necessary services you intend to provide a patient are covered under the patient's benefit plan?		
• Is this clearly spelled out in the contract or a policy manual that you have reviewed?		
• Does the MCO stand by this information or does it reserve the right to reverse itself?		

10. Does the Contract (or Administrative Manual) Clearly Designate Any and All Services and Procedures Subject to Prior Authorization Requirements?

Items to Consider	Contract Review	Assessment (keep as is, modify, or negotiate)
• If not, physicians should insist on getting this information in writing.		
• Does the MCO provide for an efficient and reliable mechanism to obtain prior authorization, which is available 24 hours a day/7 days a week?		

11. How Does the MCO Verify That a Patient Is Enrolled in a Plan?

Items to Consider	Contract Review	Assessment (keep as is, modify, or negotiate)
• When a patient comes into your office, is there a quick and efficient mechanism to verify that the patient is covered by the MCO and to determine whether the patient is an enrollee covered by an MCO plan (eg, telephone line or Web site)?		
• Is this clearly spelled out in the contract or a policy manual that you have reviewed? See the suggested contract language on verification of eligibility in the managed care contract issues link at http://www.aap.org/moc/.		
• Does the MCO stand by this information or does it reserve the right to reverse itself?		

12. In Which Products Are You Required to Participate?

Beware of all products that force physicians to participate in current and future health plans offered by the carrier without the opportunity for the physician to determine whether to participate.

Items to Consider	Contract Review	Assessment (keep as is, modify, or negotiate)
• Does the contract allow you to select which products you participate in? Or does the contract require you to participate in "all products"?		
• Does the contract allow you to terminate one product or does termination in one product automatically terminate your participation in all products?		

13. Does the Contract Allow the MCO to "Rent" You to Other Entities?

This relates to so-called silent preferred provider organizations (PPOs) where a physician signs a discounted fee-for-service contract with an MCO and then without informing the physician, the MCO "sells" or "rents" its physician network to a third party, such as a third-party administrator. The third party gets the advantage of whatever discount the MCO has negotiated with the physician. By taking discounts without negotiation or physician consent, silent PPOs violate fair business practice and do not provide any return benefits to the physician. Instead those deep discounts given to the payer result in profits that are shared with the MCO.

Items to Consider	Contract Review	Assessment (keep as is, modify, or negotiate)
• Does the contract include vague or broad definitions of the term "payer" or "participating entities"? These are signals that the contract may permit silent PPO activity. Pediatricians are cautioned against "silent PPOs" and should clarify this with the MCO.		
• Are there provisions that require the physician to agree to participate in all networks? Ensure the contract stipulates that the PPO network provides for increased patient referrals in return for discounts. One way to protect yourself from the "silent PPO" is to insert a clause in the contract that says if anyone wishes to have access to these discounted fees, then they must abide by all the terms and conditions of the agreement, which, in addition, means referring a lot of patients.		
• Review the contract with the model contract language regarding silent PPOs at http://www. aap.org/moc/.		

14. Does the Contract Require Compliance With a Prescription Drug Formulary?

Item to Consider	Contract Review	Assessment (keep as is, modify, or negotiate)
• If so, what flexibility do you have to go off-formulary when your medical judgment dictates a non-formulary drug?		

15. How Can You Terminate the Contract?

Items to Consider	Contract Review	Assessment (keep as is, modify, or negotiate)
• What are the provisions for terminating if the MCO breaches the contract? What notice must be given to the other party before the agreement can be terminated?		
• Make sure that the governing law be that of the state in which the physician practices. Some contracts contain provisions stating that the law of the state in which the document was drafted will govern contract disputes.		
• If the payer wants to make unilateral changes to the contract, can the contract be terminated if the change is unacceptable?		
• Is the MCO obligated to provide notice of your rights to terminate every year?		
• Does the contract automatically renew annually (aka "evergreen" contract)? If it is an "evergreen" contract, what provisions are there for terminations or for renegotiating? If the contract is favorable to the physician then the term of the contract should be as long as possible. And, on the other hand, if you are unsure about the contract, then the period should be as short as possible.		

16. Are Pediatric Medical and Surgical Subspecialists and Children's Hospitals Members of the Panel(s) That Contract With the MCO?

Items to Consider	Contract Review	Assessment (keep as is, modify, or negotiate)
• Are there restrictions on referrals? What paperwork and documentation needs to be completed? Will this extra administrative burden be too costly?		
• Does the MCO limit the follow-up visits with the subspecialist and require the patient to follow up with the primary care physician for the problem you sent the patient to the subspecialist for?		
• Be aware of contracts that actively encourage physicians to accept responsibility for care that you are not appropriately trained to perform.		

17. What Mechanism Is in Place for the MCO to Add New Procedures, Technical Advances, and Immunizations to Their List of Covered Services in a Timely Manner?

Items to Consider	Contract Review	Assessment (keep as is, modify, or negotiate)
• Are there provisions for carrier coverage and payment of new services and procedures?		
• If so, ensure that the practice is not at risk while the carrier determines coverage and payment. This has been especially true for new immunizations recommended by the Advisory Committee on Immunization Practices (ACIP) and AAP *Red Book* Committee in recent years, as there has been a time lag for carriers to update their claims systems for payment for new vaccines. Negotiate for payment on addition to the immunization schedule and therefore recommendation by ACIP and AAP. See the Vaccine Addendum at http://www.aap.org/moc/.		

18. What Are the Provisions Related to Collecting Co-payments, Co-insurance, and Deductibles?

You may have difficulty collecting payment from families depending on the carrier contract provisions. This is very important as consumer-driven health plans and healthcare savings accounts (HSAs) proliferate. These large-deductible health plans will require more payment from the patient and less from the health plan.

Items to Consider	Contract Review	Assessment (keep as is, modify, or negotiate)
• Are there any restrictions to collecting fees at the time of service? Check to make sure that there are no obstacles to collecting payments during the visit.		
• If you are not allowed to collect at the time of service, then reconsider the contract. Being prohibited from collecting payment due at the time of service would be financially burdensome to any business and add to the cost of the medical services provided. Consider renegotiating the payment methodology without a discount if this occurs to offset the economic hardship this creates.		
• If there are co-payments, co-insurance, or deductibles applied to preventive services and immunizations, you may have difficulty providing the AAP-recommended schedule of preventive services. Inform the carrier that these services are cost-effective and should be covered as first-dollar coverage. Advocate at the local level by contacting your AAP chapter and state medical society to introduce legislation to protect preventive services.		
• Examine the impact of increased patient payment responsibilities to your accounts receivable. What process is available or allowed from the MCO to collect payment at the time of service? For example, in an HSA product, is there a debit card so you will be paid at the time of service? If there are credit card fees, will the MCO or the patient pay those fees?		

19. Does the Contract Contain a Hold Harmless Clause?

Hold harmless and indemnification clauses often place the burden on physicians to pay the MCO for any costs or losses incurred in defending claims arising as a result of the physician's action or inaction. As a result, the physician is accepting responsibility for not only the health care professional's own negligent or willful acts or omissions but also that of the MCO. Many professional liability insurance policies do not cover such indemnification agreements. If the MCO refuses to remove the hold harmless clause, alternative language that releases both parties from liability can be appropriate. Consult your malpractice carrier for specifics.

Items to Consider	Contract Review	Assessment (keep as is, modify, or negotiate)
• Are there provisions that require the pediatrician to pay the MCO for any costs or losses incurred in defending claims as a result of the physician's action or inaction?		
• If the MCO refuses to remove the hold harmless clause, is there alternative language that can be included that releases both parties from liability?		
• Are there provisions in your malpractice coverage that address indemnification agreements?		

20. Does the Contract Have an "Escape Clause" With Regard to New Patients?

In most agreements, the physician must agree not to treat the patients of the MCO differently than other patients. If the practice is over capacity, then the demands of the patients will be difficult to meet. The contract should allow refusal of new patients for legitimate business reasons.

Items to Consider	Contract Review	Assessment (keep as is, modify, or negotiate)
• Is there a requirement that the physician always accept MCO patients as long as the physician is accepting new patients in general?		
• Are there identified circumstances in which the physician may determine not to accept new MCO patients?		
• Does the contract allow refusal of new patients for legitimate business reasons?		
• Has a membership projection been provided by the MCO?		

21. What Are the Claims Filing Requirements?

Contracts usually will limit the period allowed for filing claims and have a vague description of a clean claim. Both need to be defined in the contract.

Items to Consider	Contract Review	Assessment (keep as is, modify, or negotiate)
• What are the timely filing requirements?		
• Are there provisions to allow for an extension of the filing period due to situations beyond your control (ie, incorrect insurance information provided by the patient, unknown secondary carrier, acts of nature, etc)?		
• How is a clean claim defined? Do not let the carrier arbitrarily define what is meant be a clean claim, and make sure it is explicitly defined in the contract.		

22. What Are the Requirements of Physician Availability?

It is important to identify any specific requirements regarding availability by the physician.

Items to Consider	Contract Review	Assessment (keep as is, modify, or negotiate)
• What are the allowances for on-call coverage?		
• Are there requirements for the physician to participate in educational or training programs with the MCO?		

23. How Can the Physician-Patient Relationship Be Terminated?

There are some situations in which the physician-patient relationship has deteriorated to the point that continuing the relationship could expose the physician to potential liability. Your contract must allow you to dismiss patients from your practice or you could be forced to continue in relationships that could put you at risk.

Items to Consider	Contract Review	Assessment (keep as is, modify, or negotiate)
• What provisions are included in the contract to dismiss an MCO-covered patient from the physician's practice?		
• Does the contract specify reasons for termination, specific approval by the MCO, and documentation requirements?		

24. Does Your Contract Allow You to Write Off or Discount Patient Fees?

Sometimes patients experience financial hardship or have an unforeseen complication that causes their bill to be higher than expected. You must reserve the right to unilaterally write off fees for legitimate business reasons in accordance with your written financial policy.

Items to Consider	Contract Review	Assessment (keep as is, modify, or negotiate)
• Does the contract prevent the physician from writing off fees?		
• What recourse is allowed to the physician should the family be unwilling or unable to pay their fees?		
• Does the contract provide protection to the physician should the family threaten litigation if the physician is prevented from writing off fees?		

25. What Are the Malpractice Insurance Requirements?

Before signing a contract, the specific dollar amount of coverage needs to be defined. Otherwise the physician may be forced to carry excess coverage that they had not intended to carry.

Item to Consider	Contract Review	Assessment (keep as is, modify, or negotiate)
• Is the MCO contract provision for malpractice coverage in line with your state's malpractice laws?		

26. What Are the Provisions for Access to Medical Records?

Most contracts allow the MCO access to the physician's patient records. Look out for provisions that allow the MCO access to records that are not appropriate for their review.

Items to Consider	Contract Review	Assessment (keep as is, modify, or negotiate)
• Does the contract allow access to records that are not appropriate for MCO review (ie, records of patients not part of that MCO, personal financial data, or personnel files)?		
• Are there provisions stipulating how the carrier is to request access to records?		
• Will the carrier pay for costs incurred to review records?		

27. Does the MCO Require That Physicians Use Certain Practice Protocols?

Items to Consider	Contract Review	Assessment (keep as is, modify, or negotiate)
• Does the contract identify the protocols?		
• Do the protocols provide a standard of care?		
• For areas in which the physician does not agree with the carrier protocols, what is the process to override them based on the physician's standards? It may be helpful to reference the AAP policy statements and clinical practice guidelines at http://aappolicy.aappublications.org/.		

28. How Do You Plan to Monitor Compliance by the Carrier With the Contract?

Identify methods to monitor compliance and steps to take to deal with noncompliance.

Items to Consider	Contract Review	Assessment (keep as is, modify, or negotiate)
• Identify contract provisions on compliance, appeals, and arbitration and review by an outside entity.		
• Make a spreadsheet of the top 50 codes and all the immunizations and the MCO fee schedules. Check every explanation of benefits (EOB) to ensure compliance with the contract.		
• Use your practice management software to find any outliers.		
• Maintain good relationships with the medical directors and contracting staff.		
• Appeal denials with thorough documentation.		
• Consider electronic medical records to increase immunization rates and to document coding compliance.		

Determining the Value of a Buy-in for New Partners and a Buyout for Retiring Partners

When determining the value of a buy-in for prospective partners or a buyout for retiring partners, it is good to first determine the overhead for your practice. This will provide necessary data to determine the 2 different values.

There are a number of methods to determine overhead for a practice. One formula includes

1. Fixed expenses (eg, rent, professional liability insurance) divided equally among physicians.
2. Variable expenses (office overhead [not including the previous 2 expenses] such as staff salaries and vaccines). These expenses are based exclusively on straight productivity. For example, if Dr A generates 26% of total practice professional charges, Dr A pays 26% of the variable expenses.

Another method involves dividing overhead into the following 3 categories:
1. General office expenses (eg, staff, supplies) divided by production
2. Facility expenses (eg, rent, building overhead) divided equally
3. Direct expenses (eg, malpractice, disability, medical insurance, meetings) paid directly by the individual physician

Both formulas can be applied to practices that have physicians with mid to high levels of productivity. Expenses are shared equally, but high producers do not subsidize the practice styles of the others.

When partners join a practice, they will buy into the practice, sometimes over time. Some practices ask for a trial year of employment prior to the buy-in. Using a similar method, retiring partners can be bought out over time.

The Buy-in Amount

There are several factors to consider when determining the buy-in amount. The first is the goodwill factor of the practice. According to an article in *Medical Economics* (http://medicaleconomics.modernmedi-cine.com/memag/article/articleDetail.jsp?id=112446), this can account for 70% to 90% of the value of the practice, depending on whether the value for

accounts receivable (A/R) is included in the calculation.[1] The goodwill value depends on the market and other (often local) factors. The article in *Medical Economics* states that current trends indicate a decrease in goodwill values as hospitals seek to sell primary practices.[1] This is a reverse of a trend seen in the 1990s when primary care practices were being purchased.

The second factor to determining the buy-in amount is the value of the physical properties of the practice, including furniture and hardware. Finally, the third value to be determined is A/R.

Once the total buy-in figure is determined, the new partner pays into the value over time. For example, one practice uses a 5-year period to allow for the buy-in. The new partner is often considered a full partner at the start of the buy-in and has an equal voice in practice decisions. Whatever additional income above the buy-in amount that is generated by the new partner will be considered the new partner's income. The more productive the partner is, the more income the partner receives.

The Buyout Amount

There are several methods to determine the buyout amount. One practice calculates the average annual income from the retiring partner's last 3 years in practice. This amount is paid out to the retiree over 60 equal monthly payments. For example, if the retiring partner's average annual income was $200,000, the retiring partner would receive $3,333 monthly for 5 years. Using this example, one can see that it is very helpful to have a new partner buying into the practice at the same time a retiring partner is departing.

During the buyout process, there are 2 situations for which a practice must prepare. First, in the event that funds come into the practice for the retiring physician **after** he or she leaves (eg, withholds, A/R for that physician), the income will go to the practice and **not** the retiring partner. All parties should understand this. The second situation that may arise is the retiring partner wanting to gradually slow down during the last years of practice, rather than leaving directly from full-time practice. If this situation is approved for the retiring partner, obviously he or she will not be as productive as if working full time. This should result in a modified buyout that reflects the decrease in income coming from the retiring partner during the last years in practice.

Reference

1. Terry K. What's your practice worth? *Med Econ.* 2003;80:106–110, 113

Establishing a Pediatric Concierge Medicine Practice

Scott R. Serbin, MD, FAAP

Concierge medicine (also known as fee-based or retainer medicine) was initiated by 2 Seattle, WA, internists in 1996. There are now more than 300 concierge-style physicians in the United States. I initiated the first pediatric concierge practice in 2004.

Basically, concierge medicine entails limiting the practice to a much smaller number of patients, providing those patients with a much greater level of service, and charging a fee to be a member of the practice

Although there are many variations in the manner in which current concierge physicians have structured their practices, they all accomplish the same thing—the physician is responsible for far fewer patients, resulting in much more attentive care for the patient and a dramatically calmer environment for the physician.

The advantages for the physician of a concierge-style practice are
- Enjoy the practice of medicine—don't feel constantly rushed.
  - Able to listen to everything the parent and patient wish to discuss.
  - Thorough examination (including waiting for the child to feel comfortable and not cry during the examination).
  - Able to explain all aspects of recommendations.
  - Learn the natural course of illnesses—next-day callbacks.
  - Able to review current literature and query specialists.
  - Increase compassion and empathy.
  - Decrease risk of medical error.
- Increase autonomy in practice decisions (business and clinical).
- Increase time for family and self.
- Potential for increased income.

The disadvantages for the physician are
- Risk.
  - Insufficient patient demand
  - Regulatory environment—insurance companies, government
- Increased accessibility—must be readily available to patients.

If a physician desires to convert to a concierge style of practice, there are many tasks to accomplish. Because this is obviously a major undertaking, seeking professional advice should be considered. This may come in the form of a professional consultant, a lawyer, or a physician experienced in this field. With the professional's guidance, the following items need to be addressed:
- Current patient survey—assess level of interest in a concierge style of practice.
- Insurance company participation—an important decision, though physicians have been successful with and without.
- Menu of services—typical amenities include
  - House calls
  - Extended appointments
  - Same-day appointments
  - 24/7 physician availability
  - Physician pager or cell phone access
- Fee structure.
- Membership agreement (contract).
- Letter to current patients advising of change in practice.
- Letter to referral sources (eg, obstetricians, midwives).
- List of alternative providers versus sale of remaining practice.
- Practice name—register.
- Business plan.
- Marketing strategy.
  - Logo
  - Practice brochure
  - Web site
  - Media notification
  - Advertising

In addition, there are many logistical issues to consider in converting to a concierge-style practice, including
- Office design—do not need nearly as large a space.
- Employees—do not need nearly as many.
- Answering service versus machine.
- Cell phone versus pager.
- Copy charts for transfers—in-house versus outsource.
- Electronic medical record.

- Call coverage.
- Printing company—business cards, stationery, envelopes, clinical forms.
- Notify workers' compensation carrier—decreased payroll.
- Notify malpractice insurance carrier—ask about part-time rate.
- Enhance niche services—for example, sports medicine, development, adolescent.
- Increase printed materials—American Academy of Pediatrics Patient Education Online (http://patiented.aap.org/) Web site.
- Increase office aesthetics—paint, new carpet, new furniture.
- Retrain staff—retail orientation, not medical.
- Tracking system—laboratory tests, radiographs, specialist reports.
- House call supplies.

Physicians, and others, have expressed 2 chief concerns about the practice of concierge medicine. One is that it is elitist, and the other is that it restricts access to care. The additional expense does skew the patient population toward the more affluent; I have been surprised by the many individuals of average means who choose to join this type of practice. The best analogy is parochial schools. Many people of average means choose to send their children to parochial schools because this type of education is important to them. Likewise, parents choose to pay to join a concierge pediatric practice because they value the service amenities and personalized care a concierge pediatrician can provide.

As for restricting access to care, for those of us who practice in areas with many other pediatricians, there will always be other options besides concierge medicine. Even in areas with significant penetration of concierge practices, such as Orlando, FL, and Seattle, WA, the number of concierge physicians remains a very small percentage of available physicians. This will always be a niche type of practice.

The reality is that concierge medicine is simply another option in an already multitiered health care system. As with most other aspects of our society, you get what you pay for. Patients who desire more time with their physician and a greatly enhanced level of service can opt to pay for this. This additional expenditure represents discretionary spending on the part of the consumer—no additional insurance or government spending is required.

My personal experience with this method of health care delivery over the past 3+ years has been extraordinary. My level of satisfaction in being a pediatrician has never been greater. My patients' level of satisfaction has also been overwhelming, as demonstrated by a better than 99% retention rate (and the multitude of baked goods I am given after house calls). Although financially my practice struggled at first, now the practice is doing extremely well.

If anyone desires further information or guidance on this subject, I can be reached at 412/366-1266 or by e-mail at pinnaclepediatrics@yahoo.com.

Guaranteeing Adequate Payment From Medicaid for Rural Pediatric Practices: The Rural Health Clinic Program

Francis Rushton, MD, FAAP

Our practice in rural South Carolina has been designated a Rural Health Clinic (RHC) for the past decade. It astonishes me how many of my colleagues have not jumped through the appropriate hoops to become one. Rural Health Clinic rules guarantee that offices will be paid the actual cost of doing business for Medicaid patients, including an appropriate salary for the providers. They are designed for practitioners who want to be available for all children in the community and still make ends meet economically. Our practice is 60% Medicaid, reflecting the general make-up of the pediatric population in South Carolina, and the RHC program has been a boon.

Eligibility Requirements

Unfortunately, the program is only available to pediatric practices in rural areas that meet certain health care shortage requirements. Most states have offices of rural health that can tell you whether you are eligible. But once designated, an office site maintains RHC status forever, whether the health care provider shortage continues or not.

To qualify, there must be at least one mid-level provider, usually a nurse practitioner, within the practice site. There can be as many doctors and other health professionals as desired. There is a loophole in the law, however. If a practice is on an island (ours is), no matter how many bridges there are to connect you to the rest of the world, a nurse practitioner is not required. But we like our nurse practitioner and keep her anyway.

Setting up an RHC usually involves hiring an outside consultant to do the legwork for you. One will need a policy manual and is subject to surprise inspections that are generally a nuisance and not helpful. But the bureaucratic burden is surprisingly minimal and not noticed after the first year or two. Rural Health Clinics are administratively much simpler than Federally Qualified Health Centers.

Advantages

The major advantage is that an office is guaranteed the actual costs of seeing patients. Each year a reconciliation is required. A practice must add up its legitimate expenses and divide by the legitimate number of patient visits. That is the per-patient rate, no matter whether the patient is there for an ear recheck or an hour of counseling. There is a state cap on the rate, but this generally is not a problem for all but the most inefficient of practices.

A second advantage for our practice is that it enabled us to afford in-house mental health counseling. Our state Medicaid rates for mental health services were too low, but our credentialed counselor is able to survive on our office RHC rate.

It's unfortunate that the program is not available to all practice sites, but it does serve as an opportunity for pediatricians concerned about rural populations that are frequently underserved and subject to health disparities. For more information, contact your local state office for rural health or the Rural Health Special Interest Group (http://www.aap.org/sections/socp/sigRH.html) of the American Academy of Pediatrics Council on Community Pediatrics.

"Getting Big" With an Independent Practice Association

Geoffrey Simon, MD, FAAP

The advantage of organizational size is common across many business models, allowing increased leverage in negotiations, greater purchasing power, and savings in scalable business infrastructure. An alternative to growth through mergers or expansion is participation in an independent practice association (IPA), a third-party physician-directed joint venture designed to allow contract negotiations and other collaborative activities by individual practices, while maintaining separate tax IDs. The IPA allows small practices to maintain financial and cultural autonomy, at a relatively low cost, in capital investment and on-going expenses, while, at the same time, exercising many of the advantages of a larger organization.

There are 3 basic types of IPAs: financial risk sharing, messenger model, and clinically integrated organizations. The financial risk sharing IPA was the most common early model, and initially emerged in the 1980s as a collaborative model to manage captitated contracts. The organization would contract with a health maintenance organization (HMO) to manage a capitated risk pool to pay physician members who provided service to HMO patients. This model was extremely prevalent in markets with significant HMO penetration, particularly on the west coast. However, many of these organizations collapsed under poor management, particularly as increases in pharmacy benefits and subspecialist fees outpaced the shared payment pool.

As the insurance market changed in the late 1990s and fee-for-service insurance products emerged as the dominant product, the messenger model organization, either as an IPA or physician hospital organization (PHO), became the most common third-party entity involved in contracting. Under the messenger model, there is no financial risk sharing by practices. The IPA simply acts as a third party in contract negotiations to relay offers between insurance companies and member practices. It cannot negotiate or collectively bargain on behalf of its members, and must relay all contracts for members to consider as individual practices. A variation of this is the modified messenger model, where individual practices can predefine a fee threshold they will accept, such as a percentage of the

Resource-Based Relative Value Scale. In this case, only contract offers at or above the threshold will be relayed back to the practice, and thresholds cannot be set collectively.

In markets that are primarily fee for service, the clinically integrated IPA holds the most promise for primary care pediatricians, particularly if it is limited to primary care pediatrics rather than being multi-specialty. The key function of the organization that allows it to operate legally is an active and productive quality and utilization management program that measurably affects patient care costs and outcomes. The IPA acts as a third party to negotiate managed care contracts collectively for its members, under the premise that any additional payments above market fees are offset by cost savings and patient care outcomes that would only be achievable by the joint venture. This differs from the messenger model in that this model actively represents and negotiates on behalf of the network with single signature power, and that the contracting functionality is a by-product to support the mission of clinical integration. By remaining specialty specific, pediatrician shareholders can better control the activities that are specific to pediatric practice.

This type of IPA also can achieve significant value for its members beyond contracting and delegated credentialing. In monitoring contract compliance, sentinel underpaid claims across a network of more than 100 physicians are easier to detect than in an individual practice. Benchmark data on costs and revenues provide market-specific information to facilitate business analysis and planning. Periodic patient satisfaction surveys with both network- and practice-specific analyses identify patient-service issues and help facilitate patient loyalty in a competitive market. A practice administrators' association within the network provides a forum for administrators to solve common problems and become active participants in implementing programs on the local practice level. The ability to collect network data also allows group purchasing for insurance products. By establishing itself as a risk purchasing group, implementing an active risk management program, and collecting aggregate claims data that reflect a positive history, the IPA becomes an attractive organization for malpractice insurers to underwrite. The advantages to members are not only in negotiated discounts, but in belonging to a larger risk pool. A single claim has much less impact on a premium pool of more than 100 physicians. Additionally, whether for malpractice, health, or disability insurance, the service provided to a purchasing group with several million dollars in premium is inherently greater than what an individual practice can demand.

In considering IPA participation, practices must be keenly aware of laws and regulations concerning physician joint ventures, particularly the antitrust statutes that are enforced by the Federal Trade Commission (FTC). The FTC's stated goal is to ensure provider competition in the marketplace with a net benefit for the health care consumer in terms of costs, access, and quality. The FTC has described areas of safe harbor for IPAs that it considers "unlikely to raise anticompetitive concerns." Unfortunately, there are not specific guidelines defining what is allowable, with the FTC evaluating each organization individually "under the rule of reason." The FTC has recently pursued IPAs and PHOs with increased aggressiveness, handing out more than 20 negative decisions in the past 3 years. Most of these organizations have been messenger models that were in violation for collective bargaining, for threatening collective refusal of a contract, or for representing such a large percentage of the physician market that it would negatively affect patient access and cost. In the instances where clinically integrated IPAs have had a negative decision, these were primarily multi-specialty organizations that included a significant majority of specialists and subspecialists

within a market. Furthermore, the clinical integration activities typically were implemented only within primary care, which the FTC felt did not significantly affect the cost and care delivered by the specialists. Very few organizations have proactively requested an opinion from the FTC, and the FTC's opinions, with few exceptions, have deemed the proposals to be anticompetitive and unacceptable. As such, most successful IPAs have not pursued FTC approval but, rather, have structured themselves based on the published safe-harbor scenarios and attempted to avoid behaviors that the FTC has previously cited as illegal. For more information on FTC guidelines, go to www.ftc. gov/bc/healthcare/index.htm.

Despite the antitrust burdens, the clinically integrated pediatric IPA is an attractive option to "get big" no matter what your practice's current size. The advantages include low start-up costs, preservation of practice autonomy, specialty- and market-specific business support, and the ability to participate in an established network of quality physicians that has greater leverage with negotiations and purchasing. The inherent weaknesses of this type of organization are that there are no guarantees of contracting advantages, it is often volunteer dependent, large projects can be difficult and costly to coordinate among so many separate practices, and ongoing support for the IPA is dependent on practices perceiving a net value through participation. The keys to success are good planning with appropriate legal counsel, selecting quality practices that will actively participate, and ensuring appropriate funding to achieve the organization's goals.

Editor's note: Before embarking on a merger of practices or formation of an IPA network, the pediatrician should seek competent legal counsel.

Operating Principles of Large Groups

Budd Shenkin, MD, FAAP

Bayside Medical Group is a network of 9 small offices of 1 to 4 clinicians in the San Francisco East Bay. We have grown to this size by small steps over 20 years, starting as a solo practice, then establishing new offices, and twice purchasing existing practices. At our recent National Conference & Exhibition Section on Administration and Practice Management (SOAPM) symposium on larger group practices, I presented some of the principles that have sustained us.

Overall, we have tried to make our size work for us by maintaining the personal relationships and clinician autonomy of a small practice, while being able to afford professional management. It is easy enough to say, but we have had to be aware that the opposite can happen just as easily—without constant tending and thoughtful administrative decisions, we can become bureaucratic, lose our autonomy, and lose intimate and personal relationships with patients and with each other. Strong administration is required. It is a pervasive debilitating conceit of physicians that only clinical care deserves to be honored and reimbursed, and that administration is just "pushing paper." We in SOAPM know that nothing could be further from the truth.

People (patients, staff, and clinicians) are all different. One size never fits all. We strive to make the organization bend to the needs of our clinicians. Many need part-time employment; most want just to practice medicine and not be administrators managing employees and chasing accounts receivable. Some of the clinicians want students; others do not. In many ways, our clinicians are like various plants, some needing more attention than others, some needing more sunlight, and most needing convivial colleagues who are emotionally mature. It is helpful for an administrator to think of himself or herself as a gardener, and to try to produce and nurture these conditions.

All organizations face the issue of clinician pay. Bayside has done well with reimbursement by productivity, using the simple measure of receipts—no relative value units, and no base salary, just receipts (after an initial period of employment with salary). This

method automatically rewards a popular, hard-working, and efficient clinician; someone with more deliberate habits accordingly gets paid less. Productivity reimbursement is simple and fair.

We are organized as a corporation with a single owner. Other similar organizations have either a small group of partners as owners, or everyone as a partner with a small group of managing partners. Concentration of governance is essential for decision-making. At the same time, extra recompense is warranted for extra work, extra skills and, in some cases, extra investment and extra risk.

As professionals, clinicians need and want autonomy. The productivity formula enables them to choose their own pace. Together, clinicians can decide on clinical issues, such as immunization schedules, developmental screening procedures, etc. A time-off schedule is always important; we solicit time-off requests prior to making each schedule, and facilitate trade-offs. Clinicians can decide on initiatives, such as giving patient lectures, taking obstetricians to lunch, and e-prescribing from laptops in the examination room. The role of the organization is to support these worthy efforts.

Getting administration in tune with clinicians is probably the single-most important issue. There is probably no way to do this properly without clinicians, themselves, being administrators, which takes skill, training, and time. But, no matter how much clinician skill is there, talented administrators are essential. Our chief administrators have MBAs and have had substantial medical organization experience. We have in-house capacity for billing, accounting, information technology, and human resources.

In addition, over the years we have accumulated a bank of consultants who have developed intimate knowledge of Bayside while working with other organizations as well. We have relied most prominently on our attorney (who does work only with health care organizations), our practice consultant (who works with many small health care organizations), our tax accountant, and our financial operations consultant. In addition, we have our sign painter, our floor-coverings specialist, several real estate brokers, our publicity consultants, and others.

No matter how big an organization becomes, the essence of any practice organization remains the people who compose it. Working together concordantly, cliché though it may be, turns out to be the most crucial element in a successful practice.

The Road to Market Power: Models for Pediatric Practices to Aggregate and Grow

Herschel R. Lessin, MD, FAAP, Norman "Chip" Harbaugh, MD, FAAP

Small practices may have an uncertain economic future. There are many ways to get bigger to survive.

The field of pediatrics is undergoing a sea of change in its ability to respond to the current economic and political climate. Managed care companies are consolidating and wielding their almost total market penetration to reduce payments and erect hurdles for pediatricians. Costs are being shifted to patients and there is a rise in patient-directed accounts. In the past, small group practices have been able to weather these changes. Going forward, however, they will face increasing challenges. They will be too large to be a boutique, but too small to develop a real infrastructure. They will be large enough to develop large group problems, but too small to develop large group solutions. As pediatric practice changes, practice models must change as well. Therefore, it is important to consider going BIG.

What Is Going BIG?

By going BIG or cooperating with other pediatricians, practices can reap many benefits. They may enact group purchasing or joint ventures and share calls. This may be enough in some markets. However, the greatest benefits can be seen only with real aggregating under several models that allow physicians to legally develop greater market power but require much closer practice integration. When this is done, practices can negotiate fees, have central billing and management, discuss fees, and develop a professional structure for running the business of medicine.

Given the advent of retail-based clinics and health savings accounts and continued inadequate reimbursement, large groups are necessary to maintain clinical quality, keep control of medicine, and gain economic leverage. Large groups or corporations come in several different types.
- Organic growth to a large size
- Full asset merger
- Groups without walls
- Independent practice associations (IPAs)

Pediatricians must realize that their colleagues are not really the competition. The competition is in how the medical economic pie is divided among employers, payers, and physicians. Getting BIG gives pediatricians much more leverage when trying to compete in this era of inadequate, inequitable payments for services.

Deciding to Go BIG

In every business, there are recurrent themes. People are different, personal relationships are vital, and your organization must adapt to be responsive to these various needs. Successful physician organizations must focus on competence and quality, rather than personal control.

With Whom Do I Choose to Go BIG?

Deciding with whom you can successfully work is the key. The more integrated the organization (full asset merger) the more important this becomes. Less integrated organizations (groups without walls or IPAs) require less loss of personal control. Practice culture and economics must be closely examined for compatibility and flexibility. Good advice from accountants, bankers, lawyers, and practice management consultants is vital.

While there are many models, there is no perfect model. The landscape will determine the best model for the practice. Assessing, maintaining, and improving quality initiatives will be vital to the success of the practice.

Benefits, Challenges, and the Future

Going BIG means higher revenue, more clout, improved quality, control over hassle factors, positive increase in lifestyle with more time off and a better income, and diversification of services. On the other hand, it entails organization and planning, managing start-up issues, changing practice cultures, management problems, compensation, debt, and increased overhead. While the future of medicine is changing, it will be important to work with your peers to build something larger and continue to offer high-quality services. Pediatricians will need to stick together to continue to lead the profession and field of pediatrics.

Visit http://practice.aap.org/content.aspx?aid=2207 to view the PowerPoint presentation.

For more information, contact American Academy of Pediatrics staff in the Division of Pediatric Practice at DOPP@aap.org or call 800/433-9016, ext 4784.

Section 4

Employment/Personnel

The Interview

Excerpt from Launching Your Career in Pediatrics Handbook: Finding the Job

Once you have identified a practice opportunity, you will start the interviewing process. It is important to know that the interview is for the person hiring for the position and the person seeking the position. The interviewer will use this meeting as a way to determine if you are a good fit with the practice's mission, staff, and position. The interview is also an opportunity for you to examine the practice to determine if it is a good fit for you. Therefore, it is important to prepare for the interview beforehand and come with questions about the practice and community that can help you make this decision.

Five Steps of the Interview
1. Get acquainted. Are you compatible?
2. Find out about the practice goals, philosophy, lifestyle, and working relationships.
3. Ask questions about the practice.
   - Number of patients seen (per year, per day)
   - Staffing ratios
   - Income and financial stability
   - Partnership opportunities and procedure
   - Marketing techniques to gain patients
   - Comfort with technology
   - Payer mix
   - Others
4. Assess practice and candidate attributes.
5. Negotiate a deal.

Depending on your location and the location of the interview, the first encounter will be by phone, by e-mail, or in person. When arranging an interview, determine who you will be interviewing with, if your expenses for travel will be covered, and what the expectation is from you.

Tips for the Interview
- Dress professionally for this interview. Business attire is most appropriate, even in a casual practice.
- Bring your curriculum vitae along as well as any other information about yourself that you feel would be helpful.

- Make eye contact with your interviewer and listen carefully to the questions. Be sure that you answer all of the questions completely.
- Talk with the partners and also the staff. If possible, speak with some of the patients about what they like about the practice.
- As you begin your questions, do not start by discussing salary. It is better to understand the practice structure and responsibilities before getting into financial questions.
- If the interview will occur by phone, be sure you schedule this at a time when there are no disturbances. Be sure that there is no background noise.

Following are some questions that you may wish to ask the interviewer about the position or practice.

Interview Questions
Following is a useful checklist to take when going in for an interview with a prospective practice. Keep in mind that most interviews proceed from the informal (eg, getting to know each other, seeing if the new physician is a good fit) to the more formal (eg, contract negotiations). Keep the checklist in the back of your mind, but avoid coming across as too forward or pushy. Remember that the group may have a set of criteria by which you are being evaluated as well.

- How is the practice organized? Is it a partnership or corporation, or are the physicians all employed?
- Who makes up the group? Are they all general pediatricians? Are there family or nurse practitioners? Is everyone working full time? Who are the actual physicians participating in the call rotation? What are the responsibilities of each physician who takes calls? What is the call rotation schedule?
- Are there hospital responsibilities? Do these involve nursery calls or inpatient admissions? Does the group use area hospitalists?
- What kind of nursing support does each physician have? Will each doctor have a medical assistant, licensed practical nurse, or registered nurse, or do they share a pool of nurses?

- How does the office flow? Will each physician have a set of examination rooms or does everyone use a common set of rooms? How are patients checked in and out?
- What is a typical workday for each physician? How do they schedule well and follow-up visits versus acute visits?
- Who triages patient phone calls? What is expected of physicians with regard to returning patient calls?
- What laboratory or radiology support does the group have? If laboratory tests or radiographs are done within the facility, how does the practice bill for these?
- What kind of medical record system does the practice have (electronic vs paper)? Are there plans to convert to an electronic medical record if paper is still being used? How user-friendly is the system?
- What is the physician payment rate? What is the basis of this scale (eg, salary, seniority, productivity, patient load, call load, combination)?
- What benefits are offered to physicians? Do these include health coverage, malpractice liability, other insurance coverage, and retirement funds? If transferring from another practice, will the group offer tail coverage?
- What constitutes terms of separation, termination, and contractual breach? Are there any restrictive covenants (eg, geographic practice restrictions)?
- Does the practice have any relationship with area hospitals or universities?
- Will you be responsible for any administrative or management responsibilities?
- What will be your clinical duties (eg, calls, coverage)?
- What will your office schedule be? Hospital rounding?
- Will you need to attend deliveries? Cover the emergency department?
- Will your schedule include weekends, evenings, or holiday coverage?
- Is there a phone triage or answering service at night?
- What office space is available? Staff-provider ratios?
- What expenses are covered by the practice and what are your personal expenses (eg, licenses, phones or pagers, subscriptions, automobile)?
- What is the policy on vacations and sick leave?

- What is the policy on personal days and pregnancy or paternity leave?
- Is there a retirement plan? When can you participate?
- What is the arrangement for continuing medical education (CME)? Time? Expenses?
- What is the philosophy of the practice?
- What is the length of the contract? Are there renewal options?
- What privileges or affiliations are required? Board certification? Hospital privileges? Licenses? Will the practice pay for these?
- How will patients be assigned to you? Do you share patients with other providers or do you have your own patients?
- Will the practice assist with moving expenses?

Additional Tips on Interviewing

Behavior-based interviews have become popular recently, replacing loosely structured, traditional interviews. This type of interview allows employers to ask candidates questions about how they have handled previous situations in an effort to predict future behavior. Behavioral interviewing is used to assist employers in finding a good match, lower turnover rates, and increase job satisfaction and performance. Behavioral interviewing focuses on asking about a situation in the past, the action taken to address the situation, and the outcome.

Tips for Preparing for an Interview

- Be prepared. Questions will be based on your past experience. Therefore, have specific examples and situations prepared to share. If this job will be based on seeing patients, be prepared to answer questions such as, "Tell me about a time when you encountered a difficult patient who was unhappy with his or her service."
- Beware of questions that ask for your mistakes or personal failings. Don't answer them in a way that will make the employer doubt your abilities. You can discuss something that was difficult, but end on a positive note by relating how you managed it.
- Allow time to think of an appropriate answer, even if it requires a few moments of silence.
- Answer each question concisely, with one example. Let interviewers ask if they want elaboration or another example.
- Rehearse answers to potential questions ahead of time.

Here are some examples of interview questions using the behavioral interviewing model.

- Tell me about a project or an idea that was successful mostly because of your efforts.
- Think of a time when you had to make an important decision without enough information. Explain your decision-making process.
- Tell me about a time when you encountered a difficult patient who was unhappy with his or her service.
- Tell me about a time when something unexpected happened that changed the way you planned your day.
- Tell me about a situation in which you had to overcome or manage an obstacle to accomplish your objectives.
- Give me an example of a situation in which you found a new or an improved way of doing something significant.
- Tell me about a time when you had to work with a colleague who has a different work style or ethic. How did you handle a situation in which you disagreed with that colleague?

After the interview, it is important to send a personal note of thanks for the time the practice spent with you. Also, follow up with appropriate questions and requests for further information in a timely manner. If the practice offers you a job, you are ready to move to the next level—reviewing the contract.

Negotiating an Agreement

Excerpt from Launching Your Career in Pediatrics Handbook: Finding the Job

Once a position has been offered to you, it is time to negotiate an agreement. Following are points to consider when negotiating an agreement:

1. Status
   a. Will you be a salaried physician or full partner?
   b. If you will not be a full partner, will the opportunity be offered to you at a future date? If so, at what cost?
   c. How will expenses, profits, and losses be divided or managed? Know what your limits will be concerning openness relating to financial accounting of the firm, even if you are not a partner or an owner.
2. Involvement
   a. Will you have a voice in the administration and management of the practice? If so, to what extent, and with what limitations (eg, staffing, purchases, addition of new physicians, policy changes, site changes)?
3. Insurance
   a. Does the practice cover your malpractice insurance? What type of policy? Are health, life, and disability insurance included? Who will pay for these? What is the amount?
   b. Will tail insurance for malpractice be provided?
4. Duties and assignments
   a. What will your duties be?
   b. What will your on-call, referral, coverage, and house-call schedules be?
   c. What will your office schedule be?
   d. How are weekends, evenings, and holidays rotated?
   e. How many hours per week and per year will you be required to work?
   f. Is there additional compensation for hours worked beyond the required amount?
   g. Will you be required to take emergency department or hospital calls?
   h. Will you be attending deliveries?
   i. How will hospital rounds be rotated?
5. Office space
   a. Will you have your own office space?
   b. Will staff be shared within the offices or will specific staff be assigned to you?
   c. Will you be required to furnish your own office space?
6. Business-related expenses
   a. What expenses will you be personally responsible for?
   b. What expenses will you be expected to pay and in what proportion?
   c. Who pays for licenses, dues, pagers, journal subscriptions, and automobile expenses?
7. Office supplies, marketing, and advertising
   a. Will the group pay for the expenses of adding you to the practice, such as announcement cards, business cards, door plaques, stationary, advertising, and changing of indoor or outdoor signage?
8. Leaves, vacations, and paid time off
   a. What are the vacation and sick leave plans?
   b. Are personal days allowed? In what quantity? Are these paid?
   c. Is there pregnancy leave or paternity leave, and is this time paid?
   d. Will the number of days off or vacation weeks increase after the first year of the contract?
9. Retirement/death planning
   a. Is there a retirement plan and how does it function?
   b. Is there a contingency plan in the event of your death or the death or incapacity of a member of this group?
   c. Is there a 401(k) plan, and how soon can you participate?
10. Continuing education
    a. Are time or funds allotted for CME?
    b. Will travel expenses be paid?
    c. Can time be taken off without penalty for CME or to be involved in speaking?
    d. Is involvement in professional organizations encouraged?
11. Practice philosophy
    a. What are the philosophies of the existing group about medical care, employee relations, expenses, and the like?
    b. Are you in agreement with these philosophies?

12. Salary and compensation calculations and payment
    a. How are salaries computed and when are they paid?
    b. Is there a percentage of the fees that you will be paid over and above a certain amount?
    c. Are there bonuses given, and under what circumstances are they given?
    d. Do you receive a share of income from income-producing assets (eg, laboratory)? If compensation is based on productivity, what is the formula used, and are there minimum (base) guarantees and maximum ceilings?
    e. If you are required to submit reports to justify the payment due you, what information must you submit? Who must have access to this information?
    f. If a hospital is subsidizing your first year of practice or your practice setup, is repayment expected and, if so, on what schedule and at what percent interest?

13. Termination/withdrawal
    a. What is the termination or withdrawal policy? How much notice must be given once you decide to leave? Can you be fired or dismissed from the group, and under what circumstances? What rights do you have to dispute your termination or rectify the situation?

14. Restrictive covenants
    a. What is the noncompetition policy of the group (restrictive covenant) should you decide to leave? Would there be a certain radius from the office within which you could not practice and for what period? What would the penalties be for a breach of contract? Look for these 4 parts: geographic area, time restriction, monetary penalty, and schedule of penalty payments.

15. Moonlighting and other outside activities
    a. What is the policy addressing moonlighting and other outside activities?
    b. Are you permitted to keep funds received from outside sources?

16. Length of contract and renewal clauses
    a. What is the length of the contract?
    b. What are the renewal stipulations?

17. Privileges, affiliations, and certifications
    a. What privileges or affiliations will be required?
    b. Is board certification required within a certain period after beginning work?

    c. Are there any obligations, implied or specified, to admit to certain hospitals or use certain medical facilities?
    d. Will you need to have licensure in more than one state?

18. Practice location
    a. At what site will you be required to work (if there are satellite offices)?
    b. Does the group do contract work at a well-child clinic, hospital nursery coverage, or group home coverage?

19. Disability
    a. What is the policy should you become ill or disabled and unable to practice for a length of time?

20. Moving expenses
    a. How much, if any, of your moving or relocation expenses will be paid, for what specific expenses, and how will these expenses be paid (prepaid or by a specific date)?

21. Accounts receivable and patients
    a. Who retains ownership (property) or fees that are charged or collected by the practice—you, the practice, or your employer?
    b. Who will be doing the billing—an outside party, the practice, or perhaps the hospital?

22. Patient base
    a. How will patients be assigned to you (ie, how will you get your fair share of patients)? Are patients considered your patients or patients of the practice?
    b. Where will referrals come from?

Note: It is very important for a lawyer to review any contract before signing.

Resources

- "Pediatricians and the Law: Careful Review of Employment Contract Sets Graduates Off on Right Foot": http://aapnews.aappublications.org/cgi/content/full/26/5/17
- Employment Contracts: A Practice Management FAQ: http://practice.aap.org/content.aspx?aid=2107&nodeID=1003
- Sample Employment Contract: http://practice.aap.org/content.aspx?aid=2100

Job Descriptions for Front and Back Office Staff

Each pediatric practice needs competent staff to ensure that the office runs smoothly and efficiently. As a pediatrician, it is important to know when it is appropriate to delegate work so that the work and the practice are successful.

A job description is essential in providing employees a basic understanding of what is expected of them. These written job descriptions establish lines of authority and define the duties of each position. Pediatric offices typically employ 2 types of staff, front office and back office. Front office staff are generally responsible for managing the business aspect of the practice. Jobs may include a sign-in receptionist, file clerk, bookkeeper, insurance clerk, and sign-out clerk. Back office staff customarily handle the clinical aspects of the practice. Frequently, these are nurses (various levels), medical assistants, and laboratory personnel.

Although the jobs and responsibilities vary, the job descriptions should be in a similar format. Each job description should include the following sections:

1. Position and Title—including supervisory responsibilities
2. Basic Functions—overview of job content and the nature of position
3. Duties and Responsibilities—major activities associated with the job
4. Qualifications—education and experience
5. Principal Working Relations—working alone or with others
6. Standards of Performance—qualitative and quantitative

Job descriptions are also instrumental in recruitment, selection of qualified candidates, training, and reducing conflicts. While it is important to adhere to job descriptions, it is also important to be flexible about the basic functions because too much detail inhibits flexibility and creativity. Job descriptions should be evaluated periodically and changed as the conditions and needs of the practice change.

Finally, a job description can be used to assist with performance appraisals. This provides the employer and employee an opportunity to identify strengths and weaknesses, a basis for a salary review, communication, and job feedback.

This Information Was Adapted From the Following Resources

American Academy of Pediatrics. *Management of Pediatric Practice*. 2nd ed. Elk Grove Village, IL: American Academy of Pediatrics; 1991:47–53

American Academy of Pediatrics. *A Guide to Starting a Medical Office*. Norcross, GA: Coker Publishing, LLC; 1997:76–86

Additional Resources

"An Employment Contract Model for Joining a Medical Practice," Robert I. Freedman, Esq; Medscape; September 18, 2007
Need to register to access article

For the official employment resource for the American Academy of Pediatrics, visit http://www.pedjobs.org/.

Sample job descriptions can be found on *Practice Management Online* at http://practice.aap.org/samplepersonneldocs.aspx.

If you need more information, contact American Academy of Pediatrics staff in the Division of Pediatric Practice at dopp@aap.org or call 800/433-9016, ext 4784.

Physician Salaries and Loan Repayment Options

Excerpt from Launching Your Career in Pediatrics Handbook: Getting Started

Salary

The region of the country where you practice will likely determine your lifestyle and practice income. Surveys of pediatric salaries show that incomes are highest in the Midwest and Southeast, with the lowest salaries in the Northeast and on the West Coast. US Department of Labor Bureau of Labor Statistics

(Based on 2008 Data) (http://www.bls.gov/oes/current/oes291065.htm).

For general pediatricians—annual mean wage: $153,370; annual median wage: $146,040. The following table lists state/commonwealth annual mean wage and annual median wage:

State/Commonwealth Wage	Annual Mean Wage	Annual Median
Alabama	$171,100	a
Alaska	$165,570	$161,720
Arizona	$152,820	$148,890
Arkansas	$152,600	$143,150
California	$156,830	$148,190
Colorado	$166,300	$159,530
Connecticut	$144,990	$134,480
Florida	$154,790	$150,590
Georgia	$155,890	$152,060
Hawaii	$172,030	a
Idaho	$147,840	$149,980
Illinois	$115,900	$99,920
Indiana	$139,820	$132,130
Iowa	$199,500	a
Kansas	$154,010	$152,020
Kentucky	$204,610	a
Louisiana	$156,710	$148,060
Maine	$155,290	$152,700
Maryland	$125,880	$121,230
Massachusetts	$145,830	$145,450
Michigan	$153,520	$145,400
Minnesota	$170,860	$162,390
Mississippi	$182,990	a
Missouri	$150,290	$140,670
Montana	$110,570	$55,150

State/Commonwealth Wage	Annual Mean Wage	Annual Median
Nebraska	$167,060	$135,320
Nevada	$175,330	$159,490
New Hampshire	$151,950	$144,640
New Jersey	$156,100	$141,650
New Mexico	$158,930	$154,690
New York	$139,430	$130,580
North Carolina	$164,270	$153,790
North Dakota	$139,970	$133,290
Ohio	$149,800	$138,310
Oklahoma	$183,530	a
Oregon	$171,890	$163,140
Pennsylvania	$149,960	$137,280
Puerto Rico	$81,430	$62,300
Rhode Island	$168,760	$160,230
South Carolina	$147,080	$148,220
South Dakota	$171,370	$159,140
Tennessee	$154,010	$150,260
Texas	$153,330	$150,570
Utah	$171,730	$165,480
Vermont	$113,740	$107,900
Virginia	$142,230	$136,490
Washington	$158,080	$136,490
West Virginia	$179,560	a
Wisconsin	$167,330	$161,280

Annual wages have been calculated by multiplying the hourly mean wage by 2,080 hours; where an hourly mean wage is not published, the annual wage has been directly calculated from the reported survey data.

[a]This wage is equal to or greater than $80 per hour or $166,400 per year. Data extracted on June 1, 2009.

According to the Medical Group Management Association *Physician Compensation and Production Survey: 2008 Report Based on 2007 Data,* the national mean for general pediatricians was $196,936 and the national median was $183,265.

Salary References and Additional Resources

- AAP *Socioeconomic Survey of Pediatric Practices:* http://eweb.aap.org/pub75856
- The 2002 AAP Periodic Survey provides an overview of pediatrician's characteristics: http://www.aap.org/research/periodicsurvey/ps43soci.htm#pract1
- "Pediatricians Leading the Way: Integrating a Career and a Family/Personal Life Over the Life Cycle," *Pediatrics,* February 2006: http://pediatrics.aappublications.org/cgi/content/extract/117/2/519
- "Pediatrician Workforce Statement," *Pediatrics,* July 2005: http://aappolicy.aappublications.org/cgi/content/full/pediatrics;116/1/263
- "The Pediatrician Workforce: Current Status and Future Prospects," *Pediatrics,* July 2005: http://pediatrics.aappublications.org/cgi/content/full/116/1/e156
- 2007 Survey of Primary Care Physicians, Merritt Hawkins & Associates®: http://www5.mgma.com/ecom/Default.aspx?tabid=138&action=INVProductDetails&args=3823&pck=true
- In 2007, Merritt Hawkins & Associates conducted a survey of primary care physicians' salaries, overhead costs, job market, and career satisfaction. Of the 10,000 randomly selected primary care physicians (national physician database), 2,000 were pediatricians.
- Physician Compensation Survey—In Practice Three Plus Years, Physician Search (http://www.physicianssearch.com/physician/salary2.html)

Loan Repayment Options

As the cost of higher education continues to rise, so does the amount of loan debt. Many members of the American Academy of Pediatrics emerge from medical school or pediatric residency with a balance of more than $125,000 in student loans.

It is important to obtain qualified advice before entering into any loan repayment or employment agreement. There are many government programs that offer repayment programs. It is essential to learn about the commitments and expectations before entering into any formal agreement. Examine the source of funding and the fine print, and consult mentors on your faculty and in your student affairs office before entering into any commitments *(Pediatrics 101: A Resource Guide from the American Academy of Pediatrics,* http://www.aap.org/profed/Peds101book.pdf).

The following resources provide general information as a starting point for research. Consult with your college financial aid officer and other qualified advisors before committing to any financial arrangement.

Loan Repayment Resources

- Association of American Medical Colleges
    - (MD)2: Monetary Decisions for Medical Doctors
    - A database of state and other loan repayment/forgiveness scholarship programs with an interactive guide to information from state health departments, medical schools, federal programs, and military agencies
    - A chart showing tuition and student fees for first-year medical students, 2004 to 2005 (log-in required)
- National Institutes of Health
    - Pediatric Research Loan Repayment Program—in return for a 2-year commitment to your research career, the National Institutes of Health will repay up to $35,000 per year of your qualified repayable education debt plus an additional 39% of the repayments to cover your federal taxes, and may reimburse state taxes that may result from these payments.
    - Student Loan Consolidation—information on loan consolidation programs.
- Indian Health Service Loan Repayment Program Service Center
    - Applicants sign a 2-year agreement and provide full-time clinical practice at the Indian Health Service facilities or approved Indian health programs. In exchange, a portion to all of their educational loans will be repaid.
- National Health Service Corps
    - Applicants will serve on an interdisciplinary team to focus on community health. In exchange, applicants will receive job placement assistance, a competitive loan repayment program, an opportunity to join the National Health Service Corps Ready Responders as a US Public Health Service commissioned officer, and preceptorship and mentoring.

Salaries: Medical Office Administrators and Office Managers

Following are resources on identifying the average salaries for pediatric office managers.

US Department of Labor Bureau of Labor Statistics Medical and Health Services Managers (based on 2004 data)

http://www.bls.gov/oco/ocos014.htmUS

This resource provides an overview of the field of medical and health service management. It also provides the ranges of salaries for a variety of medical and health service managers. The salaries vary by the size of the facility as well as the level of responsibility. Median annual earnings for medical and health service managers were $67,430. The middle 50% earned between $52,530 and $88,210. The lowest 10% earned less than $41,450 and the highest 10% earned more than $117,990.

"How Do Your Staff Salaries Compare?" Medical Economics, August 5, 2005

http://medicaleconomics.modernmedicine.com/ memag/article/articleDetail.jsp?id=172911

This article provides an overview of a 2004 survey by the Professional Association of Health Care Office Management. This article also provides salary ranges for other positions within the medical office (eg, nurses, certified medical assistants, receptionists). According to this article, pediatric office managers earn an average salary of $50,755 per year and $7,840 in fringe benefits.

Medical Group Management Association Management Compensation Survey: 2007 Report Based on 2006 Data

http://www5.mgma.com/ecom/Default.aspx?tabid= 138&action=INVProduct Details&args=2754

According to this survey, for office managers, national salary mean is $50,648; the national median is $48,868 (see Table).

Definitions

Administrator: The top nonphysician professional administrative position with less authority than a chief executive officer (CEO). Maintains broad responsibilities for all administrative functions of the medical group, including operations, marketing,

finance, managed care/third-party contracting, physician compensation and reimbursement, human resources, medical and business information systems, and planning and development. Typically oversees management personnel with direct responsibilities for the specific functional areas of the organization, and reports to the governing body of the organization.

Assistant Administrator: Provides assistance to the CEO and/or administrator with the management of one or more functional areas of the medical practice such as administration, managed care, human resources, marketing, patient accounting, or operations. Has a more limited scope of responsibility than a chief operating officer. A medical group may have multiple assistant administrators. Responsible for assisting the CEO or administrator in accomplishing organizational objectives, and usually reports to the senior administrative officer.

Office Manager: Manages the nonmedical activities of a larger medical practice. Typically found in a practice that does not have an administrator. The focus of this position usually rests on the daily operations of the organization. May oversee some financial activities, such as billing and collections, and usually reports to the administrator or business services director. Copyright © 2007 Medical Group Management Association. All Rights Reserved. Used with permission.

Total Compensation[a]			
Job Title	Count	Mean	Median
Administrator (26 or more MDs)	83	$142,137	$135,000
Administrator (7–25 MDs)	303	$113,380	$103,960
Administrator (6 or fewer MDs)	302	$84,620	$80,000
Assistant Administrator	92	$95,837	$84,583
Office Manager	395	$50,648	$48,868

[a]These numbers reflect the salary of an office manager across a wide range of specialties and may not represent an accurate mean and median for an office manager working specifically in pediatrics. The Management Compensation Survey: 2007 Report Based on 2006 Data breaks down the level of experience, level of education, range of total medical revenue, range of medical revenue, and more.

Staff Salaries

Following are resources to assist pediatricians in locating the average salaries of the health care professionals in their field.

US Department of Labor Bureau of Labor Statistics (Based on 2007 Data)

http://www.bls.gov/oes/2007/may/naics4_621500. htm#b29-0000

Position	Median	Mean	Mean Annual
Licensed Practical and Licensed Vocational Nurses	$18.24	$18.72	$38,940
Medical Assistants	$13.19	$13.59	$28,270
Medical Records and Health Information Technicians	$14.08	$15.12	$31,450
Medical Secretaries	$14.02	$14.54	$30,240
Nursing Aids (Certified Nursing Assistants)	$11.14	$11.50	$23,920
Physician Assistants	$37.72	$37.41	$77,800
Receptionists and Information Clerks	$11.91	$12.24	$25,460
Registered Nurses	$28.85	$30.04	$62,480

Data extracted from www.bls.gov/oes/current/naics3_621000. htm#b31-0000 on January 23, 2009.

Salaries of Nurse Practitioners

The *Journal of Pediatric Health Care* provides an overview of nurse practitioner salaries titled "Pediatric Nurse Practitioner Salary and Practice: Results of a Midwest Metropolitan Survey."

Visit http://practice.aap.org/content.aspx?aid=2339 for physician salaries.

Visit http://practice.aap.org/content.aspx?aid=2014 for practice manager and administrator salaries.

Section 5

Finance and Payment

2010 RBRVS: What Is It and How Does It Affect Pediatrics?

The Centers for Medicare & Medicaid Services (CMS) implemented the Medicare Resource-Based Relative Value Scale (RBRVS) physician fee schedule on January 1, 1992. The Medicare RBRVS physician fee schedule replaced the Medicare physician payment system of "customary, prevailing, and reasonable" charges under which physicians were paid according to the historical record of the charge for the provision of each service. The current Medicare RBRVS physician fee schedule is derived from the "relative value" of services provided and based on the resources they consume. The relative value of each service is quantifiable and is based on the concept that there are 3 components of each service: the amount of physician work that goes into the service, the practice expense associated with the service, and the professional liability expense for the provision of the service. The relative value of each service is multiplied by geographic practice cost indices (GPCIs) for each Medicare locality and then translated into a dollar amount by an annually adjusted conversion factor. The dollar amount derived from this calculation is the Medicare payment amount for the provision of a particular service. It is critical to note that 77% of public and private payers, including Medicaid programs, have adopted components of the Medicare RBRVS to pay physicians, while others are exploring its implementation. For more information on RBRVS, go to http://aappolicy.aappublications.org/cgi/reprint/pediatrics;122/6/1395.pdf.

Elements of the RBRVS

Physician Work (Work)

The physician work component of the Medicare RBRVS physician fee schedule is maintained and updated by CMS with input from the American Medical Association (AMA)/Specialty Society Relative Value Scale Update Committee (RUC). The RUC is composed of 29 members, consisting of 23 representa-

tives from major medical specialty societies, as well as representatives from the AMA, the American Osteopathic Association, the Health Care Professionals Advisory Committee, the Practice Expense Subcommittee, and the *Current Procedural Terminology (CPT®)* Editorial Panel. The American Academy of Pediatrics (AAP) holds one of the 23 seats designated for medical specialty society representation. CMS reviews and, if necessary, modifies the RUC-recommended relative value units (RVUs) of physician work and establishes payment policy, which is published in the Federal Register (http://www.cms.hhs.gov/PhysicianFeeSched/).

The physician work component represents approximately 52% of the total RVUs for each service. Physician work is divided into pre-service, intra-service, and post-service periods that equal the total value of work for each service. The total value of physician work contained in the Medicare RBRVS physician fee schedule for each service consists of the following components:
- Physician time required to perform the service
- Technical skill and physical effort
- Mental effort and judgment
- Psychological stress associated with physician's concern about the iatrogenic risk to the patient

Practice Expense (PE)

The PE component represents approximately 44% of the total RVUs for each service. In 2002 an initial 4-year transition to resource-based PE RVUs was completed. A second 4-year transition using a revised PE methodology started in 2007 and will be completed in 2010. Starting in 2010, there will be a third 4-year transition utilizing 2 new PE revisions: 1) CMS will utilize the results of the Physician Practice Information Survey, sponsored by the AMA and 72 medical specialty societies and health professional organizations; and 2) CMS will adopt an assumption that diagnostic imaging equipment such as CT and MRI are in use 90 percent of the time that an office is open instead of 50 percent of the time.

CMS uses many sources and methodologies to determine practice expense RVUs. Beginning in 1998, some CPT codes were assigned two (2) practice expense RVUs: a lesser one for procedures performed in a facility (ie, a hospital, skilled nursing facility, or ambulatory surgical center) and a greater one for procedures/services performed at a non-facility site (ie, physician's office or patient's home). This policy continues for 2010.

Professional Liability Insurance (PLI) (Malpractice)

Professional liability insurance (malpractice) expense relative values amount to approximately 4% of the physician fee schedule payment. CMS replaced the cost-based PLI relative values with resource-based PLI RVUs in 2000. The end result of its computations was to retain the same total PLI RVUs as they were under the charge-based system.

Medicare Global Period

On the Medicare physician fee schedule, each CPT code is assigned a designation in the Medicare "global period" column. Medicare global periods define the post-operative period for procedures and affect how follow-up services are reported for a given CPT code.

The Medicare global period designations are defined in the chart below

Components of a Medicare global period including the following:
- Pre-operative visits: Pre-operative visits after the decision is made to operate beginning with the day before the day of surgery for major procedures and the day of surgery for minor procedures
- Intra-operative services: Intra-operative services that are normally a usual and necessary part of a surgical procedure
- Complications following surgery: All additional medical or surgical services required of the surgeon during the post-operative period of the surgery because of complications that do not require additional trips to the operating room

Payers that adopt Medicare's RBRVS RVUs should also be following Medicare policy with respect to Medicare global periods.

Geographic Practice Cost Indices (GPCIs)

The GPCIs reflect the relative costs associated with physician work, practice, and PLI in a Medicare locality compared to the national average relative costs.
- Cost of Living GPCI: Applied to physician work relative values
- Practice Cost GPCI: Applied to PE relative values
- PLI Cost GPCI: Applied to PLI relative values

Medicare Global Period Designation	Definition	Explanation (Example)
000	0-day Medicare global period	Payment for a 0-day global code includes the procedure/service plus any associated care provided on the same day of service (eg, **54150**)
010	10-day Medicare global period	Payment for a 10-day global code includes the procedure/service plus any associated follow-up care for 10 days (eg, **24640**)
090	90-day Medicare global period	Payment for a 90-day global code includes the procedure/service plus any associated follow-up care for 90 days (eg, **25600**)
XXX	The Medicare global period concept does not apply	Payment for an **XXX** code includes only the procedure/service (eg, **90471**)
ZZZ	Code related to another service that is always included in the Medicare global period of another service	Payment for a **ZZZ** code includes only the procedure/service; **ZZZ** codes are usually add-on codes to XXX codes (eg, **90472**)
YYY	The global period is to be set by the carrier	This designation is usually reserved for unlisted surgery codes (eg, **24999**)

2010 Geographic Practice Cost Indices (GPCIs) By Medicare Locality			
Medicare Locality	**Work**	**Practice Expense**	**Professional Liability Insurance**
Alabama	0.982	0.853	0.496
Alaska	1.500*	1.090	0.646
Arizona	0.988	0.957	0.822
Arkansas	0.961	0.846	0.446
Anaheim/Santa Ana, California	1.034	1.269	0.811
Los Angeles, California	1.041	1.225	0.804
Marin/Napa/Solano, California	1.034	1.265	0.432
Oakland/Berkeley, California	1.053	1.286	0.425
San Francisco, California	1.059	1.441	0.414
San Mateo, California	1.072	1.433	0.394
Santa Clara, California	1.083	1.294	0.377
Ventura, California	1.027	1.265	0.766
Rest of California	1.007	1.058	0.549
Colorado	0.986	0.992	0.641
Connecticut	1.038	1.185	0.980
District of Columbia + Maryland/Virginia Suburbs	1.047	1.218	1.032
Delaware	1.011	1.046	0.678
Fort Lauderdale, Florida	0.989	1.018	2.250
Miami, Florida	1.000	1.069	3.167
Rest of Florida	0.973	0.939	1.724
Atlanta, Georgia	1.009	1.014	0.836
Rest of Georgia	0.979	0.883	0.829
Hawaii/Guam	0.998	1.161	0.665
Idaho	0.967	0.883	0.546
Chicago, Illinois	1.025	1.080	1.940
East St Louis, Illinois	0.989	0.919	1.793
Suburban Chicago, Illinois	1.017	1.068	1.629
Rest of Illinois	0.975	0.880	1.219
Indiana	0.986	0.918	0.599
Iowa	0.965	0.870	0.434
Kansas	0.969	0.882	0.557
Kentucky	0.969	0.860	0.652
New Orleans, Louisiana	0.986	1.044	0.956
Rest of Louisiana	0.970	0.878	0.892
Southern Maine	0.980	1.025	0.492
Rest of Maine	0.962	0.893	0.492
Baltimore/Surrounding Counties, Maryland	1.012	1.057	1.086
Rest of Maryland	0.994	0.982	0.874
Metropolitan Boston	1.029	1.291	0.764
Rest of Massachusetts	1.007	1.106	0.764
Detroit, Michigan	1.036	1.040	1.906
Rest of Michigan	0.998	0.923	1.083

*The Medicare Improvements for Patients and Providers Act of 2008 (MIPPA) established a 1.500 work GPCI for Alaska

2010 Geographic Practice Cost Indices (GPCIs) By Medicare Locality, continued			
Medicare Locality	**Work**	**Practice Expense**	**Professional Liability Insurance**
Minnesota	0.992	0.983	0.245
Mississippi	0.959	0.854	0.808
Metropolitan Kansas City, Missouri	0.990	0.945	1.188
Metropolitan St Louis, Missouri	0.993	0.931	1.075
Rest of Missouri	0.949	0.821	0.997
Montana	0.950	0.847	0.673
Nebraska	0.959	0.890	0.245
Nevada	1.002	1.026	1.083
New Hampshire	0.982	1.039	0.462
Northern New Jersey	1.057	1.228	1.116
Rest of New Jersey	1.042	1.126	1.116
New Mexico	0.973	0.890	1.096
Manhattan, New York	1.064	1.298	1.010
New York City Suburbs/Long Island, New York	1.051	1.289	1.235
Poughkeepsie/ Northern New York City Suburbs, New York	1.014	1.077	0.822
Queens, New York	1.032	1.239	1.220
Rest of New York	0.997	0.921	0.425
North Carolina	0.972	0.925	0.634
North Dakota	0.947	0.844	0.387
Ohio	0.993	0.927	1.232
Oklahoma	0.964	0.850	0.627
Portland, Oregon	1.002	1.015	0.472
Rest of Oregon	0.968	0.927	0.472
Metropolitan Philadelphia, Pennsylvania	1.016	1.097	1.617
Rest of Pennsylvania	0.993	0.925	1.081
Puerto Rico	0.904	0.694	0.250
Rhode Island	1.013	1.088	0.996
South Carolina	0.975	0.906	0.446
South Dakota	0.942	0.864	0.420
Tennessee	0.978	0.889	0.608
Austin, Texas	0.992	0.984	0.969
Beaumont, Texas	0.984	0.875	1.346
Brazoria, Texas	1.019	0.922	1.223
Dallas, Texas	1.009	1.001	1.110
Fort Worth, Texas	0.998	0.953	1.110
Galveston, Texas	0.991	0.959	1.223
Houston, Texas	1.016	0.986	1.345
Rest of Texas	0.968	0.879	1.065
Utah	0.977	0.907	1.026
Vermont	0.968	0.983	0.489
Virginia	0.982	0.942	0.657

2010 Geographic Practice Cost Indices (GPCIs) By Medicare Locality, continued			
Medicare Locality	**Work**	**Practice Expense**	**Professional Liability Insurance**
Virgin Islands	0.997	0.978	1.009
Seattle (King County), Washington	1.014	1.085	0.706
Rest of Washington	0.987	0.974	0.693
West Virginia	0.973	0.827	1.353
Wisconsin	0.988	0.921	0.409
Wyoming	0.956	0.842	0.889

Medicare Conversion Factor (CF)

The Medicare CF is a national value that converts the total RVUs into payment amounts for the purpose of paying physicians for services provided. Since January 1, 1998, there has been one Medicare CF, as specified by the Balanced Budget Act of 1997. Anesthesia has a separate CF, but is paid using a different formula. The Medicare CF is updated annually. Medicare conversion factors in past years have been $36.6137 (2000), $38.2581 (2001), $36.1992 (2002), $36.7856 (2003), $37.3374 (2004), $37.8975 (2005), $37.8975 (2006), $37.8975 (2007), $38.0870 (2008), and $36.0666 (2009).

2010 Medicare CF = $36.0666

[NOTE: President Obama signed the Department of Defense Appropriations Act of 2010 which provided for a zero percent (0%) update to the 2010 Medicare Physician Fee Schedule for a two month period, January 1, 2010 through February 28, 2010.]

Additional components of the Medicare RBRVS physician fee schedule factored into the payment structure include the following:

- Medicare Economic Index (MEI): The allocation of RVUs to pools for physician work, PE, and professional liability insurance have been revised to correspond with the MEI. Work is now allocated 52% of the total RVUs, PE is 44%, and PLI is 4%.
- Health Professional Shortage Areas (HPSAs): Incentive payments for physician services provided to patients in HPSAs, which are medically underserved communities, urban and rural locations that have a documented shortage of medical professionals.
- Nonparticipating Physicians: Reduced payments for physicians, called "nonparticipating" physicians, who do not accept Medicare "assignment."

The law sets the payment amount for nonparticipating physicians at 95% of the payment amount for participating physicians (ie, the fee schedule amount).

- Budget Neutrality: Statutory guidelines indicate that revisions to the RVUs for physician services may not alter physician expenditures within the Medicare RBRVS physician fee schedule by more than $20 million from the principal expenditures that would have resulted if the RVU adjustments were never initiated. In 2007 and 2008 the Medicare program applied a separate budget neutrality adjustment factor to the physician work RVUs to ensure Medicare budget neutrality in light of work RVU increases tied to the 2005 Five-Year Review. However, by virtue of the Medicare Improvements for Patients and Providers Act of 2008, starting in 2009 CMS is required to maintain Medicare budget neutrality exclusively via annual adjustments to the Medicare CF.

How to Use the RBRVS

CMS publishes RVUs for *CPT* codes in the Federal Register. To calculate the Medicare physician payment for a service, the RVUs for each of the 3 components of the Medicare RBRVS physician fee schedule are multiplied by their corresponding GPCIs to account for geographic differences in resource costs. The sum of these calculations is then multiplied by a dollar CF. When determining payment, it is important to take into consideration all the mechanisms within the Medicare RBRVS physician fee schedule incorporated into the final payment for physician services. Please note that third-party payers other than Medicare may not use all of the elements of the RBRVS to determine physician payment. For example, they may use their own CF or not factor in the GPCIs.

Example: Level 3 office visit for the evaluation and management of an established patient in Marco Island, Florida ("Rest of Florida" Medicare Locality).

[Remember that in order for the physician to code **99213,** the appropriate history, physical examination, and medical decision-making must be documented.]

The following RVUs, GPCIs, and Medicare CF are based on the information provided by CMS in the *Federal Register* on November 25, 2009.

CPT Code 99213		Location: Marco Island, Florida ("Rest of Florida" Medicare Locality)	
Work RVUs	0.97	Work GPCI	0.973
Non-facility PE RVUs	0.80	PE GPCI	0.939
PLI RVUs	0.05	PLI GPCI	1.724

Method 1 (Non-Geographically Adjusted and Using Non-Medicare CF)

This is an example of a physician payment mechanism in a non-facility setting that takes into consideration the total RVUs from the Medicare RBRVS but excludes all other components of the physician fee schedule. Often the total RVUs are multiplied by a payer-specific CF that is not associated with the Medicare CF.

Step 1
Add together the physician work, non-facility PE, and PLI RVUs to obtain the total non-facility RVUs for the office visit.
- Total non-facility RVUs for *CPT* code **99213** =
- Work RVUs + Non-facility PE RVUs + PLI RVUs
- (0.97) + (0.80) + (0.05) = 1.82

Step 2
Multiply the total Medicare RVUs for *CPT* code **99213** by a non-Medicare, payer-specific primary care CF (which may or may not be different than the 2010 Medicare CF of $36.0666).

For example: Payer-specific primary care CF = $38.00

- Total physician payment for the provision of *CPT* code **99213** by this third-party payer =
- (Total Medicare RVUs) x (Payer CF)
- (1.82) x (38.00) = $69.16

Note: In some cases, payers will not use the Medicare total RVUs for a service in their calculation of physi-

cian payment. Instead, they may apply their own relative value adjustments.

Method 2 (Geographically Adjusted and Using Medicare CF)

This is an example of the Medicare RBRVS physician fee schedule payment in a non-facility setting for *CPT* code **99213** in Marco Island, Florida. The following example assumes that a physician has accepted assignment and is practicing in an area of the country that does not have a shortage of medical professionals.

Step 1
Multiply the physician work, non-facility PE, and PLI RVUs by the appropriate GPCIs; add the figures thus obtained to get the total geographically adjusted RVUs for the office visit.
- Total non-facility RVUs for *CPT* code **99213** (geographically adjusted) =
- (Work RVUs x Work GPCI) + (Non-facility PE RVUs x PE GPCI) + (PLI RVUs x PLI GPCI)
- (0.97 x 0.973) + (0.80 x 0.939) + (0.05 x 1.724)
- (0.94381) + (0.7512) + (0.0862) = 1.78121

Step 2
Multiply the total geographically adjusted RVUs by the Medicare CF to obtain the physician payment for the office visit.
- 2010 Medicare CF = $36.0666
- Total Medicare payment for the provision of *CPT* code **99213** in Marco Island, Florida =
- Total geographically adjusted RVUs for *CPT* code 99213 x 2010 Medicare CF
- (1.78121 x $36.0666 = $64.24)

In this example, a physician practicing in Marco Island, Florida would receive $64.24 for providing the level 3 established patient office visit for a Medicare beneficiary.

To apply Method 2 using your own GPCIs, access the 2010 RBRVS Conversion Spreadsheet at http://www.aap.org/visit/RBRVSConversionSpreadsheet.xls.

A table that provides RVUs for a series of *CPT* codes commonly reported by pediatricians has been included at the end of this document. Please refer to this table to determine Medicare RVUs for other pediatric services and procedures.

Concluding Remarks

In today's rapidly changing health care environment, it is crucial to understand the Medicare RBRVS physician fee schedule. Many third-party payers, including Medicaid programs, private carriers, and managed care organizations are using variations of the Medicare RBRVS to determine physician payment rates. In order for a physician to succeed in the changing marketplace, measurements of the costs involved in providing services will need to be ascertained; these costs include physician income and benefits, PEs, PLI premiums, as well as the frequency of services provided. Once this information is determined and the appropriate RVUs for each service are obtained, a physician will be able to calculate the costs involved in the provision of each service, as well as the average cost per service provided and per member per month estimates.

CPT Code	Work RVUs (wRVUs)	Non-facility (NF) Practice Expense (PE) RVUs	Facility (F) Practice Expense (PE) RVUs	PLI RVUs	Total NF RVUs	Total F RVUs	100% Medicare (NF)	100% Medicare (F)	Medicare Global Period
Office or Other Outpatient Services, New Patient									
99201	0.48	0.57	0.18	0.03	1.08	0.69	$38.95	$24.89	XXX
99202	0.93	0.88	0.35	0.06	1.87	1.34	$67.44	$48.33	XXX
99203	1.42	1.19	0.50	0.10	2.71	2.02	$97.74	$72.85	XXX
99204	2.43	1.61	0.82	0.16	4.20	3.41	$151.48	$122.99	XXX
99205	3.17	1.91	1.05	0.20	5.28	4.42	$190.43	$159.41	XXX
Office or Other Outpatient Services, Established Patient									
99211	0.18	0.34	0.06	0.01	0.53	0.25	$19.12	$9.02	XXX
99212	0.48	0.57	0.17	0.03	1.08	0.68	$38.95	$24.53	XXX
99213	0.97	0.80	0.32	0.05	1.82	1.34	$65.64	$48.33	XXX
99214	1.50	1.15	0.49	0.08	2.73	2.07	$98.46	$74.66	XXX
99215	2.11	1.46	0.70	0.11	3.68	2.92	$132.73	$105.31	XXX
Office or Other Outpatient Consultations*									
99241	0.64	0.66	0.24	0.05	1.35	0.93	$48.69	$33.54	XXX
99242	1.34	1.10	0.51	0.10	2.54	1.95	$91.61	$70.33	XXX
99243	1.88	1.46	0.71	0.13	3.47	2.72	$125.15	$98.10	XXX
99244	3.02	1.96	1.14	0.16	5.14	4.32	$185.38	$155.81	XXX
99245	3.77	2.30	1.38	0.21	6.28	5.36	$226.50	$193.32	XXX
Prolonged Physician Service With Face-to-Face Patient Contact; Outpatient									
99354	1.77	0.74	0.60	0.09	2.60	2.46	$93.77	$88.72	ZZZ
99355	1.77	0.72	0.57	0.09	2.58	2.43	$93.05	$87.64	ZZZ
Preventive Medicine Services, New Patient									
99381[N]	1.19	1.27	0.42	0.06	2.52	1.67	$90.89	$60.23	XXX
99382[N]	1.36	1.33	0.48	0.07	2.76	1.91	$99.54	$68.89	XXX
99383[N]	1.36	1.31	0.48	0.07	2.74	1.91	$98.82	$68.89	XXX
99384[N]	1.53	1.37	0.55	0.08	2.98	2.16	$107.48	$77.90	XXX
99385[N]	1.53	1.37	0.55	0.08	2.98	2.16	$107.48	$77.90	XXX

CPT Code	Work RVUs (wRVUs)	Non-facility (NF) Practice Expense (PE) RVUs	Facility (F) Practice Expense (PE) RVUs	PLI RVUs	Total NF RVUs	Total F RVUs	100% Medicare (NF)	100% Medicare (F)	Medicare Global Period
Preventive Medicine Services, Established Patient									
99391[N]	1.02	1.05	0.36	0.05	2.12	1.43	$76.46	$51.58	XXX
99392[N]	1.19	1.11	0.42	0.06	2.36	1.67	$85.12	$60.23	XXX
99393[N]	1.19	1.10	0.42	0.06	2.35	1.67	$84.76	$60.23	XXX
99394[N]	1.36	1.16	0.48	0.07	2.59	1.91	$93.41	$68.89	XXX
99395[N]	1.36	1.17	0.48	0.07	2.60	1.91	$93.77	$68.89	XXX
H1N1 Influenza Immunization Administration									
90470[I]	0.20	0.42	0.42	0.01	0.63	0.63	$22.72	$22.72	XXX
Immunization Administration									
90471	0.17	0.41	N/A	0.01	0.59	N/A	$21.28	N/A	XXX
90472	0.15	0.14	0.06	0.01	0.30	0.22	$10.82	$7.93	ZZZ
90473[R]	0.17	0.22	0.05	0.01	0.40	0.23	$14.43	$8.30	XXX
90474[R]	0.15	0.10	0.05	0.01	0.26	0.21	$9.38	$7.57	ZZZ
Immunization Administration Under Age 8 With Physician Counseling									
90465	0.17	0.41	N/A	0.01	0.59	N/A	$21.28	N/A	XXX
90466	0.15	0.14	0.06	0.01	0.30	0.22	$10.82	$7.93	ZZZ
90467[R]	0.17	0.22	0.09	0.01	0.40	0.27	$14.43	$9.74	XXX
90468[R]	0.15	0.13	0.05	0.01	0.29	0.21	$10.46	$7.57	ZZZ
Hydration, Therapeutic, Prophylactic, and Diagnostic Injections and Infusions and Chemotherapy and Other Highly Complex Drug or Highly Complex Biologic Agent Administration									
96360	0.17	1.30	N/A	0.02	1.49	N/A	$53.74	N/A	XXX
96361	0.09	0.32	N/A	0.01	0.42	N/A	$15.15	N/A	ZZZ
96365	0.21	1.61	N/A	0.03	1.85	N/A	$66.72	N/A	XXX
96366	0.18	0.38	N/A	0.01	0.57	N/A	$20.56	N/A	ZZZ
96367	0.19	0.70	N/A	0.01	0.90	N/A	$32.46	N/A	ZZZ
96368	0.17	0.35	N/A	0.01	0.53	N/A	$19.12	N/A	ZZZ
96372	0.17	0.41	N/A	0.01	0.59	N/A	$21.28	N/A	XXX
96373	0.17	0.32	N/A	0.01	0.50	N/A	$18.03	N/A	XXX
96374	0.18	1.26	N/A	0.02	1.46	N/A	$52.66	N/A	XXX
96375	0.10	0.50	N/A	0.01	0.61	N/A	$22.00	N/A	ZZZ
Vision and Hearing Screening									
99173[N]	0.00	0.06	N/A	0.01	0.07	N/A	$2.52	N/A	XXX
99174[N]	0.00	0.70	N/A	0.01	0.71	N/A	$25.61	N/A	XXX
92551[N]	0.00	0.28	N/A	0.01	0.29	N/A	$10.46	N/A	XXX
92552	0.00	0.59	N/A	0.01	0.60	N/A	$21.64	N/A	XXX
Developmental Testing									
96110	0.00	0.19	N/A	0.01	0.20	N/A	$7.21	N/A	XXX
96111	2.60	0.89	0.79	0.12	3.61	3.51	$130.20	$126.59	XXX
Medication Management									
90862	0.95	0.58	0.28	0.03	1.56	1.26	$56.26	$45.44	XXX

CPT Code	Work RVUs (wRVUs)	Non-facility (NF) Practice Expense (PE) RVUs	Facility (F) Practice Expense (PE) RVUs	PLI RVUs	Total NF RVUs	Total F RVUs	100% Medicare (NF)	100% Medicare (F)	Medicare Global Period
Care Plan Oversight									
99339[B]	1.25	0.76	N/A	0.06	2.07	N/A	$74.66	N/A	XXX
99340[B]	1.80	1.02	N/A	0.09	2.91	N/A	$104.95	N/A	XXX
Physician Telephone and Online E/M Services									
99441[N]	0.25	0.12	0.08	0.01	0.38	0.34	$13.71	$12.26	XXX
99442[N]	0.50	0.21	0.18	0.03	0.74	0.71	$26.69	$25.61	XXX
99443[N]	0.75	0.29	0.26	0.04	1.08	1.05	$38.95	$37.87	XXX
99444[N]	0.00	0.00	0.00	0.00	0.00	0.00	$0.00	$0.00	XXX
Physician Medical Team Conference									
99367[B]	1.10	N/A	0.38	0.06	N/A	1.54	N/A	$55.54	XXX
Newborn Care Services									
99460	1.17	N/A	0.37	0.06	N/A	1.60	N/A	$57.71	XXX
99461	1.26	1.08	0.44	0.06	2.40	1.76	$86.56	$63.48	XXX
99462	0.62	N/A	0.20	0.03	N/A	0.85	N/A	$30.66	XXX
99463	1.50	N/A	0.58	0.08	N/A	2.16	N/A	$77.90	XXX
99464	1.50	N/A	0.43	0.08	N/A	2.01	N/A	$72.49	XXX
99465	2.93	N/A	1.01	0.15	N/A	4.09	N/A	$147.51	XXX
Initial Hospital Care									
99221	1.89	N/A	0.59	0.13	N/A	2.61	N/A	$94.13	XXX
99222	2.57	N/A	0.81	0.15	N/A	3.53	N/A	$127.32	XXX
99223	3.79	N/A	1.19	0.20	N/A	5.18	N/A	$186.82	XXX
Subsequent Hospital Care									
99231	0.76	N/A	0.26	0.04	N/A	1.06	N/A	$38.23	XXX
99232	1.39	N/A	0.45	0.07	N/A	1.91	N/A	$68.89	XXX
99233	2.00	N/A	0.64	0.10	N/A	2.74	N/A	$98.82	XXX
Discharge Day Management									
99238	1.28	N/A	0.54	0.06	N/A	1.88	N/A	$67.81	XXX
99239	1.90	N/A	0.76	0.08	N/A	2.74	N/A	$98.82	XXX
Observation Care									
99217	1.28	N/A	0.54	0.06	N/A	1.88	N/A	$67.81	XXX
99218	1.28	N/A	0.42	0.07	N/A	1.77	N/A	$63.84	XXX
99219	2.14	N/A	0.69	0.10	N/A	2.93	N/A	$105.68	XXX
99220	2.99	N/A	0.97	0.14	N/A	4.10	N/A	$147.87	XXX
Prolonged Physician Service With Face-to-Face Patient Contact; Inpatient									
99356	1.71	N/A	0.59	0.08	N/A	2.38	N/A	$85.84	ZZZ
99357	1.71	N/A	0.59	0.08	N/A	2.38	N/A	$85.84	ZZZ
Physician Standby Services									
99360X	1.20	N/A	0.42	0.06	N/A	1.68	N/A	$60.59	XXX

CPT Code	Work RVUs (wRVUs)	Non-facility (NF) Practice Expense (PE) RVUs	Facility (F) Practice Expense (PE) RVUs	PLI RVUs	Total NF RVUs	Total F RVUs	100% Medicare (NF)	100% Medicare (F)	Medicare Global Period
Critical Care Services									
99291	4.50	2.41	1.24	0.25	7.16	5.99	$258.24	$216.04	**XXX**
99292	2.25	0.86	0.62	0.12	3.23	2.99	$116.50	$107.84	**ZZZ**
Pediatric Critical Care Patient Transport									
99466	4.79	N/A	1.52	0.24	N/A	6.55	N/A	$236.24	**XXX**
99467	2.40	N/A	0.77	0.12	N/A	3.29	N/A	$118.66	**ZZZ**
Inpatient Pediatric and Neonatal Critical Care									
99468	18.46	N/A	5.22	0.93	N/A	24.61	N/A	$887.60	**XXX**
99469	7.99	N/A	2.36	0.40	N/A	10.75	N/A	$387.72	**XXX**
99471	15.98	N/A	4.76	0.80	N/A	21.54	N/A	$776.87	**XXX**
99472	7.99	N/A	2.39	0.40	N/A	10.78	N/A	$388.80	**XXX**
99475	11.25	3.03	3.03	0.56	14.84	14.84	$535.23	$535.23	**XXX**
99476	6.75	1.82	1.82	0.34	8.91	8.91	$321.35	$321.35	**XXX**
Initial and Continuing Intensive Care Services									
99477	7.00	N/A	2.15	0.28	N/A	9.43	N/A	$340.11	**XXX**
99478	2.75	N/A	0.97	0.14	N/A	3.86	N/A	$139.22	**XXX**
99479	2.50	N/A	0.79	0.13	N/A	3.42	N/A	$123.35	**XXX**
99480	2.40	N/A	0.76	0.12	N/A	3.28	N/A	$118.30	**XXX**
Moderate (Conscious) Sedation Provided by the Same Physician Performing the Diagnostic or Therapeutic Service									
99143[c]	0.00	0.00	0.00	0.00	0.00	0.00	$0.00	$0.00	**XXX**
99144[c]	0.00	0.00	0.00	0.00	0.00	0.00	$0.00	$0.00	**XXX**
99145[c]	0.00	0.00	0.00	0.00	0.00	0.00	$0.00	$0.00	**ZZZ**
Moderate (Conscious) Sedation Provided by a Physician Other Than the Health Care Professional Performing the Diagnostic or Therapeutic Service									
99148[c]	0.00	0.00	0.00	0.00	0.00	0.00	$0.00	$0.00	**XXX**
99149[c]	0.00	0.00	0.00	0.00	0.00	0.00	$0.00	$0.00	**XXX**
99150[c]	0.00	0.00	0.00	0.00	0.00	0.00	$0.00	$0.00	**ZZZ**
After Hours and Emergency Services									
99050[B]	0.00	0.00	0.00	0.00	0.00	0.00	$0.00	$0.00	**XXX**
99051[B]	0.00	0.00	0.00	0.00	0.00	0.00	$0.00	$0.00	**XXX**
99058[B]	0.00	0.00	0.00	0.00	0.00	0.00	$0.00	$0.00	**XXX**
Allergen Immunotherapy									
95115	0.00	0.26	N/A	0.01	0.27	N/A	$9.74	N/A	**XXX**
95117	0.00	0.32	N/A	0.01	0.33	N/A	$11.90	N/A	**XXX**
Orthopedic Procedures									
23500	2.21	2.84	2.84	0.29	5.34	5.34	$192.60	$192.60	**090**
24640	1.25	1.68	0.85	0.15	3.08	2.25	$111.09	$81.15	**010**
25600	2.78	3.99	3.34	0.36	7.13	6.48	$257.15	$233.71	**090**

CPT Code	Work RVUs (wRVUs)	Non-facility (NF) Practice Expense (PE) RVUs	Facility (F) Practice Expense (PE) RVUs	PLI RVUs	Total NF RVUs	Total F RVUs	100% Medicare (NF)	100% Medicare (F)	Medicare Global Period
Otolaryngologic Procedures									
69200	0.77	2.27	0.64	0.08	3.12	1.49	$112.53	$53.74	000
69210	0.61	0.63	0.21	0.06	1.30	0.88	$46.89	$31.74	000
69401	0.63	1.46	0.62	0.06	2.15	1.31	$77.54	$47.25	000
Pulmonary Procedures									
94640	0.00	0.37	N/A	0.01	0.38	N/A	$13.71	N/A	XXX
94664	0.00	0.38	N/A	0.01	0.39	N/A	$14.07	N/A	XXX
Radiologic Procedures									
76885	0.74	2.93	N/A	0.04	3.71	N/A	$133.81	N/A	XXX
76886	0.62	2.20	N/A	0.02	2.84	N/A	$102.43	N/A	XXX
Urologic Procedures									
51701	0.50	1.11	0.24	0.04	1.65	0.78	$59.51	$28.13	000
54150	1.90	2.59	0.74	0.16	4.65	2.80	$167.71	$100.99	000
54160	2.53	3.76	1.43	0.18	6.47	4.14	$233.35	$149.32	010
54161	3.32	N/A	2.07	0.24	N/A	5.63	N/A	$203.05	010
54162	3.32	4.01	2.08	0.24	7.57	5.64	$273.02	$203.42	010
Dermatologic Procedures									
10060	1.22	1.50	1.10	0.09	2.81	2.41	$101.35	$86.92	010
10120	1.25	2.08	1.01	0.12	3.45	2.38	$124.43	$85.84	010
17110	0.70	2.02	1.01	0.06	2.78	1.77	$100.27	$63.84	010
17111	0.97	2.26	1.15	0.09	3.32	2.21	$119.74	$79.71	010
17250	0.50	1.34	0.39	0.05	1.89	0.94	$68.17	$33.90	000
Health and Behavior Assessment/Intervention									
96150	0.50	0.11	0.10	0.01	0.62	0.61	$22.36	$22.00	XXX
96151	0.48	0.11	0.10	0.01	0.60	0.59	$21.64	$21.28	XXX
96152	0.46	0.10	0.09	0.01	0.57	0.56	$20.56	$20.20	XXX
96153	0.10	0.03	0.02	0.01	0.14	0.13	$5.05	$4.69	XXX
96154	0.45	0.10	0.09	0.01	0.56	0.55	$20.20	$19.84	XXX
96155	0.44	0.16	0.16	0.02	0.62	0.62	$22.36	$22.36	XXX
Medical Nutrition Therapy									
97802	0.53	0.26	0.22	0.02	0.81	0.77	$29.21	$27.77	XXX
97803	0.45	0.24	0.19	0.02	0.71	0.66	$25.61	$23.80	XXX
97804	0.25	0.10	0.10	0.01	0.36	0.36	$12.98	$12.98	XXX
Education and Training for Patient Self-Management									
98960[B]	0.00	0.65	N/A	0.01	0.66	N/A	$23.80	N/A	XXX
98961[B]	0.00	0.31	N/A	0.01	0.32	N/A	$11.54	N/A	XXX
98962[B]	0.00	0.23	N/A	0.01	0.24	N/A	$8.66	N/A	XXX

CPT Code	Work RVUs (wRVUs)	Non-facility (NF) Practice Expense (PE) RVUs	Facility (F) Practice Expense (PE) RVUs	PLI RVUs	Total NF RVUs	Total F RVUs	100% Medicare (NF)	100% Medicare (F)	Medicare Global Period
Counseling Risk Factor Reduction and Behavior Change Intervention									
99401[N]	0.48	0.48	0.17	0.02	0.98	0.67	$35.35	$24.16	**XXX**
99402[N]	0.98	0.67	0.35	0.05	1.70	1.38	$61.31	$49.77	**XXX**
99403[N]	1.46	0.85	0.52	0.07	2.38	2.05	$85.84	$73.94	**XXX**
99404[N]	1.95	1.03	0.70	0.10	3.08	2.75	$111.09	$99.18	**XXX**
99406	0.24	0.12	0.08	0.01	0.37	0.33	$13.34	$11.90	**XXX**
99407	0.50	0.19	0.16	0.02	0.71	0.68	$25.61	$24.53	**XXX**
99408[N]	0.65	0.27	0.23	0.03	0.95	0.91	$34.26	$32.82	**XXX**
99409[N]	1.30	0.50	0.46	0.07	1.87	1.83	$67.44	$66.00	**XXX**

Note: Information for table extracted from the *Federal Register,* November 25, 2009

* While payment for consultations (including *CPT* codes **99241-99245**) was eliminated in the Medicare program effective January 1, 2010, please note:
   • Consultation codes are <u>not</u> being deleted from *CPT* nomenclature
   • Consultation codes will remain on the RBRVS fee schedule with their established values
   • It is a *Medicare payment policy* and may not be adopted by other payers. However, if non-Medicare payers *do* choose to adopt this policy, it is imperative that they also make the budgetary accommodations as have been done in the Medicare program. The Medicare funds saved in not paying for consultations have been used to increase the 2010 RBRVS relative value units for other evaluation and management (E/M) codes, including the new and established office visit codes **(99201-99215)** and the initial hospital care codes **(99221-99223).** Non-Medicare payers that follow the Medicare consultation policy must also utilize the higher RVUs for these non-consultation E/M codes.

The Academy is currently working with non-Medicare payers to discourage adoption of the Medicare consultation policy. For more information, please see the AAP Position on Medicare Consultation Policy at http://www.aap.org/moc/reimburse/codingrbrvsresources.htm.

Key:
Work RVUs = Physician work RVUs
Non-facility PE RVUs = PE RVUs for services provided in a non-facility (eg, physician's office) setting
Facility PE RVUs = PE RVUs for services provided in a facility (eg, hospital) setting
PLI RVUs = Professional liability insurance RVUs
Total non-facility RVUs = Sum of the work, non-facility PE, and PLI RVUs
Total facility RVUs = Sum of the work, facility PE, and PLI RVUs
100% Medicare = Non-geographically adjusted Medicare payment (either non-facility (NF) or facility (F))
Medicare global period = Medicare global periods define the post-operative period for procedures and affect how follow-up services are reported for a given *CPT* code

[B] =	Bundled Medicare service; if RVUs are shown, they are not used for Medicare payment
[C] =	Medicare carrier-priced service; individual payer payment policies apply
[I] =	Not valid for Medicare purposes; Medicare uses another code for the reporting of these services
[N] =	Non-covered Medicare service; if RVUs are shown, they are not used for Medicare payment
[R] =	Restricted coverage; special coverage instructions apply; if the service is covered and no RVUs are shown, it is carrier-priced
[X] =	Medicare statutory exclusion; if RVUs are shown, they are not used for Medicare payment

Note: AAP works with the RUC and CMS to have values assigned and published for all CPT codes

For further information, please contact the Division of Health Care Finance and Quality Improvement at dhcfqi@aap.org. For updated information, please refer to the AAP Pediatric Coding Newsletter *(coding.aap.org) and* Practice Management Online *(practice.aap.org).*

Developed by the Committee on Coding and Nomenclature, with contributions by Linda Walsh and Becky Dolan.

Important note: Given the relative frequency with which code and valuation revisions occur, articles related to coding may not reflect the most current information available. Please check the online version of this article at http://practice.aap.org/content.aspx?aid=2310 and the *AAP Pediatric Coding Newsletter* at http://coding.aap.org for updated guidance. This version was created on January 4, 2010.

Because the American Academy of Pediatrics (AAP) is not able to verify the accuracy of the facts relating to a patient encounter, we cannot be held responsible for any coding decisions that you make based on the guidance you receive from the AAP. It is your responsibility to only code for what you do during a patient encounter.

Top 10 Underutilized *CPT* Codes in Pediatrics

1. **99214** and **99215** (established patient office or other outpatient services) represent only 20% and 5%, respectively, of all evaluation and management codes submitted in pediatric claims. If you meet the requirements set forth by *Current Procedural Terminology (CPT®)* and have the appropriate documentation, you should bill for what you do, even if that is a fourth- or fifth-level visit.

2. **99241, 99242, 99243, 99244,** and **99245** (office or other outpatient consultations) are underused in pediatrics. Did you know that these codes would be appropriate to use for a preoperative visit? Just make sure that you follow up with the requesting physician (ie, the surgeon) with a written report. Many times, this requirement can be fulfilled with the completion of a hospital's standard preoperative form.

3. Are you using modifier **25** when a patient presents with a significant, separate problem or illness that is found during the course of a preventive medicine service visit? If you perform 2 significant, separately identifiable evaluation and management (E/M) services during the course of a single visit, you should attach modifier **25** to the office or other outpatient service code and list that in addition to the preventive medicine service code. Make sure to keep your office notes separate (either on a separate sheet of paper or separated by a line on a single sheet of paper) and to link the appropriate *International Classification of Diseases, Ninth Revision, Clinical Modification (ICD-9-CM)* code (diagnosis) to each visit. For example, the preventive medicine service may be linked to **V20.2** (routine infant or child health check), while the office or other outpatient service may be linked to **380.12** (acute swimmers' ear).

4. Certain traumas may require you to perform E/M, as well as additional procedures. Are you getting credit for your work? An example is when a patient presents as a victim of suspected child abuse. You are required to perform a complete E/M service in addition to an anogenital exam with colposcopic magnification (**99170**). Therefore, you should report both the E/M service and the colposcopy, making sure that you append modifier **25** to the E/M code to red flag the fact that you performed a significant, separately identifiable E/M service in addition to the colposcopy during a single visit.

5. What if a patient is rushed to your office with severe trauma? Do you see that patient right away, essentially on a walk-in basis, and make all other patients wait? If you do, you should be billing for "service(s) provided on an emergency basis in the office, which disrupts other scheduled office services" (**99058**) in addition to the E/M code.

6. What if a patient comes to your office after your regularly scheduled office hours? You should make sure that you are billing for **99050** (services provided in the office at times other than regularly scheduled office hours, or days when the office is normally closed) *in addition* to the E/M code.

7. Do you have regularly scheduled office hours for Sundays? Did you know that you can charge for it? **99051** (service[s] provided in the office during regularly scheduled evening, weekend, or holiday office hours, in addition to basic service) can be reported *in addition* to the E/M code.

8. Nursemaids' elbow is a common occurrence in the pediatric population. Do you know that you can code for the treatment of it? Additionally, code **24640** (closed treatment of radial head subluxation in child, nursemaid elbow, with manipulation) may be reported *in addition* to an E/M code if a significant, separately identifiable E/M service is provided. If this is the case, attach the modifier **57** (decision for surgery) or the modifier **25** (significant, separately identifiable E/M service) to the associated E/M code. Furthermore, you should note that Medicare assigns code **24640** a 10-day global period. This means that if a patient returns for follow-up within 10 days of the initial visit and their carrier follows Medicare global periods, you should not charge them for the portion of the visit that deals with the elbow recheck.

9. Do you have a patient who receives home health care? You can bill for care plan oversight! Care plan oversight codes (**99339** and **99340**) are reported separately from codes for office or other outpatient, hospital, home, nursing facility, or domiciliary services. **99339** (individual physician

supervision of patient [patient not present] requiring complex and multidisciplinary case modalities involving regular physician development and/or revision to care plans, review of subsequent reports of patient status, review of laboratory and other studies, communication [including telephone calls] with other health care professionals involved in the patient's care, integration of new information into the medical treatment plan and/or adjustment of medical therapy, within a calendar month; 15–29 minutes) and **99340** (30 minutes or more) should be billed once per month, based on the total amount of time spent on the aforementioned services. It might be a good idea to develop a permanent log sheet for the patient's chart to keep track of the total time spent on the case; a few minutes here and there can really add up!

10. Do you spend a lot of time on the phone or via e-mail communicating with your patients? While the track record of payment for non–face-to-face services is somewhat sketchy, it is still a good idea to bill for what you do. Physician case management is a process whereby a physician is responsible for direct care of a patient and for coordinating and controlling access to or initiating and/or supervising other health care services needed by the patient. Whether you communicate with the patient via phone **(99441–99443)** or e-mail **(99444),** you are providing care for the patient and should bill for your services.

Important note: Given the relative frequency with which code and valuation revisions occur, articles related to coding may not reflect the most current information available. Please check the online version of this article at http://practice.aap.org/content.aspx?aid=1904 and the *AAP Pediatric Coding Newsletter* at http://coding.aap.org for updated guidance.

Because the American Academy of Pediatrics (AAP) is not able to verify the accuracy of the facts relating to a patient encounter, we cannot be held responsible for any coding decisions that you make based on the guidance you receive from the AAP. It is your responsibility to only code for what you do during a patient encounter.

Anatomy of a New Code: The *CPT* and RUC Survey Processes

The *CPT* Process: So You Want a New Code

Best Reasons for New Codes

1. New clinical service or technical procedure not found in the current version of *Current Procedural Terminology (CPT®)* and not sufficiently represented or reported with existing *CPT* codes
2. Change of an existing service or procedure when the existing *CPT* code no longer adequately describes the service or the typical patient (or the associated physician work or practice expense)
3. When the *CPT* code generally used for a service or procedure does not represent the technical difficulty or physician work when dealing with a specific population (eg, neonates)

How to Start: The AAP CPT *Code Development Process*

1. Define the service or procedure and the "typical patient" as clearly as possible. Consult with other American Academy of Pediatrics (AAP) sections or specialties that may also have an interest in the idea for a new code or who may be affected by the proposed change to gather support. Early in the process, review the American Medical Association (AMA) *CPT* code application to note the information you will need to find when you discuss your idea with others. A copy of the application is available at http://www.ama-assn.org/ama/pub/category/3866.html or from AAP staff (800/433-9016, ext 7931).
2. Establish the relative prevalence or frequency of the proposed procedure or service. Preferably, there should be some broad institutional experience and geographic distribution. If this is a cutting-edge procedure performed primarily at one facility, it is not likely to find its way into *CPT*. Furthermore, if the code proposal is accepted by *CPT*, we will be required to survey at least 30 physicians who are familiar with the procedure/service. *If we are unable to identify a sufficient number of qualified physicians who are willing to complete the AMA/Specialty Society Relative Value Scale Update Committee (RUC) survey, the Committee on Coding and Nomenclature (COCN) may likely choose not to proceed with the proposal until a critical mass of those able to be surveyed has been identified.*

3. Develop a written "clinical vignette" describing the typical patient and the service. Developing an effective vignette is vitally important because this vignette will also be used during the RUC process to establish physician work and practice expense. References from the literature may prove to be helpful in establishing the frequency, scope, and relative difficulty (eg, complications) of the procedure.
4. Obtain input from your colleagues (eg, fellow AAP section members, adult specialty society) throughout this process. The AAP COCN staff and the COCN member who serves as a liaison to your AAP section are available to assist in the development and refinement of the vignette and the completion of the *CPT* proposal application.
5. Where members of other professional societies also provide the service to the typical patient, we must consider whether those groups will support this application, and actively seek their assent before we submit the proposal to the AMA. *In the case of pediatric subspecialty services, the support of the associated adult specialty society is frequently essential if there is to be a successful application. While the AAP will provide support in contacting other professional societies and requesting their support, it is our experience that this support is best obtained by members of the relevant AAP section who may have professional relationships within that adult specialty society.*
6. If the request for a new code is being driven by special technical considerations related to a specific population (and altered physician work effort for that population), the vignette must be able to establish a meaningful and objective difference (anatomic, physiologic, etc) from the general population. It has been our experience in efforts to establish "pediatric codes," or age distinctions in generic codes, that we must be prepared to provide clear evidence for the difference between the 2 groups (eg, infants vs adults). Medical literature can also be helpful in providing the evidence for this distinction.

7. The completed vignette and *CPT* application should be submitted to COCN for review. The COCN will determine whether the vignette and application provide a reasonably compelling case for the proposed code, and whether it would be feasible to move forward with the application. The COCN will also edit and further refine the proposal (if needed) in preparation for submission to the AMA. It should be noted that if COCN does not support submission of the proposal, the author(s) will not be able to submit the proposal as representatives of the AAP. Rather, they will be limited to submitting the proposal as individuals.

The AMA CPT Process

1. Once complete, the application is submitted by COCN to AMA *CPT* staff for their review in preparation for consideration by the *CPT* Editorial Panel (Figure 1), a 16-member panel of physicians from various specialties, representatives from private payers, and the Centers for Medicare & Medicaid Services (CMS).

2. On the completion of AMA staff review, the proposal is sent to all AMA member medical specialty societies for their review and comment in advance of the *CPT* Editorial Panel meeting. Because all specialty societies are not represented on the *CPT* Editorial Panel, this provides each society with an opportunity to offer its support (or disapproval) and comment on the proposal. The comments of the specialty society advisors are shared with the sponsoring society and the *CPT* Editorial Panel.

3. The AAP *CPT* advisor then formally presents the proposal to the panel at a quarterly *CPT* Editorial Panel meeting. In certain circumstances, we may require the presence of a knowledgeable member of the authoring section to assist in the presentation of the proposal to the *CPT* Editorial Panel.

4. The vote of the panel generally results in 1 of the following 3 outcomes: (a) approval of the proposal, (b) rejection of the proposal, or (c) postponement of the proposal until a future meeting. The third outcome may allow for further refinement of the proposal and negotiation of support from other societies. The panel is also empowered to make editorial changes in the proposed descriptor of an accepted code.

5. Approved codes are then referred to the RUC for determination of the new *CPT* code's value.

The RUC Process: Establishing the Value of New CPT Codes

1. Your new *CPT* code is next referred to the RUC for the assignment of a relative value, based on physician work and practice expense (Figure 2). The RUC is larger than the *CPT* Editorial Panel, representing many specialty societies including the AAP, nonphysician providers, hospitals, payers, and CMS.

2. Like *CPT*, prior to presentation at the RUC, all AMA member medical societies are notified of the new or modified code. Societies are given the option to participate in the survey to determine the physician work and practice expense related to the code, or the opportunity to comment on the survey results prior to the RUC meeting.

3. The sponsoring society (eg, the AAP) and all other interested societies then conduct a survey of the new code using the same clinical vignette developed for the *CPT* proposal. Because the Resource-Based Relative Value Scale (RBRVS) contains separate components of physician and practice expense, physicians are asked to complete a survey that measures both at the practice level. The RUC requires a minimum of 30 respondents for the survey results to be accepted as credible. (Note: While a survey is required to be completed for the physician work component, it is not required for the direct practice expense component. Rather, an expert panel consensus is an acceptable alternative means of developing direct practice expense recommendations.)

4. The COCN then analyzes the completed survey data and establishes relative value unit (RVU) recommendations for physician work and direct inputs for practice expense. The AAP RUC advisor then presents the survey results and the final AAP recommendations to the RUC. In certain circumstances, we may require the presence of a knowledgeable member of the involved section to assist in the presentation of the proposal and survey results to the RUC.

5. The RUC deliberates on the physician work RVU and practice expense recommendations from the survey. The RUC may choose to (a) approve the proposed values, (b) reject the proposed values, or (c) send the issue to a facilitation committee where a different (usually lower) value is negotiated. If the RUC is unable to approve or negotiate

Figure 1. The CPT Process

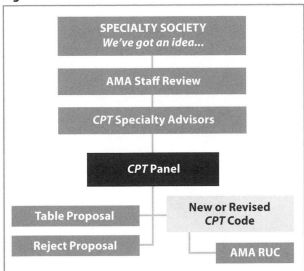

Current Procedural Terminology (CPT) © 2003 American Medical Association. All Rights Reserved.

Figure 2. The RUC Process

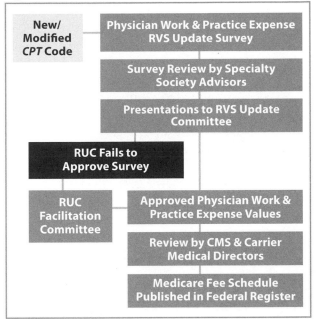

Current Procedural Terminology (CPT) © 2003 American Medical Association. All Rights Reserved.

an acceptable value for the physician work and/or practice expense, it may choose to (a) request that the sponsoring society conduct another survey and re-present at a future meeting, (b) refer the code back to *CPT* for further refinement, or (c) refer the code to CMS for valuation.

6. The RUC-approved values for physician work are then referred to CMS for its consideration. In general, more than 90% of RUC-approved values are accepted by CMS. The CMS also establishes final values for the practice expense components approved by the RUC, as well as a value for the professional liability insurance (malpractice) expense component.

7. The CMS-approved values are then published as part of the final rule in the *Federal Register*. Pending public comment, the values subsequently become part of the RBRVS Medicare physician fee schedule.

Completing a RUC Survey: Your Survival Guide

If you are selected to complete a survey—feel honored! You have the opportunity to properly value an important pediatric service, an opportunity that may never happen again. The information provided below will be helpful in understanding the survey process.

Physician Work

Physician work includes the following elements:
a. Time it takes to perform the service
b. Mental effort and judgment
c. Technical skill and physical effort
d. Psychological stress associated with risk of adverse outcome

1. Physician work does **not** include those services provided by support staff (eg, registered nurse, licensed practical nurse, billing staff, technicians, or receptionists).

2. Physician work is valued by examining the services given to the patient during 3 distinct periods—the preservice period (prior to the face-to-face contact), the intra-service period (the face-to-face time or the actual procedure), and the post-service period (services provided after the patient contact including the completion of records and even a time for a follow-up call to the patient).

3. A list of *CPT* reference codes is then compared with the service being surveyed, allowing a comparison of time and the estimation of complexity/intensity on a 1 to 5 scale. At least some of the codes on this reference list will be familiar to the surveyed physician and, therefore, should allow a good comparison. One considers the following components of physician work:

a. Mental effort and judgment, which relates to the
   1. Number of possible diagnoses and/or number of management options to be considered
   2. Amount or complexity of medical records, diagnostic tests, and/or other information that must be reviewed
   3. Urgency of medical decision-making
b. Technical skill and physical effort, which includes the
   1. Technical skill required
   2. Physical effort required
c. Psychological stress, which encompasses
   1. The risk of significant complications, morbidity, and/or mortality
   2. How the outcome depends on the skill and judgment of the physician
   3. The estimated risk of a malpractice suit with a poor outcome
   4. To complete the physician work portion, one then estimates the new code's work RVU and provides an estimate of the number of times the procedure has been performed by the surveyor. Finally, the surveyor is asked to comment whether the vignette used for the survey is "typical" for the service.

Direct Practice Expense

Certain practice expenses are deemed "direct" by CMS, and survey data are solicited for this component as well. Direct practice expense includes clinical staff time, medical supplies, and medical equipment used in performing the patient service. Administrative staff expenses and other "indirect" practice expenses are accounted for through specialty-specific hourly expenses as determined by CMS.

1. The site of service is defined as the setting where the main component of the service is provided. Services can be provided in
   a. In-office settings: Includes physician offices, freestanding imaging centers, independent pathology laboratories.
   b. Out-of-office settings: Includes all other settings (hospitals, ambulatory surgical centers, nursing homes, community mental health centers, state or local public health centers, rural health clinics, etc). The RUC typically does not recognize the presence of practice expense in out-of-office settings.

2. Clinical staff time. This is the time spent by health care professional clinical staff who are employed/contracted by the physician to provide clinical activities, and who cannot bill separately. These clinical activities include reviewing and/or obtaining a history, room/equipment preparation, patient examination, charting, review of laboratories, patient education, room/equipment cleaning, follow-up phone calls.
   a. Administrative activities performed by office staff are not included (eg, scheduling, registration, pre-certification, report to referring physician, billing and collection, etc).
   b. Preservice work is included, including work performed days before the procedure such as a preoperative workup.
      • Does not include consult evaluation where decision to provide procedure was made or other distinct evaluation and management (E/M) services.
   c. Intra-service refers to work related to the actual time the service occurs.
   d. Post-service refers to clinical staff efforts related to post-procedure work during global period.
      • Does not include unrelated E/M services during the postoperative period or other unrelated services provided by the same physician.

3. Medical equipment and supplies include
   a. Expendable or disposable medical supplies such as examination table paper, gloves, gown, etc
   b. Durable medical equipment
   c. Procedure-specific equipment (eg, electrocardiogram machine, colposcope, fiberoptic light)
   d. Medical equipment overhead (eg, stethoscope, blood pressure monitor) used in virtually all services and valued less than $500
   e. Does not include clinical supplies that can be billed for separately (eg, vaccines) or administrative or office supplies

To complete this section of the survey, the respondent is asked to identify a *CPT* code that uses similar resources as the surveyed code.

For further information regarding the *CPT* and RUC processes, please contact the Division of Health Care Finance and Practice at 800/433-9016, ext 7931.

Developed by Steven E. Krug, MD, FAAP, member of the COCN.

Practice Finance Checklist

This tool provides a basic overview of tips to ensure the financial health of your practice.

On a Daily Basis

- Compare the patient visits with payments received.
- Review the missing report to catch any patients who missed appointments.
- Review the payments and charges totaled during the midday and end of day.
- Compare the end-of-day strep and flu tests with actual charges to ensure that each test used was charged.
- Compare the clinical documentation of vaccines with the billing to ensure that all vaccines that were used were also charged.
- Audit the charge slips and the health record to ensure all charges are captured and billed correctly. This can also be conducted on a weekly basis.

On a Monthly Basis

- Review charges, payments, and adjusters per payer (by insurance company, personal, collections, medical record charges). Be sure that the payments are correct according to the contracts.
- Compare payments of common *Current Procedural Terminology* codes with similar payments from the previous month. This can ensure that certain codes are paid at the same rate or have not been bundled, deleted, or decreased.
- Compare total monthly charges and payments with the same month from the previous year.
- Compare year-to-date charges with payments.
- Review monthly expenses.
- Payer mix (by insurance company and personal)
  - Percent of charges
  - Relative value percent
  - Percent of deposit
- Review the evaluation and management coding curve by provider.
- Review the trends by month for the past year.
- Evaluate the number of newborns, transfers, and inpatients.
- Review results of the annual budget monthly against budget for variances and possible problem areas.
- Have practice accountant review the finances.

On a Quarterly Basis

- Review budget by line item and visits, charges, receipts, productivity, and payer mix.
- Have practice accountant review the finances.

On an Annual Basis

- Review and renegotiate payer contracts.
- Review each revenue and expense item within the chart of accounts.
- Review contracts for major line item costs such as rent, telephone, and insurance (eg, health, liability, property).
- Have practice accountant review the finances.

Tips

- Consider using a credit card with rewards for all bills. Some reward cards provide cash back. This can save money, especially if you use them to purchase vaccines. This is also a cost-effective way to manage payables.
- Consider working with your hospital systems purchasing contract to order medical and laboratory supplies.
- Consider using a group purchasing organization for vaccine purchase and supplies. Visit http://practice.aap.org/content.aspx?aid=2381 for additional information.
- Request that various medical suppliers bid on a package of the most frequently used supplies.
- Do as much as possible electronically, including billing, claims, remittance postings, and bill paying.
- Be aware of the amount of overtime paid to staff, costs incurred by the physicians, and medical and office supplies.

Coordination of Benefits: Tips for Reducing Payment Delays and Improving Accounts Receivable

One of the major reasons for delays in claims processing is the need for information to support coordination of benefits (COB). Coordination of benefits (COB) applies to a person who is covered by more than one health plan. The COB provision and regulations require that all health plans and other payers (eg, Medicaid and Medicare) coordinate benefits to eliminate duplication of payment and assist patients to receive the maximum benefit to which they are entitled. By adhering to the COB provisions, the health plans and other payers can determine which plan will pay for a claim first. The health plan or payer obligated to pay a claim first is called the "primary" payer and the other plan or payer is termed "secondary." Together, the primary and secondary payers coordinate payments for services up to 100% of the covered charges at a rate consistent with the benefits. When information about all potential sources of coverage is not available to plans and payers, claims will generally be "pended" and remain unpaid until complete COB information is on file.

Top reasons for COB-related delays in payment include (1) incomplete or inaccurate COB information on file with the plan or payer and (2) failure to attach the explanation of benefits (EOB) from the primary payer when billing the secondary payer. In addition, one of the leading reasons for claim denials is failure to submit complete and clean claims. The following tips are designed to assist physicians/providers and their billing staff to reduce payment delays attributed to COB-related problems.

1. Ask All Patients About Secondary Insurance Coverage

Have an office procedure to collect and/or confirm primary and secondary insurance information at each visit. Ask patients to provide the following information about their spouse and/or dependents: social security number, birth date, group/policy number for other medical coverage (if applicable), and Medicare or Medicaid ID card (if applicable). Collect this information at the time the appointment is booked to allow time for your staff to confirm eligibility prior to the visit.

2. Know What Plans and Payers Need to Pay Claims

Although each plan and payer may have slightly different requirements, there are some requirements that are nearly universal. For example, nearly all plans require a copy of the EOB from the primary payer prior to paying a claim as the secondary payer. Most plans and payers publish their requirements, and the information should be available in physician/provider manuals, online, and by contacting physician/provider representatives.

3. Determine Primary and Secondary Payers

It is important for physicians/providers to determine primary and secondary payers so that claims can be sent to the primary payer first. Some plans will be able to tell physicians/providers whether they are primary or secondary at the time the physician/provider contacts the plan to verify eligibility. Typically, the following rules are used by plans and payers to determine the primary and secondary payer:

- The payer covering the patient as a subscriber will be the primary payer.
- If the patient is a dependent child, the payer whose subscriber has the earlier birthday in the calendar year will be the primary payer. This is known as the Birthday Rule.

4. Attach EOB From Primary Payer When Submitting Claim to Secondary

Secondary payers must have a copy of the EOB provided by the primary payer to process and pay a claim. Make attaching an EOB to claims filed with secondary payers a part of your routine office procedure.

A Special Consideration for Medicare Claims

Many health plans receive Medicare claims automatically when they are the secondary payer. In this case, the explanation of Medicare benefits (EOMB) will indicate that the claim has been automatically crossed over for secondary consideration. Physicians/providers should look for this indication on their EOMBs and should not submit a paper claim to the secondary payer. A paper claim submitted in this circumstance would be coded as a duplicate and rejected by the secondary payer.

A committee representing health plans and health care physicians/providers prepared this document. Organizations that participated in the development of this document include American Academy of Family Physicians, American College of Obstetricians and Gynecologists, American Academy of Dermatology Association, Bethesda Healthcare System, Piedmont Hospital, Group Health Incorporated, and Health Alliance Plan. America's Health Insurance Plans and the Healthcare Financial Management Association convened the committee.

The Business Case for Pricing Vaccines and Immunization Administration

One of the goals of the American Academy of Pediatrics (AAP), shared by the American Academy of Family Physicians (AAFP) and the Centers for Disease Control and Prevention (CDC) Advisory Committee on Immunization Practices (ACIP) is to promote maximum immunization coverage for all infants, children, adolescents, and young adults. If that goal is to be achieved, physicians must be reimbursed for the full costs (direct and indirect) of providing the immunization. As new vaccines are introduced into the AAP, AAFP, and ACIP schedule, how should the practicing pediatrician price them to ensure recovery of direct and indirect costs and what payments are appropriate from the insurers? To answer this question, we must first accept the fact that a pediatric practice is really a small business and must run on sound, generally accepted business principles to remain viable. These new vaccines have become increasingly expensive, necessitating a more business-like approach. What does this mean? For universal purchase states, this only means getting an acceptable immunization administration fee, as there are no direct vaccine purchase costs. But as we will see below, there are indirect costs in maintaining vaccines that need to be recovered.

Vaccine-Related Expenses

1. Purchase price (acquisition cost) of the vaccine: This is the amount paid by the physician for the vaccine. A public source on the manufacturer's price for vaccines can be accessed on the CDC vaccine price list for the private sector at http://www.cdc.gov/vaccines/programs/vfc/cdc-vac-price-list.htm.
2. Personnel costs for ordering and inventory: Medical office staff (clinical and administrative) time to monitor vaccine stock, place orders, negotiate costs and delivery and payment terms, and monitor storage procedures (locks, alarms, temperature controls, etc).
3. Storage costs: Since the vaccines must be stored at a specific temperature, there are equipment costs: refrigerator(s), freezer(s), locks, alarm systems, temperature monitoring devices, generators for continued electrical supply (all of which are depreciated).

4. Insurance to insure against loss of the vaccine.
5. Wastage/nonpayment: There is an estimated wastage/nonpayment of at least 5% (this should be accurately accounted for in each office). This includes drawing up the vaccine and having the patient/family reconsider; and subsequent nonpayment as well as nonpayment despite collection efforts.
6. Lost opportunity costs: The cost that is often forgotten is the cost of the money invested in vaccine inventory. A recent inventory at a 10-provider, 3-location pediatric group showed that they had $100,000 in vaccine inventory. Any business that invested that money in a product would expect a reasonable return on investment and so should every pediatric practice.

Immunization Administration Expenses

This service is separately reportable from the vaccine product. Some payers mistakenly believe that inadequate vaccine payments can be made up by nominal immunization administration fees. However, these are 2 separate expenses.

The Centers for Medicare & Medicaid Services (CMS) uses its Medicare Resource-Based Relative Value Scale (RBRVS), which assigns relative value units (RVUs) to services based on the resources used. The RVUs of a *Current Procedural Terminology (CPT®)* code take into account the physician work, practice expenses, and professional liability insurance expenses associated with that service.

1. Physician work: The total value of physician work contained in the Medicare RBRVS physician fee schedule includes
   - Physician time required to perform the service
   - Technical skill and physical effort
   - Mental effort and judgment
   - Psychological stress associated with the physician's concern about the iatrogenic risk to the patient
2. Practice expense: Medicare RBRVS uses both direct and indirect practice expenses to determine practice expense RVUs, including resources used within the facility or physician's office (or patient's home) in providing the service. The practice expense component of the immunization administration fee includes: (1) clinical staff time

(RN/LPN/MA blend), including time for vaccine registry input, refrigerator/freezer temperature log monitoring/documentation, and refrigerator/freezer alarm monitoring/documentation); (2) medical supplies (1 pair non-sterile gloves, 7 feet of examination table paper, 1 Occupational Health and Safety Administration–compliant syringe with needle, 1 CDC information sheet, 2 alcohol swabs, 1 band-aid); and (3) medical equipment (exam table, dedicated full size vaccine refrigerator with alarm/lock [commercial grade], and refrigerator/freezer vaccine temperature monitor/alarm).

3. Professional liability insurance expense: The professional liability insurance RVUs assigned to a code are based on CMS historic malpractice claims data.

These 3 components are combined to create a total RVU (see Table below). Under Medicare RBRVS, the injectable pediatric immunization administration codes (**90465** and **90466**) and the non–age-specific immunization administration codes (**90471** and **90472**) have the same RVU while the oral/intranasal pediatric (**90467** and **90468**) and non–age-specific

(**90473** and **90474**) codes are similarly valued. With the 2009 Medicare conversion factor of 36.0666, this translates to $20.92 for **90465** and **90471**; $10.46 for **90466** and **90472**; $13.71 for **90467** and **90473**; $10.10 for **90468**; $10.28 for **90468**; and $9.02 for **90474** on the 2009 Medicare RBRVS physician fee schedule.

So what should be the final price for a vaccine that ensures recovery of direct and indirect costs? If you are receiving adequate immunization administration fees, then the vaccine charge should stand on its own. Payment needs to cover the purchase price, the office expenses as noted above, and a return on the investment for the dollars invested in vaccine inventory. When you add this up, we estimate that the total costs of providing the vaccine is approximately 17% to 28% above the direct vaccine purchase price. If the immunization administration fee is less than appropriate, then this either needs to be renegotiated or additional costs moved into the vaccine charge.

Insurers understand business principles including the concept of return on investment and expect it in their business. There is no reason we should accept their

2009 Medicare Relative Value Units for Immunization Administration					
CPT Code and Description	Physician Work RVUs	Practice Expense RVUs (Non-facility)	Professional Liability Insurance RVUs	Total RVUs	Total RVUs x 2009 Medicare Conversion Factor (36.0666) = Medicare Fee
90465 Immunization administration under age 8 with physician counseling, one injection	0.17	0.40	0.01	0.58	$20.92
90471 Immunization administration, one injection	0.17	0.40	0.01	0.58	$20.92
90466 Immunization administration under age 8 with physician counseling, each additional injection	0.15	0.13	0.01	0.29	$10.46
90472 Immunization administration, each additional injection	0.15	0.13	0.01	0.29	$10.46
90467 Immunization administration under age 8 by intranasal/oral route, first administration	0.17	0.20	0.01	0.38	$13.71
90473 Immunization administration by intranasal/oral route, first administration	0.17	0.20	0.01	0.38	$13.71
90468 Immunization administration under age 8 by intranasal/oral route, each additional administration	0.15	0.12	0.01	0.28	$10.10
90474 Immunization administration by intranasal/oral route, each additional vaccine	0.15	0.09	0.01	0.25	$9.02

refusal to recognize it in our business by paying only the vaccine purchase price. They pass on their increased costs to their purchasers to maintain profitability. We have a legitimate business case to make for adequate payment for vaccines and immunization administration and we must all make it.

For information on the AAP private payer advocacy, contact Lou Terranova at lterranova@aap.org or at 800/433-9016, ext 7633

© by the American Academy of Pediatrics (Revised 11/08). May be reproduced with appropriate attribution to the American Academy of Pediatrics

Current Procedural Terminology (CPT®) 5-digit codes, nomenclature, and other data are copyright 2008 American Medical Association (AMA). All Rights Reserved.

Important note: Given the relative frequency with which code and valuation revisions occur, articles related to coding may not reflect the most current information available. Please check the online version of this article at http://practice.aap.org/content.aspx?aid=1808 and the *AAP Pediatric Coding Newsletter* at http://coding.aap.org for updated guidance.

Because the American Academy of Pediatrics (AAP) is not able to verify the accuracy of the facts relating to a patient encounter, we cannot be held responsible for any coding decisions that you make based on the guidance you receive from the AAP. It is your responsibility to only code for what you do during a patient encounter.

When Is It Appropriate to Report 99211 During Immunization Administration?

Abstract: Code 99211 should not be reported for every nurse-only vaccine administration patient encounter. Rather, careful consideration needs to be given regarding the significance and medical necessity for such a visit.

When vaccines are given in the pediatric office, questions often arise concerning the reporting of evaluation and management (E/M) services performed during the same visit where vaccines are administered. The answer always depends on whether the provider performs a *medically necessary and significant, separately identifiable E/M visit, in addition to the immunization administration.* If such a service is performed, an E/M code is reported, most likely from the **99201– 99215** code family (office or other outpatient service), in addition to the appropriate code for immunization administration **(90465–90468** or **90471–90474)** plus the code for the vaccine product(s). In such cases, payers may require that modifier **25** (significant, separately identifiable E/M service by the same physician on the same day of the procedure or other service) be appended to the E/M code to distinguish it from the actual administration of the vaccine.

The identification of a significant, separately identifiable service for E/M codes usually involves the performance and documentation of the key components (ie, history, physical examination, and medical decision-making) or time. However, the reporting of code **99211** is unique among E/M codes in having no key component requirements. The *Current Procedural Terminology (CPT®)* descriptor for code **99211** states, "Office or other outpatient visit for the evaluation and management of an established patient, that may not require the presence of a physician. Usually, the presenting problem(s) are minimal. Typically, 5 minutes are spent performing or supervising these services." Therefore, how this concept is defined when the E/M code in question is **99211** needs further clarification.

To address this issue, it becomes important to determine the following:
- What services are included in the immunization administration codes?
- What additional services are required to appropriately report a **99211?**
- What are the documentation requirements for a **99211?**

What Services Are Included in the Immunization Administration Codes?

The following services are included in the immunization administration *CPT* codes:
- Administrative staff services, such as making the appointment, preparing the patient chart, billing for the service, and filing the chart
- Clinical staff services, such as greeting the patient, taking routine vital signs, obtaining a vaccine history on past reactions and contraindications, presenting a Vaccine Information Statement (VIS) and answering routine vaccine questions, preparing and administering the vaccine with chart documentation, and observing for any immediate reaction

The relative value units (RVUs) for the injectable immunization administration codes **(90465–90466** and **90471–90472)** were significantly increased in 2005. Additionally, equivalent RVUs were published for the intranasal and oral immunization administration codes **(90467–90468** and **90473–90474)** in 2006. These increases can be attributed to the fact that Centers for Medicare & Medicaid Services (CMS) views many of the services that are included under code **99211** as part of the immunization administration codes. Accordingly, the RVUs for code **99211** have essentially been "built" into the RVUs for the immunization administration codes.

The immunization administration codes are valued on the Medicare physician fee schedule (Resource-Based Relative Value Scale [RBRVS]). See chart below.

What Additional Services Are Required to Appropriately Report a 99211?

The E/M service must exceed those services included in the immunization administration codes. In addition, there are 2 principles to keep in mind. They are as follows:
1. The service must be medically necessary.
2. The service must be separate and significant from the immunization administration.

When the provider (usually the nurse) evaluates, manages, and documents the significant and separate complaint(s) or problem(s), the additional reporting of **99211** is justified. In such circumstances, the nurse typically conducts a brief history and record review along with a physical assessment (eg, indicated vital signs and observations) and provides patient education in helping the family or patient manage the problem encountered. These nursing activities are all directly related to the significant, separate complaint, and unrelated to the actual vaccine administration.

What Are the Documentation Requirements for a 99211?

All reported E/M codes must meet documentation requirements as outlined in *CPT* guidelines or in the CMS Documentation Guidelines. For most of the E/M services that physicians perform, this means that some designated combination of the key components of history, physical examination, and medical decision-making must be met and clearly documented. Alternatively, if more than 50% of the time spent during the E/M service is spent in counseling or coordinating care, time becomes the "key" or controlling factor in selecting a code.

Code 99211 is the one E/M service typically provided by the nurse and not the physician. As such, its documentation requirements differ. There are no required key components typical of the physician services noted above. Further, the typical time published in *CPT* for **99211** is 5 minutes. The American Academy of Pediatrics (AAP) encourages documenting the date of service and reason for the visit, a brief history of any significant problems evaluated or managed, any examination elements (eg, vital signs or appearance of a rash), a brief assessment and/or plan along with any

counseling or patient education done, and signatures of the nurse and supervising physician.

While not required, it may help payers to better understand the medical necessity of the nurse E/M service if it is linked to a different *International Classification of Diseases, Ninth Revision, Clinical Modification (ICD-9-CM)* code than the one used for the vaccine given when appropriate. Further, encounter documentation should be a separate entry from the charting of the vaccine itself (product, lot number, site and method, VIS date, etc, which usually are all recorded on the immunization history sheet). Each practice should consider developing protocols and progress note templates for vaccine services.

Finally, if the nurse provides the **99211** visit, it is reported under the physician's name/tax ID number, making it inherently an "incident-to" service. In such situations, it is a service restricted to established patients and requires the supervising physician's "direct supervision," which is defined by the CMS as the physician being physically present in the office suite (not in the patient's room) and immediately available to provide assistance. Most "nurse" E/M services are carried out under a protocol of orders developed by the physician for the particular service and should be fully documented in the record. As always, the physician supervising the care should sign the chart entry.

Coding Information From *CPT* and CMS

The American Medical Association provides some instruction on the correct reporting of **99211** at the

CPT Code	Work RVUs	Non-facility Practice Expense RVUs	Malpractice RVUs	Total Non-facility RVUs	2008 Medicare Non-facility Payment
90465	0.17	0.38	0.01	0.56	$21.33*
90466	0.15	0.12	0.01	0.28	$10.66
90467	0.17	0.17	0.01	0.35	$13.33
90468	0.15	0.11	0.01	0.27	$10.28
90471	0.17	0.38	0.01	0.56	$21.33
90472	0.15	0.13	0.01	0.29	$11.05
90473	0.17	0.18	0.01	0.36	$13.71
90474	0.15	0.09	0.01	0.25	$9.52

RVUs = relative value units
*Sample conversion for **90465**
Medicare 2008 conversion factor = $38.0870
0.56 RVUs x $38.0870 = $21.33

time of immunization administration in its *CPT Assistant* (October 1999 and April 2005). *CPT* reaffirms the nature of a reportable E/M service as significant and separate from the immunization administration itself.

CMS also provides direction for reporting **99211** during visits where only the nurse sees the patient and gives an injection. Under CMS Medicare payment policy, it is not correct to report an E/M service if the nurse services are only related directly to the injection itself. In that vein, CMS significantly increased its fee for immunization administration in 2005, providing reimbursement for the typical activities of the nurse as listed above under the immunization administration codes.

One of the ways in which CMS Medicare payment policy is enforced is via the National Correct Coding Initiative (NCCI) edits. Version 12.0 (January 2006) of the NCCI edits introduced edits that prohibit the Medicare reporting of **99211** with the immunization administration codes under any circumstances. The AAP immediately appealed the edits, requesting at the very least that a modifier override be allowed (ie, modifier **25** appended to code **99211** to indicate that a significant, separately identifiable E/M is being provided). The AAP has continued to advocate for this change.

While private payers often follow CMS lead in such coding guidance, it should be noted that some private payers and state Medicaid agencies do not use Medicare RBRVS or the NCCI edits and have their own reporting guidelines and payment policies for nurse visits. As with other services that are high in volume, the AAP encourages pediatricians to query payers when developing office policies on reporting nurse services, and carefully review the explanation of benefits returned from all payers after these claims are processed.

Coding Examples

VIGNETTE #1

A 7-month-old girl visits your office to be immunized against influenza and is seen only by your nurse. The nurse takes a brief history and learns the infant has a cough without change in appetite, sleep, or activity level. He takes vital signs and assesses that the infant has no contraindications to getting the vaccine, and discusses the office practice protocol for the management of the respiratory problem with the mother.

Additionally, the nurse documents that the patient meets the current guidelines for vaccination and has no contraindications to the immunization per the Centers for Disease Control and Prevention (CDC) guidelines. Next, he reviews the VIS with the mother and obtains consent for the immunization. The nurse then administers the influenza vaccine.

The encounter would be reported as follows:

CPT	ICD-9-CM
99211-25 (E/M service)	**786.2** (cough)
90657 (influenza vaccine)	**V04.81** (need for prophylactic vaccination and inoculation against certain viral diseases; influenza)
90471 (immunization administration)	**V04.81** (need for prophylactic vaccination and inoculation against certain viral diseases; influenza)

An example of written documentation for this **99211** encounter follows (the actual vaccine data with lot number and site/route and VIS date are recorded on a separate immunization record):

The patient is here for the influenza vaccine. Mother reports a cough for several days without any fever. She is eating well and there has been no wheezing or rapid breathing. Her temperature is 98.7°F and respiratory rate is 38/minute—she appears well. The symptomatic treatment of the cough per protocol was discussed and the mother was instructed to call or return if the problem worsened.

She has no allergies to foods or history of reactions to past vaccines. The risks and potential side effects of the hepatitis B vaccine were discussed after the VIS was given, and the mother was informed of the correct dosage of an antipyretic should fever or fussiness occur afterwards. An influenza vaccine was given.

K. Brooks, LPN/R. Dunn, MD (signatures/date)

VIGNETTE #2

A 5-year-old is brought in by the mother for a catch-up measles-mumps-rubella (MMR) vaccine. She says the child is fine and has already been counseled on the vaccine and has no concerns. The nurse proceeds to review the vaccine history, presents the VIS, and receives an order for the vaccine from the physician. She then administers and documents the vaccine. In this situation, the service is only vaccine related and no significant or separate E/M service is provided. Therefore, the only services reported are the immunization administration and the vaccine product code.

The encounter would be reported as follows:

CPT	ICD-9-CM
90707 (MMR vaccine)	**V06.4** (need for prophylactic vaccination and inoculation against combinations of diseases; measles-mumps-rubella [MMR])
90471 (immunization administration)	**V06.4** (need for prophylactic vaccination and inoculation against combinations of diseases; measles-mumps-rubella [MMR])

VIGNETTE #3

A 4-month-old patient had an illness with high fever at her preventive medicine visit 2 weeks ago, and now returns to see your nurse for her second hepatitis B vaccine. The nurse performs an interval history, finding the symptoms from the earlier illness had resolved. She then confirms that the infant is afebrile by taking the infant's temperature, and makes the observation that the infant is playful. After assessing that the patient is currently in good health, she confirms that there are no contraindications to the immunization per the CDC guidelines. Next, the nurse reviews the VIS with the father, antipyretic dosage for weight, and gets the father's consent for the immunization. The nurse then administers the hepatitis B vaccine, observes for immediate reactions, and schedules the third hepatitis B immunization visit for 2 months later.

This encounter would be reported as follows:

CPT	ICD-9-CM
99211-25 (E/M service)	**V67.59** (follow-up examination; following other treatment; other)
90744 (hepatitis B vaccine)	**V05.3** (need for other prophylactic vaccination and inoculation against single diseases; viral hepatitis)
90471 (immunization administration)	**V05.3** (need for other prophylactic vaccination and inoculation against single diseases; viral hepatitis)

An example of written documentation for this **99211** encounter follows (the actual vaccine data with lot number and site/route and VIS date are recorded on a separate immunization record):

The patient is here for a missed hepatitis vaccine and has had no fever for 7 days, is eating again, and seems to be well per father. Past vaccines have been well tolerated. Her temperature now is 98.7°F and she appears well. The risk and potential side effects of the hepatitis vaccine were discussed after the VIS was given and the parent was informed of the correct dosage of an antipyretic should fever or fussiness occur afterwards. The night call system was explained and the access number given.

K. Brooks, LPN/R. Dunn, MD (signatures/date)

NOTE: Some payers may *inappropriately* deny claims that link code **99211** to a "V" *ICD-9-CM* code. Neither *CPT* nor *ICD-9-CM* guidelines* prohibit such reporting when the *ICD-9-CM* code reported is the most specific one available to describe the patient encounter. Furthermore, *CPT* guidelines clearly outline the requirements for reporting a given level E/M code. If the key components of history, physical examination, and medical decision-making or time requirements (when greater than 50% of the visit is spent counseling/coordinating care) are met for a given code, the physician is correct in the reporting of that code. *CPT* guidelines do not make the reporting of a certain level E/M code contingent on the patient exhibiting certain symptoms or falling under a particular diagnosis. *CPT* guidelines correctly recognize that there can be considerable variation in the treatment of a patient with a particular diagnosis and that it is inappropriate to validate the legitimacy of a reported E/M code by the presence of a certain diagnosis(es). Claims adjudication processes that prohibit the reporting of "V" *ICD-9-CM* codes with anything other than preventive medicine services *CPT* codes are inconsistent with *CPT* and *ICD-9-CM* guidelines and are counterintuitive to the continuum of care that can be provided for a patient with a given diagnosis. Further, it should be noted that the office or other outpatient services *CPT* codes (**99201–99215**) are not limited to "sick" visits only. Therefore, it is appropriate to report "V" codes or any other *ICD-9-CM* codes that most appropriately reflect the reason for the encounter with the office or other outpatient services codes.

* ICD-9-CM Official Guidelines for Coding and Reporting

C. Chapter-Specific Coding Guidelines

C18. Classification of Factors Influencing Health Status and Contact with Health Service

A. *ICD-9-CM provides codes to deal with encounters for circumstances other than a disease or injury. The Supplementary Classification of Factors Influencing Health Status and Contact with Health Services (**V01.0–V83.89**) is provided to deal with occasions when circumstances other than a disease or injury (codes **001–999**) are recorded as a diagnosis or problem. There are four primary circumstances for the use of V codes, including:*

1. *When a person who is not currently sick encounters the health services for some specific reason, such as to act as an organ donor, to receive prophylactic care, such as inoculations or health screenings, or to receive counseling on a health-related issue.*

D. *Categories of V Codes*

2. *Inoculations and vaccinations: Categories **V03–V06** are for encounters for inoculations and vaccinations. They indicate that a patient is being seen to receive a prophylactic inoculation against a disease. The injection itself must be represented by the appropriate procedure code. A code from **V03–V06** may be used as a secondary code if the inoculation is given as a routine part of preventive health care, such as a well-baby visit.*

For questions, please contact the AAP Division of Health Care Finance and Quality Improvement at dhcfqi@aap.org.

Current Procedural Terminology (CPT®) 5-digit codes, nomenclature, and other data are copyright 2008 American Medical Association (AMA). All Rights Reserved.

Important note: Given the relative frequency with which code and valuation revisions occur, articles related to coding may not reflect the most current information available. Please check the online version of this article at http://practice.aap.org/content.aspx?aid=2119 and the *AAP Pediatric Coding Newsletter* at http://coding.aap.org for updated guidance.

Because the American Academy of Pediatrics (AAP) is not able to verify the accuracy of the facts relating to a patient encounter, we cannot be held responsible for any coding decisions that you make based on the guidance you receive from the AAP. It is your responsibility to only code for what you do during a patient encounter.

Improving Mental Health Services in Primary Care: Reducing Administrative and Financial Barriers to Access and Collaboration

Background

The Statistics

Approximately 70% of children and adolescents who are in need of treatment do not receive mental health services. Of those who seek treatment, only 1 in 5 children use mental health specialty services. Thus approximately 75% to 85% fail to receive specialty services, and most of these children fail to receive any services at all.[1] For the families that seek services, 40% to 50% terminate treatment prematurely because of lack of access, lack of transportation, financial constraints, child mental health professional shortages, and stigma related to mental health disorders.[1,2] Only a small proportion of these children receive treatment from mental health professionals. Most of these children receive services from primary care clinicians. In 2005, 25.3% of children 4 to 17 years of age who received nonpsychopharmacologic treatment for emotional or behavioral difficulties in the past 12 months were seen by their pediatric or general medical practice.[3]

Although many mental health disorders in children are not being diagnosed, primary care clinicians have been identifying emotional and behavioral disorders in children at an increasing rate. From 1979 to 1996, pediatrician-identified psychosocial problems rose from 6.8% to 18.7% among children 4 to 15 years of age.[3] As a result, primary care clinicians are seeing a growing population of patients with mental health needs and have taken on a greater role in prescribing psychotropic medications. Between 1987 and 1996, psychotropic drug use among children and adolescents nearly tripled, growing from 1.4% to 3.9%, or more than 2 million children.[4]

The need for primary care clinicians to treat children with emotional and behavioral disorders will only continue to increase in the future. In 2005, 16% of US children 4 to 17 years of age had parents who had talked to a health care professional or school personnel about their child's emotional or behavioral difficulties in the past 12 months.[3] The federal Bureau of Health Professions estimates that simply to maintain the current utilization rates of psychiatric care, the

nation will need 12,624 child and adolescent psychiatrists in 2020; unfortunately, only 8,312 are anticipated to be in practice at that time.[5] In addition, the child and adolescent psychiatric workforce is not anticipated to increase significantly in future years, as the number of positions in child and adolescent psychiatry residency programs has continued to decrease—from 130 in 1980 to 114 in 2002.[5]

The American Academy of Pediatrics (AAP) Pediatric Research in Office Settings Network and the American Academy of Family Physicians' Ambulatory Sentinel Practice Network study (2000) found that pediatricians are quite variable in their sense of responsibility for providing mental health care. Although most pediatricians surveyed reported it was their responsibility to identify children with a wide range of mental health or substance abuse disorders (eg, attention-deficit/hyperactivity disorder [ADHD], depression, anxiety, learning disorders), fewer than half reported they felt it was their responsibility to manage any disorder beyond ADHD.[6,7] This comfort level with managing ADHD is likely a result of a thoughtful and planned educational effort.

Key Issues for Pediatricians and Psychiatrists

Inadequate Range of Diagnostic ICD-9-CM Codes

Many time-consuming pediatric developmental and behavioral problems do not meet the criteria for a "disorder" diagnosis as specified in the *Diagnostic and Statistical Manual of Mental Disorders, 4th Edition (DSM-IV)* and the *Internal Classification of Diseases, 9th Revision, Clinical Modification (ICD-9-CM)*. These include conditions described in *The Classification of Child and Adolescent Mental Diagnoses in Primary Care: Diagnostic and Statistical Manual for Primary Care*, which emphasizes situational problems, behavioral aberrations, or concerns, which, if addressed early, might not evolve into pathology (disorders). The current array of diagnostic codes does not fully capture the wide range of developmental and behavioral problems presenting in children. Consequently, absent the codes acceptable to payers, primary care clinicians are typically not paid for their time spent identifying, treating, and managing these problems.

Mental Health Carve-outs

Given the current shortage of child psychiatrists, developmental/behavioral pediatric specialists, and child psychologists, much of the burden of treating child and adolescent behavioral disorders falls on the shoulders of primary care pediatricians. These physicians are frequently not appropriately paid for their time spent in treating and managing the care of children's mental health disorders, in large part, because of mental health "carve-outs." In many private and public insurance plans, behavioral health services, identified by the *ICD-9-CM* diagnostic codes **290–319** used to identify the treated condition, have been "carved out" from other health care expenditures. In such an arrangement, a managed behavioral health care organization pays only the contracted behavioral health specialists on its behavioral health "panel" for these services. Pediatricians typically are not credentialed to provide care in the mental health panel and, thus, are considered ineligible to bill for the mental health care services they provide in their office. This is a significant barrier to access to mental health care for many children and this suggests a subtle form of discrimination against children with identified mental

health conditions. Only through consistent and universal parity of mental health codes with physical health codes among all third-party payers will this aspect of limited access be addressed.

In addition to "diagnostic parity," "procedural parity" has been a part of the *Current Procedural Terminology (CPT)* **908xx** mental health procedure codes since their initial valuation by the Centers for Medicare & Medicaid Services for payment under the Medicare Resource-Based Relative Value Scale (RBRVS). For fairly equivalent services, in terms of time spent and complexity of the service, evaluation and management (E/M) codes have had higher RBRVS relative value units (RVUs) assigned when compared with **908xx** codes. For example (Table 1), an initial new patient consultation visit in the office setting for concerns reflecting underlying depression is worth 3.77 work RVUs for a professional using E/M consultation code **99245** (consultation, new or established patient). This is more highly valued when compared with 2.80 work RVUs earned for **90801** (psychiatric diagnostic interview examination) customarily mandated as the appropriate code for use by mental health professionals. Not only are the **908xx** codes undervalued relative to the E/M service codes, but the expected post-service work time is significantly longer for

Table 1. Valuation Comparisons of Evaluation and Management Codes and Psychiatric Services

Code	Work RVUs	Non-facility Total RVUs	RBRVS Intra-service Time (minutes)	*CPT* Time (minutes)	RBRVS Payment 2009: Non-facility[a]
99245 Consultation: new or established patient	3.77	6.28	60	80	$226.50
90801 Psychiatric diagnostic interview exam	2.80	4.24	60	Not specified	$152.92
99215 Level 5 office visit: established patient	2.00	3.46	35	40	$124.79
90807 Office visit (psychotherapy w/ E/M service) (45–50 min)	2.02	2.77	50	45–50	$99.90
99214 Level 4 office visit: established patient	1.42	2.56	25	25	$92.33
90805 Individual psychotherapy with medical E/M services	1.37	1.97	30	20–30	$71.05

Work RVUs indicates physician work RVUs; non-facility, practice-based setting; non-facility total RVUs, sum of the work, non-facility practice expense, and professional liability insurance RVUs; intra-service time, typical face-to-face time between the physician and the patient/family.

[a]Calculated using $36.0666, the 2009 Medicare conversion factor. For more information on the Medicare conversion factor, access the AAP RBRVS brochure at http://www.aap.org/visit/rbrvsbrochure.pdf.

the **90801** service (55 minutes) when compared with expected post-service work for the E/M service **99245** (20 minutes). There is more work "captured" in a code, which is also undervalued in RVUs. This certainly could be a factor in many mental health providers' decision to only accept cash payment from families and not to accept these contract terms from managed care payers.

Inadequate Benefit Packages

With the future implementation of the federal mental health parity law in 2010, many more Americans will have access to plans with equivalent mental and physical health benefits. The Paul Wellstone and Pete Domenici Mental Health Parity and Addiction Equity Act of 2008 applies to all group health plans with 50 or more employees, whether they are self-funded (regulated under ERISA) or fully insured (regulated under state law), that provide mental health or substance use benefits. However, the new law does not apply to individual health plans and health plans offered by businesses with 50 or fewer employees.

Robust implementation of the new parity law is necessary, because under current state laws, many insurance plans have policies that limit access to mental health services. These may include separate deductibles, high co-pays, and annual spending limits lower than those established for medical services. These policies impede access to mental health services for many children and add to pediatricians' burden in providing or finding needed care. Also adding to the issues, purchasers (eg, employers) often determine the scope of benefits coverage, thereby creating more barriers to pediatricians' ability to provide or refer to appropriate services.

Such limitations in mental health benefits frequently have been motivated by cost concerns. Experience has shown that improving children's access to outpatient mental health services may actually reduce the cost of mental health care. In 1992 North Carolina introduced full coverage parity of mental health and non-mental health conditions into its state health plan for state employees: a single insurance deductible, full freedom of choice of mental health providers, and only moderate management of generous benefits through a contract with Value Behavioral Health.[8] By 1998 North Carolina saw mental health payments as a percentage of total health payments decrease from 6.4% to 3.1%.[9] Mental health hospital days during this period decreased by 70%.[9] This outcome was docu-

mented also by Sturm, who studied insurance plans offering parity in behavioral health spending limits.[6] These findings support the thesis that increasing access to outpatient mental health services through parity of mental health benefits is both economically and medically beneficial.[10]

Incentives to Support Colocation of Care

Physicians have a long-established pattern of extending access to their medical services through the employment of nurse practitioners and physician assistants in their offices to treat patients under their supervision. Medicare pays for these services as being billed as services provided directly by the physician so long as they are provided according to Medicare "incident-to" regulations. Insurance companies follow the same billing conventions for medical services but do not provide similar economic incentives for psychiatric services provided by psychiatric advanced practice nurses, psychologists, and social workers employed in medical and psychiatric group practice settings, even though they meet the same "incident-to" standards. Without this incentive, there is no recognition that a psychologist employed by a child and adolescent psychiatrist and working in the same office suite delivers team-based care that improves access to care and the complexity of service. Such incentives are important to the development of models of colocated primary and mental health care.

Lack of Payment for Non–Face-to-Face Aspects of Care

Many plans do not pay for team medical conferences among professionals involved with the child's care; ongoing monitoring as aspects of mental health care; communication with other medical and nonmedical professionals, including consultants, teachers, and therapists; medical conferences; or many other non-clinical aspects of caring for these children (care plan oversight, health risk assessment, etc). There is growing evidence that non–face-to-face services are not only more cost-effective but also preferred by families because of time constraints and convenience.[11] They are also critical to care plan oversight (*CPT* codes **99339–99340),** allowing the primary care clinician to oversee all aspects of care being provided to the patient.

CPT codes for care plan oversight **(99339–99340)** have RVUs published on the Medicare RBRVS and may be reported in addition to face-to-face E/M services. Payers have been uneven about payment for these services, however. Because mental health care implicitly involves coordinated care among services in school, outpatient therapies, and the care coordinator, payment denial for this care plan oversight by behavioral managed care again suggests discrimination against the child with mental health care needs.

A very significant amount of care coordination involves telephone communication beyond the typical "post-service" work included in the E/M *CPT* codes. Frequently, telephone care involves communication with family members. In 2006 the AAP published the "Payment for Telephone Care" policy statement citing evidence that telephone care does not increase overall health care costs. Recommendations were made for pediatricians to develop office policies and procedures to ensure consistent processes for reporting telephone care, to notify the families of their patients before initiating a fee for telephone care, and to code for appropriately documented telephone calls (using *CPT* codes **99441–99443**). The AAP and American Academy of Child and Adolescent Psychiatry (AACAP) have worked nationally to obtain valuation of these 3 codes. Inclusion of values for these services on the Medicare RBRVS will allow non-Medicare payers to use these values in establishing their own fee schedules.

Lack of Payment for Sessions With Parents Alone

Children's mental health treatment is most effective when providers develop a partnership with parents and/or other caregivers. Separate meetings with parents frequently are necessary for gathering history, providing education, and working with parents to develop strategies for helping their child and dealing with challenging behavior. Often during well-child examinations, more time is needed to speak with parents without the child present. Pediatricians are increasingly communicating face-to-face with parents and counseling them on child/adolescent developmental and behavioral issues. Child and adolescent psychiatrists and psychologists have a specific valued *CPT* code for this type of service **(90846)** but have been concerned about the lack of payment for this type of session. Payment must be supported for these sessions, which is best accomplished by paying for E/M codes for pediatricians and child and adolescent psychiatrists using time as the key factor.[12]

Access to Child and Adolescent Psychiatric Specialty Treatment

Pediatricians will encounter children whose problems do not improve with initial interventions and/or children with a severe level of impairment or complex coexisting conditions that require specialty consultation and, often, specialty treatment. The AACAP publication "When to Seek Referral or Consultation with a Child Adolescent Psychiatrist" details the parameters related to this referral process.[5]

Primary care practitioners generally need consultation in the following circumstances:

1. When a child or adolescent demonstrates an emotional or behavioral problem that constitutes a threat to the safety of the child/adolescent or the safety of those around him/her (eg, suicidal behavior, severe aggressive behavior, an eating disorder that is out of control, other self-destructive behavior)
2. When a child or adolescent demonstrates a significant change in his or her emotional or behavioral functioning for which there is **no obvious or recognized precipitant** (eg, the sudden onset of school avoidance, a suicide attempt or gesture in a previously well-functioning individual)
3. When a child or adolescent demonstrates emotional or behavioral problems (regardless of severity) and the primary caregiver has serious emotional impairment or a substance abuse problem (eg, a child with emotional withdrawal whose parent is significantly depressed, a child with behavioral difficulties whose parents are going through a "hostile" divorce)
4. When a child or adolescent demonstrates an emotional or behavioral problem in which there is evidence of significant disruption in day-to-day functioning or reality contact (eg, a child/adolescent who has repeated severe tantrums with no apparent reason, a child reports hallucinatory experiences without an identifiable physical cause)
5. When a child or adolescent is hospitalized for the treatment of a psychiatric illness
6. When a child or adolescent with behavioral or emotional problems has had a course of treatment intervention for 6 to 8 weeks without meaningful improvement
7. When a child or adolescent presents with complex diagnostic issues involving cognitive, psychological, and emotional components that may be related to an organic etiology or complex mental health/legal issues

8. When a child or adolescent has a history of abuse, neglect, and/or removal from home, with current significant symptoms as a result of these actions

9. When a child or adolescent whose symptom picture and family psychiatric history suggest that treatment with psychotropic medication may result in an adverse response (eg, the prescription of stimulants for a hyperactive child with a family history of bipolar disorder or schizophrenia)

10. When a child or adolescent has had only a partial response to a course of psychotropic medication or when any child is being treated with more than 2 psychotropic medications

11. When a child younger than 5 years experiences emotional or behavioral disturbances that are sufficiently severe or prolonged as to merit a recommendation for the ongoing use of a psychotropic medication

12. When a child or adolescent with a chronic medical condition demonstrates behavior that seriously interferes with the treatment of that condition

13. When a child or adolescent is having difficulty with school performance and attempts to remediate the problem(s) by the primary care physician and school personnel have not resulted in significant improvement

Joint effort involving pediatricians, child and adolescent psychiatrists, health plan administrators, and other mental health professionals should actively plan to deal with the availability of these consultation and referral services in routine, urgent, and emergency situations.

Coordination Between the Pediatrician and the Child and Adolescent Psychiatrist or Other Treating Providers

Even in the fortunate situations in which a child or adolescent psychiatrist or mental health professionals are available, unless the mental health specialist is physically colocated within the medical home, communication between these professionals and primary care physicians is often fragmented, as previously described. Thus those providing the care are often deprived of the collegial "give and take," which enhances treatment skills and facilitates the placement of patients in the optimal therapeutic setting. For services to be effective and efficient and meet the families' needs, health care professionals must communicate and coordinate with each other as previously described.

This communication may properly involve a written report. Written summaries, which often require a full description of all the events germane to the child's mental health condition, are frequently much longer and more detailed than the usual report developed to document a physical condition or surgical procedure. Creating these documents almost always extends beyond the stated "post-service" work, and the current state of payment places the burden on the mental health provider and/or primary care clinician. There is an inherent demand for an unpaid service.

Acknowledgments
This paper was developed with guidance from members of the AAP Task Force on Mental Health and the AACAP Committee on Health Care Access and Economics.

AAP Task Force on Mental Health
*Jane Meschan Foy, MD, Chair
Terry Carmichael, MSW
Paula Duncan, MD
Barbara Louise Frankowski, MD, MPH
Darcy Gruttadaro, JD
Alain Joffe, MD, MHP
Kelly James Kelleher, MD, MPH
Penelope Krener Knapp, MD
Danielle Laraque, MD
*Thomas K. McInerney, MD
Patricia Jean O'Malley, MD
Gary Q. Peck, MD
*James M. Perrin, MD
Michael Gerard Regalado, MD
Garry Steward Sigman, MD
Leonard Read Sulik, MD
Myrtis Sullivan, MD, MPH
Jack T. Swanson, MD
*Lynn Mowbray Wegner, MD
Mark L. Wolraich, MD

*Steven E. Wegner, MD (Chair, AAP Committee on Child Health Financing)

AAP Staff
Julie Kersten Ake
Mark Del Monte, JD
Aldina Hovde, MSW
Linda Paul, MPH
Lou Terranova, MHA
Linda Walsh, MAB

AACAP Committee on Health Care Access and Economics

Michael Houston, MD, Chair
*Alan Axelson, MD
Sherry Barron-Seabrook, MD
David Berland, MD
Martin Glasser, MD
Harold Graff, MD
Anthony Jackson, MD
Lisa Ponfick, MD
*Barry Sarvet, MD
Robert Schreter, MD
Benjamin Shain, MD
Harsh K. Trivedi, MD
*Lynn Mowbray Wegner, MD, AAP Liaison

AACAP Staff

Kristin Kroeger Ptakowski

*Core group involved in the development of the white paper.

This paper was supported by the Improving Mental Heath in Primary Care Through Access, Collaboration, and Training (IMPACT) grant (G95MC05434), which was awarded to the AAP in 2005 from the US Department of Health and Human Services, Health Resources and Services Administration, Maternal and Child Health Bureau.

References

1. US Department of Health and Human Services. *Mental Health: A Report of the Surgeon General— Executive Summary.* Rockville, MD: US Department of Health and Human Services, Substance Abuse and Mental Health Services Administration, Center for Mental Health Services, National Institutes of Health, National Institute of Mental Health; 1999

2. American Academy of Pediatrics Committee on School Health. School-based mental health services. *Pediatrics.* 2004;113(6):1839–1845

3. Simpson GA, Cohen RA, Pastor PN, Reuben CA. *U.S. Children 4-17 Years of Age Who Received Treatment for Emotional or Behavioral Difficulties: Preliminary Data From the 2005 National Health Interview Survey.* Atlanta, GA: National Center for Health Statistics, Centers for Disease Control and Prevention; 2006. http://www.cdc.gov/nchs/products/pubs/pubd/hestats/children2005/children2005.htm. Accessed June 20, 2008

4. Kelleher KJ, McInerny TK, Gardner WP, Childs GE, Wasserman RC. Increasing identification of psychosocial problems: 1979–1996. *Pediatrics.* 2000;105(6):1313–1325

5. Koppelman J. *The Provider System for Children's Mental Health: Workforce Capacity and Effective Treatment.* Washington, DC: George Washington University; 2004

6. Gardner W, Kelleher KJ, Wasserman R, Childs G, et al. Primary care treatment of pediatric psychosocial problems: a study from Pediatric Research in Office Settings and Ambulatory Sentinel Practice Network. *Pediatrics.* 2000;106(4):e44. http://pediatrics.aap-publications.org/cgi/content/full/106/4/e44

7. Williams J, Klinepeter K, Palmes G, Pulley A, Foy JM. Diagnosis and treatment of behavioral health disorders in pediatric practice. *Pediatrics.* 2004;114(3):601–606

8. Data on the Mental Health Benefit. Prepared by the NC Psychological Association from data supplied by the NC State Health Plan Office. April 1999

9. Power TJ, Mautone JA, Manz PH, Frye L, Blum NJ. Managing attention-deficit/hyperactivity disorder in primary care: a systematic analysis of roles and challenges. *Pediatrics.* 2008;121(1):e65–e72. http://pediatrics.aappublications.org/cgi/content/full/121/1/e65

10. Sturm R. How expensive is unlimited mental health coverage under managed care? *JAMA.* 1997;278(18):1533–1537

11. American Academy of Pediatrics Section on Telephone Care and Committee on Child Health Financing. Payment for telephone care. *Pediatrics.* 2006;118(4):1768–1773

12. Schor EL. Rethinking well-child care. *Pediatrics.* 2004;114(1):210–216

Important note: Given the relative frequency with which code and valuation revisions occur, articles related to coding may not reflect the most current information available. Please check the online version of this article at http://practice.aap.org/content.aspx?aid=2775 and the *AAP Pediatric Coding Newsletter* at http://coding.aap.org for updated guidance.

Because the American Academy of Pediatrics (AAP) is not able to verify the accuracy of the facts relating to a patient encounter, we cannot be held responsible for any coding decisions that you make based on the guidance you receive from the AAP. It is your responsibility to only code for what you do during a patient encounter.

Current Procedural Terminology Category II Codes: Pay-for-Performance Measures

Category II *Current Procedural Terminology (CPT®)* codes were developed to simplify reporting of performance measures and eliminate the need for chart abstraction. These supplemental tracking codes are used by physicians and hospitals to report specific services that contribute to positive outcomes and high-quality care. The performance measures used to establish Category II *CPT* codes are developed by national organizations including the National Committee for Quality Assurance and the American Medical Association (AMA) Physician Consortium for Performance Improvement (PCPI) based on quality measures currently accepted and used in the health care industry.

The Centers for Medicare & Medicaid Services (CMS) led the way for pay-for-performance programs by establishing a voluntary reporting program in January 2006. As part of this program, CMS is collecting data on evidence-based quality measures for the Medicare population through the use and reporting of Healthcare Common Procedure Coding System (HCPCS) Level II codes **G8006–G8186.** For reporting performance measures to Medicare, either the appropriate Category II *CPT* code or HCPCS Level II G code is used.

Category II *CPT* codes are used for reporting purposes only and therefore do not have values assigned on the Medicare physician fee schedule (Resource-Based Relative Value Scale or RBRVS). The reporting of Category II *CPT* codes is optional, and these codes are not used in place of Category I *CPT* codes. However, they may be very beneficial to a practice, because they allow internal monitoring of performance, patient compliance, and outcomes.

Performance Measurement Codes

Category II *CPT* codes have been developed for 9 clinical conditions (including complete performance measurement sets) and 5 screening measures. The treatment of asthma is the only performance measure that currently applies to the pediatric population. If a pediatric practice cares for patients 18 years or older, it may report Category II *CPT* testing and treatment codes for hypertension, diabetes mellitus, and community-acquired bacterial pneumonia and screening codes for tobacco use and cessation. The American

Academy of Pediatrics (AAP) served as a leading organization in the development of performance measures for pediatric acute gastroenteritis, otitis media with effusion, and acute otitis externa through the AMA PCPI measure development process. The AAP also is participating in the development of measures for outpatient parenteral antibiotic therapy and adolescent major depressive disorder.

Each Category II *CPT* code describes the performance of a clinical service that is typically included in an evaluation and management (E/M) code or a test result that is part of a laboratory procedure. This is an additional reason that there are no relative value units assigned to Category II *CPT* codes.

These codes are grouped within categories based on established clinical documentation methods (eg, history, physical findings, assessment, plan). Each code identifies the specific clinical condition and performance measured. The categories are defined as follows:

Composite measures: 0001F–0015F

Several measures are grouped to facilitate reporting of a clinical condition when all included components are met.

Patient management: 0500F–0526F

These codes are used to describe utilization measures or measures of patient care provided for specific clinical purposes (eg, prenatal care, pre- and postsurgical care, referrals).

Patient history: 1000F–1137F

Patient history codes are used to describe measures for aspects of patient history and review of systems.

Physical examination: 2000F–2044F

These codes describe aspects of the physical examination or clinical assessment.

Diagnostic screening processes or results: 3006F–3354F

These codes are used to report results of clinical laboratory tests and radiologic or other procedural examinations.

Therapeutic, preventive, or other interventions: 4000F–4250F

Codes in the **4000F** range describe pharmacologic, procedural, or behavioral therapies, including preventive services such as patient education and counseling.

Follow-up or other outcomes: 5005F–5062F

These codes are used to describe the review and communication of test results to patients, patient satisfaction or experience with care, and patient functional status.

Patient safety: 6005F–6045F

Code **6005F** is used to report the rationale (eg, severity of illness and safety) for the recommended level of care (eg, home, hospital) for a patient. It identifies whether an assessment was made to determine the level of care required for patients with community-acquired pneumonia.

Structural measures: 7010F–7025F

These codes are used to identify measures that address the setting or system of the delivered care.

Category II Modifiers

Four Category II modifiers (**1P**, **2P**, **3P**, and **8P**) are used to report services that were considered but not provided because of medical reason(s), patient choice, or system reasons.

Modifier **1P** (performance measure exclusion modifier due to medical reasons) is used to report that one of the performance measures was not performed, because it was not indicated (eg, already performed) or was contraindicated (eg, because of a patient's allergy).

Modifier **2P** (performance measure exclusion modifier due to patient choice) is used to report that the performance measure was not performed because of a patient's religious, social, or economic reasons; the patient declined (ie, noncompliance with treatment); or other specific reasons.

Modifier **3P** (performance measure exclusion modifier due to system reasons) is used to report that the performance measure was not performed because the payer does not cover the service, the resources to perform the service are not available, or other reasons attributable to the health care delivery system. These modifiers are only used with Category II codes and only when allowed based on the specific reporting instructions for each performance measure.

Modifier **8P** (performance measure reporting modifier—action not performed, not otherwise specified) is used as a reporting modifier to allow the reporting of circumstances when an action described in a measure's numerator is not performed and the reason is not otherwise specified.

Tip: Make sure that the medical record includes written documentation of patient noncompliance or other reason for nonperformance of the measure.

Reporting the Codes

When reporting Category II *CPT* codes, Appendix H (located in the back of the *CPT* manual) should be used in coordination with the Category II section in *CPT*. Appendix H includes an alphabetic index of performance measures by clinical condition or topic and includes the measure developer (eg, PCPI), the performance measure, description of the measure, and the associated code. It also directs the reader to the measure developer's Web site to access the complete description of the measure.

Users should always review the description of the Category II *CPT* code in the *CPT* manual and access the measure developer's Web site for the specification documents of the performance measure. For example, specifications and requirements for reporting performance measures for asthma are located at www.physicianconsortium.org.

Each performance measure outlined in Appendix H includes a symptom or activity assessment, numerator, denominator, percentage, and reporting instructions. A patient must meet the criteria specified in the denominator (*International Classification of Diseases, Ninth Revision, Clinical Modification [ICD-9-CM]* code) to be included in the numerator (Category II code) for a particular performance measure.

Let's see how this works when using Category II *CPT* codes for patients with asthma.

Your practice elects to report Category II *CPT* codes for your asthmatic patients who meet the patient selection criteria. This performance measure will apply to all patients 5 to 40 years of age with a documented diagnosis of asthma who were evaluated during at least one office visit during the reporting year for the frequency of daytime and nocturnal asthma symptoms. You meet all the criteria in the asthma measurement set as specified by the developer of the performance measurement.

You review the applicable codes as identified under the Category II *CPT* code section and Appendix H, and because there are constant updates to the Category II *CPT* codes, you refer to the AMA Web site to access the latest information on these codes (www.ama-assn.org/go/cpt).

Code **1005F** is used to report that asthma symptoms were evaluated in the patient who meets the criteria for the asthma performance measure. There are 2 codes to report patient history assessments for asthma. Code **1038F** is reported for assessment of patients with persistent asthma (mild, moderate, or severe) and code **1039F** is reported for assessment of patients with intermittent asthma. If a patient with persistent asthma is on prescribed preferred long-term control medication or an acceptable alternative treatment, code **4015F** is reported in addition to code **1038F**. Modifier **2P** (patient noncompliance) may be reported with code **4015F**. Modifier **1P** (measure not performed due to patient allergy) may not be reported with **4015F**.

Reporting the measures to a payer (electronically or with a CMS-1500 claim form) is done the same way as reporting any *CPT* code. Report the appropriate E/M code (eg, **99201–99215**) based on the level of service performed and documented with all the appropriate *ICD-9-CM* codes that were addressed during the course of the visit. Report the Category II *CPT* code that relates to the performance measure with any applicable Category II modifier. In this case, only the *ICD-9-CM* code for asthma **(493.00, 493.02)** will be linked to the Category II *CPT* codes.

Example

An 8-year-old established patient is seen with complaints of an upper respiratory infection (URI) and follow-up for moderate, persistent asthma. He is currently on albuterol and steroids administered by a metered-dose inhaler. His last exacerbation was a month ago. A brief history of present illness with review of the respiratory; ear, nose, and throat (ENT); and constitutional systems and past history is performed. Physical examination of the respiratory, ENT, and cardiovascular systems is performed. He is advised to take over-the-counter medications for his URI, his asthma is currently stable, prescriptions are renewed, and the physician discusses the criteria for an urgent follow-up visit.

This visit would be reported as follows:

99213   Established patient; expanded history and physical examination with low-complexity medical decision-making; *ICD-9-CM* **465.9** (URI), **493.00** (asthma, unspecified)

1005F   Asthma symptoms evaluated; *ICD-9-CM* **493.00**

1038F   Persistent asthma; *ICD-9-CM* **493.00**

4015F   Persistent asthma, long-term control medication prescribed; *ICD-9-CM* **493.00**

The appropriate *ICD-9-CM* code(s) is reported and linked to the procedure(s) based on the diagnosis(es) that is addressed during the course of the visit. Only the codes for asthma **(493.00, 493.02)** would be linked to the Category II *CPT* codes.

The reporting of Category II *CPT* codes is optional at this time, and the information is used for reporting purposes only.

By the Committee on Child Health Financing and the Steering Committee on Quality Improvement and Management

Important note: Given the relative frequency with which code and valuation revisions occur, articles related to coding may not reflect the most current information available. Please check the online version of this article at http://practice.aap.org/content.aspx?aid=2401 and the *AAP Pediatric Coding Newsletter* at http://coding.aap.org for updated guidance.

Because the American Academy of Pediatrics (AAP) is not able to verify the accuracy of the facts relating to a patient encounter, we cannot be held responsible for any coding decisions that you make based on the guidance you receive from the AAP. It is your responsibility to only code for what you do during a patient encounter.

What Are Consumer-Driven Health Plans, Health Savings Accounts, and Health Reimbursement Accounts?

The following is an excerpt from the PediaLink Module "Contract Negotiation With Payers." For additional information on this module to help physicians develop a better contract, see www.pedialink.org/cme/_coursefinder/CMEdetail.cfm?aid=31177&area=liveCME.

Consumer-Driven Heath Plans

Consumer-driven health plans (CDHPs) are the fastest-growing plan design across the country. In an attempt to reduce their health care costs, employers are shifting financial responsibility to their employees by offering health plans that feature high deductibles and coinsurance obligations. Most CDHPs feature favored coverage for wellness services such as immunizations, well-child visits, and periodic checkups. Inherent in these models is the increased responsibility for the patient and family to pay a larger amount of the pediatrician's bill.

CDHPs usually base reimbursement on a fee schedule. Typically, the fee schedule applies to all in-network services, even if the plan is not paying anything for the care you have provided. The most common high-deductible plan designs have a $1,500 annual individual deductible. Once the deductible is met, the plan then pays for services at 80% of a defined reasonable and customary fee schedule. But even if the plan is not paying for your care, how much the patient is required to pay you and how much you are required to accept is still governed by your contract with the plan and fee schedule.

Health Savings Accounts

Health savings accounts (HSAs) are tax-favored savings accounts funded with pretax dollars by the individual or the employer. The individual can withdraw money from the account at any time with no penalty or taxes to pay for qualified medical expenses. An HSA can be established only in conjunction with high-deductible health insurance plans that meet Internal Revenue Service rules that set the amount of the individual and family deductible. The amount an employee can put in an HSA is capped at the amount of his or her annual deductible of his or her health insurance policy, but many people put less money aside in their HSA. Any unused funds each year remain in the account, accumulate tax-free, and can be used for future medical expenses.

Health Reimbursement Accounts

Health reimbursement accounts (HRAs) are funded by the employer and can be used by an employee as pretax dollars. These accounts can be set up independent of any specific health plan or benefit design. Moneys can be used by the employee to pay for medical expenses. HRA funds can be carried over from year to year. The amount of the contributions to the HRA varies based on the employer's discretion. The employer owns the fund, and any unused amounts may or may not be transferred on termination of employment depending on the terms of the fund. Medical spending accounts and flexible spending accounts are versions of HRAs with particular features.

Visit the following link for more information: www.pedialink.org/cme/_coursefinder/CMEdetail.cfm?aid=31177&area=liveCME

Additional Resources

- Office Financial Policy: http://practice.aap.org/content.aspx?aID=2184 (see sample on page 235)
- Options for Charging Up Front for Health Savings Accounts: http://practice.aap.org/content.aspx?aID=2251

Health Savings Account Algorithm

Do you wonder if you can charge patients who have health savings accounts (HSAs) at the time of their visit?

Because patients have an HSA does not automatically mean that the physician can bill the amount due at the point of service. This is dependent on the physician's contract with the health plan carrier, state regulations, and the amount of money in the account. To find out if you can bill at the point of service, use the algorithm below.

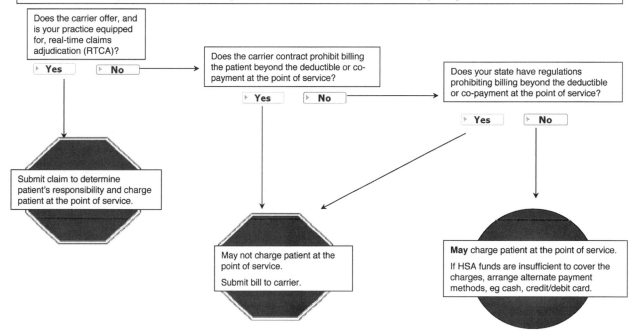

practice management online
Helping You Help Children

Health Savings Account Algorithm

Do you wonder if you can charge patients who have health savings accounts (HSAs) at the time of their visit?

Because patients have an HSA does not automatically mean that the physician can bill the amount due at the point of service. This is dependent on the physician's contract with the health plan carrier, state regulations, and the amount of money in the account.

To find out if you can bill at the point of service, complete the following questions.

This is intended as a guide and practices are urged to review their carrier contracts concerning billing under HSAs.

Does the carrier offer, and is your practice equipped for, real-time claims adjudication (RTCA)?

▸ Yes   ▸ No

Submit claim to determine patient's responsibility and charge patient at the point of service.

Does the carrier contract prohibit billing the patient beyond the deductible or co-payment at the point of service?

▸ Yes   ▸ No

May not charge patient at the point of service.

Submit bill to carrier.

Does your state have regulations prohibiting billing beyond the deductible or co-payment at the point of service?

▸ Yes   ▸ No

May charge patient at the point of service.

If HSA funds are insufficient to cover the charges, arrange alternate payment methods, eg cash, credit/debit card.

Medical Liability and Risk Management

A Liability Checklist for the Primary Care Office: "No Chinks in the Armor"

Robert A. Mendelson, MD, FAAP
Member, Committee on Medical Liability and Risk Management

Experienced pediatricians know the value of carefully evaluating their practice styles and clinic operations to find any "chinks in their protective armor" that might make their practices vulnerable to malpractice suits. This is especially important in today's health care environment with so many physicians working in troubling malpractice times.

The medical malpractice crisis that began in 2000 has remained a stubborn problem in all but 7 states—California, Colorado, Indiana, Louisiana, New Mexico, Texas, and Wisconsin. All of these states have some type of **effective tort reform.** The other 43 states are either in crisis now (21 states) or experiencing problems in limited areas (22 states). With no federal medical liability reform on the horizon and many states having existing tort reforms challenged in the courts (eg, limits on noneconomic damages and statute of limitations for minors), prudent pediatricians are looking for ways to tighten operations and change behavior to reduce medical errors and the likelihood of malpractice actions.

The proper way to approach risk management is through a process that identifies, evaluates, and addresses problems in our practices that may
1. Injure patients
2. Lead to malpractice claims
3. Cause financial loss to health care entities (especially one's own practice)

Effective risk management depends on reliable recognition of risk exposure, **determination** of its causes, **implementation** of corrective action, and **continual monitoring** of risk indicators to determine if the risk exposure is resolved.

To understand how and why malpractice claims are initiated, it is important to be familiar with the "anatomy" of a lawsuit. Four criteria must be met for a tort to be successful.

1. The existence of the physician's duty to the plaintiff (usually based on the existence of the physician-patient relationship)
2. The applicable standard of care and its violation (ie, breach of the physician's duty)
3. Damages (a compensable injury)
4. A causal connection between the violation of the standard of care and the injury

Each of these must be proved in court, and that is where many of the problems arise.

Typically, a physician-patient relationship is established by a face-to-face medical encounter, but it also can be established by non–face-to-face medical encounters, such as telephone, e-mail, or telemedicine. This aspect can be complicated and confusing. Courts have found that a subspecialist who was "curbstoned" about a particular patient by the general pediatrician can be named and sued despite never having had contact with the patient.

The applicable "standard of care" is defined as "what a reasonable practitioner in that specialty would do under the same circumstances." If the care provided to the patient does not meet this standard, it is considered a "breech of duty." In many suits, this becomes the central matter of contention with experts on both sides testifying as to whether the standard of care was met.

Finally, expert testimony is used to prove by a preponderance of the evidence whether the breech of duty was the proximate cause of injury.

But, take heart. Remember that 60% to 70% of all suits against physicians are eventually dropped or settled with no payment on the behalf of the defendant. In cases that go to court, 80% to 90% are won by the defendant physician.

According to the Physician Insurers Association of America, an association of more than 40 medical liability insurance carriers, diagnostic interview (taking the medical history) is the procedure that resulted in most claims against pediatricians both in 2005 and in the cumulative data. Of the 6,631 pediatric claims that were closed from 1985 to 2005, 48.6% involved the performance of a diagnostic interview, evaluation, or consultation. Some $221 million of the $407 million paid on behalf of pediatricians involved this procedure. By contrast, the next most prevalent procedure that resulted in claims against pediatricians was a general physical examination (16.8% of claims and 18.3% of indemnity payments).

Staying out of court is the best game plan. Following are some risk-management strategies for pediatricians:

1. **A careful, well-written, legible record** is always the best defense and is essential to practicing good medicine. Since most suits are filed months to years after the "event," remember that we don't always remember. Typically, the physician (now "defendant") may have little or no memory of the "event" because so much time has elapsed since the occurrence. The plaintiff seems to "remember exactly" what happened, what was said, what the result was, and when discussions and treatment occurred. Medical records need to be complete, accurate, timely, and never erased or altered inappropriately. If a chart correction is necessary, draw a line through the words to be changed (leaving them legible) and write or dictate a corrected note at the end of the record explaining the reason for the correction. If you are concerned that a bad outcome or vulnerable occurrence may precipitate a malpractice action, dictate a detailed narrative as soon as possible and date and time it accurately. Preparing this document while details are fresh in your mind can often serve as your "memory" when it is needed months to years later. Also, consider notifying your insurance carrier, who may consult with you, open a file, and await further developments. Early claims management can be invaluable.

2. **Review and initial all laboratory and imaging studies** and correspondence before placing them in the chart. Implement a process for alerting the physician to "panic values" and "abnormal" results as soon as the reports are received.

3. Hospital charts must be reviewed daily, especially notes from hospitalists, residents, and nurses, and all progress notes.

4. **Document important phone contacts.** Any *medically relevant* information obtained or given during a telephone call should be documented. Conversations with patients, emergency physicians, telephone triage services, and others with whom you have offered patient-management advice, such as calls regarding referrals to other physicians, probable drug reactions, changes in medication, severe injuries, and potentially serious symptoms. Have qualified, trained staff use pediatric telephone triage protocols that have been reviewed by the supervising physician. Review telephone encounter reports from after-hours call centers and answering services in a timely fashion before they are filed with telephone logs or in patient charts. Develop a system for documenting after-hours calls (eg, dictate a message on your office or mobile phone voice mail, use a PDA, or use preprinted sticky notes that can be stuck in the patient chart later). Note when delayed entries are made. Documenting the callback instructions given to parents often is as important as documenting symptoms reported to the doctor. The Section on Telephone Care suggests giving the advice, "Call me back if your child's symptoms *Persist*, if they *Change* or are *Worsening*, or if they cause you *Anxiety*. Also, I need to know if they include any of the following symptoms that are *Specific* to your child's condition." Document it using the abbreviation PCWAS. Retain telephone call logs in compliance with applicable laws.

5. Educate patients on your practice style, availability, and billing policies via a practice brochure.

6. Know your office billing practices; make sure no patient account is sent for collection without your knowledge. Not paying a bill may be a patient's way of expressing dissatisfaction with care provided. Have someone in the office contact the family *before* the account is turned over to a collection agency.

7. Continue your medical education with continuing medical education (CME), especially areas in which you feel you could use more training.

8. Use risk-management resources from the American Academy of Pediatrics (AAP), including the "Pediatricians and the Law" column in *AAP News*. A copy of *Medical Liability for Pediatricians*

(6th edition) should be available as a reference in every pediatric office. Attendance at loss-prevention workshops, whether presented by your insurer, your medical society, the AAP, or others, should be high on our list of CME priorities.

9. Practice good medicine, know your limitations, and consult and refer as needed.

10. **Listen** and talk to your patients; try to never appear rushed; consider ending each patient encounter with something like, "Is there anything else we should discuss?"

11. Don't "bad-mouth" another physician regarding care provided, particularly based on a patient's description of the event. This is the initiating incident in many malpractice suits. Remember, the patient is presenting only one subjective side of the story.

12. Notify your medical liability insurance carrier right away if patient records are requested by an attorney.

13. Long-term solutions include supporting tort reform in your state and nationally, and encouraging your colleagues to do the same.

14. Conduct a loss-prevention review of your charts from time to time. A checklist, Minimizing Medical Liability Risk with Patient Chart Audits for Pediatric Practices (http://practice.aap.org/public/Chart%20Audit%20PMO.doc), is provided as an online exclusive.

CMS Issues Final Stark Phase III Regulations

AAP Committee on Medical Liability and Risk Management

The Centers for Medicare & Medicaid Services (CMS) announced on August 27 that the long-awaited Phase III physician self-referral final rule would be published in the September 5 *Federal Register.*

According to the 516-page display copy posted by CMS, the final rule responds to comments on the March 26, 2006, Phase II interim final rule with comment period (69 Fed. Reg. 16054), which set forth the self-referral prohibition and applicable definitions, interpreted various statutory exceptions, and created additional regulatory exceptions for arrangements that do not pose a risk of program or patient abuse.

CMS said the Phase III final rule in general reduces "the regulatory burden on the health care industry through the interpretation of statutory exceptions and modification of the exceptions that were created using the Secretary's discretionary authority...."

With respect to indirect compensation arrangements, CMS explains in the final rule that the relationship between the physician and his or her physician organization is disregarded and the physician "stands in the shoes" of his or her physician organization.

According to CMS, the "effect of this new provision is that many arrangements that would have constituted indirect compensation arrangements if analyzed under Phase I and Phase II are now deemed to be direct compensation arrangements, and the indirect

compensation arrangements exception cannot be used."

Moreover, under the Phase III final rule, "many arrangements that may not have met the definition of an 'indirect compensation arrangement' under the Phase I and Phase II analysis will constitute direct compensation arrangements that must satisfy the requirements of an exception in order for the physician to make DHS referrals to the entity furnishing DHS."

CMS adds that the "stand in the shoes" provisions are applicable as of the effective date of the Phase III final rule, but that arrangements satisfying the Phase II definition of "indirect compensation arrangement" as well as other regulatory requirements as of the date the final rule is published need not be amended during the original or current renewal term of the arrangement to comply with the Phase III final regulations.

One thing is certain. This latest iteration of the Stark Regulations will take considerable legal advice and expertise to tease out the implications for physician organizations.

To view a prepublication edition of the regulations, visit http://www.cms.hhs.gov/PhysicianSelfReferral/Downloads/CMS-1810-F.pdf.

Health Insurance Portability and Accountability Act of 1996 (HIPAA) Administrative Simplification

On August 21, 1996, the Health Insurance Portability and Accountability Act of 1996 (HIPAA) was signed into law. One part of the law requires the adoption of uniform national standards for health information, establishing how information should be formatted, shared, and protected. This will affect every aspect of pediatric practice, and you should begin now to understand HIPAA. Over the next 2 years, the American Academy of Pediatrics (AAP) will develop summaries and sample materials to help you incorporate these requirements into your practice.

Protecting Health Information

Standardization of electronic transactions in health care will greatly facilitate the sharing of data, raising concerns about how the data will be protected. HIPAA required the first-ever national standards for privacy protections of health information. The privacy rule establishes significant restrictions on the use and release of medical records, describes privacy safeguard standards that must be met, gives patients several important rights, and provides for significant penalties for misuse of health information. In addition to concerns about privacy of health information, increased exchange and compilation of electronic health information raises concerns about physical and technical security. HIPAA requires the adoption of a national standard for security of electronic health information. The 1998 proposed rule describes minimum security requirements, and requires each health care organization covered by the rule to designate a security official.

Standards for Electronic Transmission

The core element of administrative simplification is to require the use of a single standardized format for 10 common health care transactions including health care claims, eligibility inquiries, referral certification and authorization, and payment. In these transactions the use of specific clinical code sets, including *Current Procedural Terminology* and *International Classification of Diseases, Ninth Revision,* is required. The use of national standard identifiers for providers, health plans, and employers will also be required. The requirement for a national identifier for individuals has been extremely controversial, and in the fall of 1998, Congress prohibited the promulgation of a national patient identifier.

Who Is Covered by HIPAA?

The AAP expects that most pediatricians will be covered by HIPAA because they submit electronic claims themselves and/or use a billing service or clearinghouse to convert paper claims to electronic format. The HIPAA Administrative Simplification provisions apply to certain covered entities
- All health plans or payers
- All health care clearinghouses
- Health care providers who electronically conduct any of the 10 HIPAA transactions or who use a clearinghouse to electronically conduct transactions on the providers' behalf

Final rules have been published on standards for electronic transactions and privacy of health information. Covered providers must comply with the transactions rule by October 16, 2002, and with the privacy rule by April 14, 2003. Proposed rules on security, national provider identifiers, and national employer identifiers were published in 1998. No other proposed or final rules have been published yet, and Department of Health and Human Services (HHS) has no expected date for publication.

Privacy of Health Information

On December 28, 2000, the HHS published a final rule on the privacy of health information under HIPAA, establishing the first national standards for the privacy of medical records. Covered providers, including most pediatricians, will have to comply with the privacy rule by April 14, 2003, as will all health care clearinghouses and large health plans. (Small plans have until April 14, 2004, to comply.) The rule applies to all individually identifiable health information held or disclosed by one of these covered entities in any form.

The privacy rule establishes significant restrictions on the use and release of medical records. Generally, patient information can only be used for purposes of treatment, payment, and health care operations, and providers must obtain general signed consent for disclosures for these purposes. Under specific guidelines established by the rule, health information can be used or disclosed without consent for purposes such as public health, health oversight, and research.

Health information cannot be used for purposes not described in the rule without explicit authorization from the individual. Disclosures of information must be limited to the minimum necessary for the purpose of the disclosure, except that the full record may be disclosed to health care providers for treatment purposes.

What Providers Must Do

The rule describes privacy safeguard standards that covered entities must meet, but it leaves detailed policies and procedures for meeting these standards to the discretion of each covered entity. Health care providers and other covered entities must
- Adopt written privacy procedures.
- Take steps to ensure that their business associates protect the privacy of health information.
- Train employees.
- Designate a privacy officer.
- Establish grievance processes.

Rights Granted to Patients

In addition to these restrictions and administrative requirements for covered entities, the privacy rule gives patients several important rights.
- Providers and health plans are required to give patients a clear written explanation of how they can use, keep, and disclose patient information.
- Patients must be able to see and get copies of their records and request amendments to their records.
- A history of most disclosures must be made accessible to patients.
- Providers and health plans generally cannot condition treatment or payment on a patient's agreement to disclose health information for non-routine uses.
- People have the right to complain to a covered entity, or to the secretary of HHS, about privacy violations.

Penalties

HIPAA provides for significant penalties for misuse of health information. Covered entities that violate the privacy rule would be subject to civil penalties of $100 per incident, up to $25,000 per person, per year, per standard; and federal criminal penalties of up to $50,000 and 1 year in prison for obtaining or disclosing protected health information; up to $100,000 and 5 years in prison for obtaining protected health infor-

mation under "false pretenses"; and up to $250,000 and 10 years in prison for obtaining or disclosing protected health information with the intent to sell, transfer, or use it for commercial advantage, personal gain, or malicious harm.

How the Privacy Rule Applies to Children and Adolescents

In general, the privacy rule allows parents to exercise privacy rights on behalf of their unemancipated minor children. If a particular health care service meets one of the following criteria, however, the health care provider is not allowed to share information concerning that service with the parent:
- The minor consents to the health care service, no other consent to that service is required by law, even if a parent's consent was obtained, and the minor has not requested that the parent be given the privacy rights for that service.
- The minor may lawfully obtain the health care service without the consent of a parent, and the minor, a court, or another person authorized by law consents to the service.
- The parent assents to an agreement of confidentiality between a provider and the minor with respect to the health care service.

Resources From the AAP

The AAP will continue its efforts to educate pediatricians about HIPAA and to advocate for HIPAA implementation that works for children's health care. More information on HIPAA is available on the AAP Member Center (www.aap.org/moc) and on *Practice Management Online* at http://practice.aap.org/hipaa.aspx.

For more information about HIPAA and its effect on pediatricians, e-mail HIPAA@aap.org, or call the AAP Division of Pediatric Practice at 800/433-9016, ext 4089.

Improve Vaccine Liability Protection

To maximize pediatrician liability protection, physicians should improve compliance with the Vaccine Injury Compensation Program (VICP). Just giving parents Vaccine Information Statements (VISs) is not enough. Chapters can help pediatricians by teaching them to use the 4 Ds—Distribute, Discuss, Document, and Dialogue—of vaccine risk communication.

Distribute

The National Childhood Vaccine Injury Act (NCVIA) requires that vaccine providers distribute a VIS for vaccines covered by the National VICP or purchased through a contract with the Centers for Disease Control and Prevention (CDC) each time the vaccine is given (even if the VIS has been given for a previous dose). Despite this federal requirement, only 6 out of 10 pediatricians report distributing a VIS with each dose of vaccine.[1]

Discuss

The VIS should be a springboard for discussing the risk communication. Pediatricians should provide oral and/or visual explanations as needed and confirm that parents understand the risks and benefits of specific vaccines. This discussion is especially important for persons unable to read, but should be implemented for all patients.

Document

The NCVIA requires the provider to document the name, address, and title of the person administering the vaccine, the date of vaccine administration, and the vaccine manufacturer and lot number of the vaccine used. Providers should also include the VIS edition date in their documentation and affirm that the VIS was distributed and discussed with the patient. To aid physicians with documentation, the American Academy of Pediatrics (AAP) has created a vaccine administration documentation form, which is available for purchase. Remember that in many liability cases "if it isn't documented, it didn't happen."

Dialogue

Sometimes parents don't want their children immunized. Pediatricians should maintain open dialogue with parents who have doubts about immunizations and over time try to establish a trusting relationship by seeking to understand their reasons for refusal. Pediatricians need to explain the risks of not vaccinating and should have them sign an informed refusal document at each visit during which vaccination is declined. A sample AAP Refusal to Vaccinate form is available on page 239.

A VIS is a 1-page, double sided information sheet produced by the CDC that explains the risks and benefits of vaccination. VISs are available through state health departments, by calling the National Immunization Information Hotline at 800/232-4636 (English and Spanish), and on the Internet at the following Web sites: www.aap.org, www.cdc.gov/nip, and www.immunize.org.

For more information on medical liability, *Medical Liability for Pediatricians,* 6th edition, is available for purchase (http://eweb.aap.org/pub39077). The manual focuses on practical approaches to avoiding liability exposure, with updated material on risk management, vaccine liability, and more. Also included are easy-to-use tools including documentation dos and don'ts and additional resources.

CDC expert speakers are available to present on VIS and other topics pertaining to immunizations. For additional information, or to request a speaker for an upcoming conference, please contact cispimmunize@aap.org.

---

1. American Academy of Pediatrics. Periodic survey #48: experiences with medical liability. Available at: http://www.aap.org/research/periodicsurvey/ps48aexs.htm. Accessed July 15, 2003

Reducing Vaccine Liability: Strategies for Pediatricians

General Background Information

The National Childhood Vaccine Injury Act (NCVIA) of 1986 was enacted to respond to public health concerns about vaccines and reduce vaccine liability. Through the NCVIA, the National Vaccine Injury Compensation Program (VICP) (http://www.hrsa.gov/vaccinecompensation/) was established to maintain an accessible and efficient forum for individuals thought to be injured by childhood vaccines. The VICP is a no-fault alternative to the traditional tort system for resolving vaccine injury claims. The VICP covers all vaccines recommended by the Centers for Disease Control and Prevention (CDC) for routine administration to children. New vaccines incorporated into the routine immunization schedule (as recommended by the CDC Advisory Committee on Immunization Practices) will be automatically included in the Vaccine Injury Table.

Settlements are based on the Vaccine Injury Table (http://www.hrsa.gov/vaccinecompensation/table.htm), which summarizes medical conditions and the time interval of onset following receipt of a covered vaccine. It was created to justly compensate those injured by vaccines while separating out unrelated claims. The Vaccine Injury Table is continually updated as more information becomes available from research on vaccine side effects.

The NCVIA mandates that all health care professionals report certain adverse events that occur following vaccination. As a result, the US Food and Drug Administration and the CDC established the Vaccine Adverse Events Reporting System (VAERS) (http://www.vaers.org/) in 1990. VAERS provides a mechanism for the collection and analysis of adverse events associated with vaccines currently licensed in the United States. Adverse events are defined as health effects that occur after immunization that may or may not be related to the vaccine. While VAERS provides useful information on vaccine safety, the data are somewhat limited. Specifically, judgments about causality (whether the vaccine was truly responsible for an adverse event) cannot be made from VAERS reports because of incomplete information.

Anyone can file a VAERS report, including health care professionals, manufacturers, and vaccine recipients or, when appropriate, parents/guardians. VAERS report forms should be used to report adverse events. Pre-addressed, postage-paid report forms can be obtained by calling 800/822-7967 or through the VAERS Web site.

Strategies to Reduce Vaccine Liability

Provide Vaccine Information Statements— It's the Law!

The NCVIA requires physicians to notify all parents and patients of the benefits and risks of vaccines through the use of Vaccine Information Statements (VISs). Despite this, only 62% of pediatricians indicated that they gave out a VIS with each dose of vaccine (Davis TC, et al. *Pediatrics.* 2001; 107:e17). According to AAP Periodic Survey #48, 6 out of 10 pediatricians report distributing VIS with every dose of each vaccine. About one-fourth do so with the first dose only, 10% sometimes do so, and fewer than 6% say they never distribute VISs.

- VISs must be *produced by the CDC* and cannot be altered. Pediatricians may add the name, address, etc, of their practice, but substantive changes are not acceptable.
- The relevant VIS must be given prior to administration of *every dose* of the vaccine (including each dose of a multidose series).
- The VISs should be supplemented with visual presentations or verbal explanations, as appropriate.
- Pediatricians must provide the *most current* VIS to parents.

For more information on VISs, visit: http://www.cdc.gov/vaccines/pubs/vis/default.htm.

Correctly Document Required Vaccine Information

The NCVIA and/or CDC requires physicians to document the
- Date of vaccine administration
- Vaccine manufacturer
- Vaccine lot number
- Name and business address of the health care professional who administered the vaccine
- VIS version date
- Date the VIS was provided to the parent/guardian

The American Academy of Pediatrics (AAP) recommends also recording the
- Site and route of administration
- Vaccine expiration date
- Statement indicating that the VIS was provided and discussed with the parent

Vaccines that are not covered by the VICP do not require VISs to be provided, unless the vaccine is obtained through a CDC contract (ie, Vaccines for Children program). Any vaccine under CDC contract requires a VIS and documentation regardless of whether it is covered by VICP. The AAP recommends using the VISs and following the same record-keeping practices with all vaccines. Table 1 provides a summary of documentation recommendations.

Be Informed About Parental Consent Requirements

While obtaining a parental signature on the VIS is optional, it is common practice for pediatricians to request that parents initial each individual VIS. Pediatricians should check with their hospital's office of legal affairs or their state's immunization program manager for current state medical consent laws addressing vaccinations since such laws vary by state.
- Parental consent for immunization is standard practice in 43 states.
- Thirty-four states require separate consent for each injection when more than one injection is required to complete a vaccination series.

Address and Document Parental Refusal to Vaccinate

There are many reasons why parents refuse to vaccinate their children. Most commonly, parents are not aware or may have no memory of the seriousness of the diseases that vaccines prevent. Therefore, their concern frequently shifts from the *risk of disease* to the *risk of vaccines*. The proliferation of an increasingly vocal anti-vaccine movement, which produces a wealth of unreliable, emotionally charged information that is easily accessible to parents has also increased concern about vaccine safety.

Another reason parents may refuse to vaccinate relates to vaccine mandates for school entry. Parents may feel that their right to make decisions for their children is taken away. An ongoing debate regarding the duty of society to protect healthy children versus the right of families to make decisions has caused efforts in more than a dozen states to rescind vaccine mandates or provide philosophical exemptions (AAP Committee on Medical Liability, 2004).

If a parent refuses a recommended vaccine and their child later develops a disease, the issue of professional liability can arise. Therefore, documentation of a parental refusal is essential. Documentation should indicate that
- The parent was informed of why the vaccine is recommended.
- The parent was informed of the risks and benefits of vaccination.
- The parent was informed of the possible consequences of not vaccinating.
- Patient educational materials were provided.

The AAP Refusal to Vaccinate Form (see page 239), which should not be considered a legal document without advice from a lawyer, may be used as a template for documentation of parental refusal.

Table 1. Guidance for Use of Vaccine Information Statements[a]	
Distribution	**Documentation in the Patient's Medical Record**
Must be provided each time a National Vaccine Injury Compensation Program (VICP)-covered vaccine is administered[b]	Vaccine manufacturer, lot number, and date of administration[b]
Given to parent, legal guardian, or patient (non-minor) to keep[b]	Name and business address of the physician administering the vaccine[b]
Must be the current version[c]	Vaccine information Statement version date and date it is provided[c]
Can provide (not substitute) other written or audio-visual materials as necessary[d]	Site (eg, deltoid area), route of administration (eg, intramuscular), and expiration date of the vaccine[d]

[a]Source: AAP Committee on Medical Liability. *Medical Liability for Pediatricians.* 6th Edition. 2004.
[b]Required under the National Childhood Vaccine Injury Act.
[c]Required under Centers for Disease Control and Prevention instructions implementing the National Childhood Vaccine Injury Act.
[d]Recommended by the American Academy of Pediatrics.

The form can be revised based on the needs of individual practices.

Pediatric Practice Resources

- AAP Committee on Medical Liability, *Medical Liability for Pediatricians*: http://eweb.aap.org/pub39077
- AAP Committee on Medical Liability Web site: http://www.aap.org/visit/comlhome.htm
- AAP Childhood Immunization Support Program (CISP) Vaccine Liability Web site: http://www.aap.org/immunization/pediatricians/liability.html
- Vaccine Injury Compensation Program Web site: http://www.hrsa.gov/vaccinecompensation/
- Vaccine Injury Table: http://www.hrsa.gov/osp/vicp/table.htm
- Vaccine Adverse Events Reporting System Web site: http://www.vaers.org

- AAP CISP Vaccine Information Statements Fact Sheet: http://www.aap.org/immunization/pediatricians/liability.html
- Immunization Action Coalition Vaccine Information Statement Web site (VISs in over 30 languages): http://www.immunize.org/vis/index.htm#index
- AAP CISP Improve Vaccine Liability Protection: The 4 D's Fact Sheet: http://www.aap.org/immunization/pediatricians/pdf/ImproveVaccineLiabilityProtection.pdf
- AAP Refusal to Vaccinate Form: http://www.aap.org/immunization/pediatricians/refusaltovaccinate.html and page 239
- AAP Committee on Bioethics Policy Statement "Responding to Parental Refusals of Immunization of Children": http://aappolicy.aappublications.org/cgi/reprint/pediatrics;115/5/1428.pdf

Risk Management Strategies for the Consultant

1. Foster relationships with referring physicians. Work with them to make sure they communicate the urgency of the referral requests and that expectations, roles, and responsibilities are clearly established prospectively.
2. If you cannot accommodate the patient within the time period needed, advise the patient and the referring physician as soon as possible so that other arrangements can be made. Document this notification.
3. Specify the records, films, and test results to be available for the appointment and who should be responsible for securing them.
4. The consultant should document the available information at the time of the consult and any gaps.
5. Document consultations with primary care physicians, even "curbside" discussions, and specify your understanding of the nature of the informal nature of the conversation.
6. Follow up with patients and send timely reports to primary care physicians.
7. Make sure the "hand-off," the transfer of care back to the referring physician, is clean and understood by all parties. Notify patients in writing of termination of care and keep good records.
8. Pay attention to cases with potential foreseeable risks.

Additional Resources

- AAP policy statements regarding medical liability and malpractice: http://practice.aap.org/content.aspx?aid=1981
- Consultation or Referral?: http://practice.aap.org/content.aspx?aid=1284
- Consultation Request Form: http://practice.aap.org/content.aspx?aid=1332
- Risk Management for the Primary Care Pediatrician: http://practice.aap.org/content.aspx?aid=1290

Managing Medical Liability Risks for Telephone Care

Excerpt from Payment for Telephone Care: A Toolkit

Pediatricians should be aware that telephone care with patients has many of the same medical liability pitfalls as office visits, and a few additional risks unique to non–face-to-face care. This chapter suggests ways to manage legal risks specific to pediatric telephone care.

Establishing a Doctor-Patient Relationship

A doctor-patient relationship may be created if a physician provides medical advice to a patient (or the parent/legal guardian of a minor patient) over the telephone. With that relationship comes a legal duty, one of the foundations for a malpractice claim. The American Academy of Pediatrics (AAP) policy statement on payment for telephone care advises pediatricians to limit telephone advice to established patients whom they have previously examined and gathered a history, and with whom they have a prior doctor-patient relationship.

Documentation of Calls

While there is some controversy over the degree to which telephone calls with patients must be documented, it is clear that any medically relevant information obtained or given during a call should be recorded. Referrals to other physicians, probable drug reactions, changes in medication, severe injuries, and potentially serious symptoms are examples of these.

After-hours calls are frequently taken "on the run" by physicians, and a system must be developed for ensuring that documentation reaches the patient's chart in a timely fashion. Some physicians leave a message on the office answering machine or with their answering service. Others dictate a message into their mobile phone (if it has that feature), and others use PDAs or inscribe notations on low-tech telephone encounter forms at the time of the call that can be pasted into a patient chart later. Delayed entries should include the time the note was entered into the chart as well as the time the call was received. If you plan to bill for telephone care, the documentation will need to be even more thorough (see Chapter 7 of *Payment for Telephone Care: A Toolkit* at http://practice.aap.org/content.aspx?aID=2266).

Documenting the call-back instructions given to parents is often as important as documenting the reported symptoms. In many cases, these can be abbreviated simply as **PCWAS**: "Call me back if your child's symptoms *Persist,* if they *Change* or are *Worsening,* or if they cause you *Anxiety.* Also I need to know if they include any of the following symptoms that are *Specific* to your child's condition." (For example, vomiting, sleepiness, or severe headache after head trauma.) It is also important to document conversations with telephone triage services, emergency department physicians, and others with whom you have offered patient-management advice.

Avoid a Wellness Bias

When a patient has been examined by you or another physician in the recent past, and little pathology was found, there is a tendency to be overly reassured by that examination. Each call must be treated in a "stand-alone" manner to be certain that new or worsening symptoms receive prompt attention. A common source of telephone liability occurs when physicians don't respond appropriately to a patient's complaints after a recent benign examination. Be wary when the patient is reported to "look much sicker" or "has much more pain" since the prior encounter.

Watch for "Hidden Agendas"

Whenever calls seem inappropriate for the time of day, the number of calls about a single symptom seem excessive, or the degree of anxiety exhibited by the parent is out of proportion for the problem, the real reason for the call may be different from the symptoms being presented. It is best to politely answer the parent's questions first, and then follow with a question like "You have called about this three times today. The symptoms don't sound serious to me. Is there something else I need to know?" The most important response from a parent is "I can't put my finger on what is wrong, but my child just isn't acting right and I really feel frightened by the way he looks."

Use Language That Is Descriptive and Unambiguous

Because the child is not actually seen over the telephone, it is sometimes necessary to develop a specialized telephone language to evaluate the severity of illness. "Trouble breathing" can mean severe dyspnea or a stuffy nose. It is preferred to ask about "straining or working hard to breathe" or "pulling to get air in and out." Similarly, learning that a febrile child has a rash may not be helpful without knowing whether it looks like "bleeding or bruising under the skin" or whether it has the sudden appearance of "red freckles."

Protect Patient Confidentiality

The Health Insurance Portability and Accountability Act of 1996 (HIPAA) regulations apply to telephone calls between patients and medical staff. Conversations with and about patients (with pharmacies, other physicians, therapists, etc) should be conducted in places where names and sensitive information will remain private. Be especially wary of answering requests for patient information from individuals who represent themselves as family members, insurance representatives, and helpful friends—especially following trauma. Before sharing information, you must be certain of the caller's identity and obtain the permission of the parent or legal guardian of the minor patient. Telephone messages left with persons other than the child's parent or legal guardian or on answering machines should be purposely vague but not cause undue anxiety.

"This is Doctor Smith calling with laboratory results. Everything looks fine. Please call me for more information." (Note: Neither the patient's name or the specific tests were mentioned.)

Recorded Messages

Recorded messages on telephone answering machines should clearly state when and how often messages are retrieved. They should note that messages about emergencies should not be left at this site.

Practice Good Medicine

This is the best but not infallible protection against malpractice actions. It is also very important to remain an ally and advocate for your patients and their families. Statements like "This sounds terrible. I don't understand why you didn't call me sooner" may be intended to let parents know that a poor outcome is not your fault. Instead you might create parental guilt, making parents want to blame someone else, and your insensitivity might place you first on that list. A much better strategy is to express empathy with anxious parents' concerns. When you do, you are more likely to be rewarded with their loyalty and gratitude. Additional information on risk management and telephone care can be found in *Medical Liability for Pediatricians,* 6th edition, from the AAP (http://eweb. aap.org/pub39077).

Section 7

Patient Management

The information that follows is a summary of Chapter 4, "Effective Communication Techniques" from *Plain Language Pediatrics: Health Literacy Strategies and Communication Resources for Common Pediatric Topics*. The entire chapter can be downloaded by visiting http://practice.aap.org/content.aspx?aid=2816.

Whether written or verbal, communication is the cornerstone of partnering with parents and patients in pediatric care. A child who doesn't know how to ask for help after a certain age, and a parent who can't understand the medication label, contribute to prolonged or worsened symptoms, and both need our help to keep children healthy.

The most important idea to remember is to practice patient-centered care. Patient-centered (or family-centered) care includes using a style of communication that gives the patient or family a larger role in the patient-doctor interaction and the decision-making process. This approach has been shown to improve not only communication and compliance, but also patient satisfaction.

Following is a brief overview of additional tips:

Use Everyday Words, or "Plain Language"

- Use plain language (sometimes called "living-room language"). This can bridge that communication gap, in writing and in conversation.

Sit Down and Allow the Patient to Talk Too

- Don't feel the need to cover as much as possible within each visit.
- Prioritize topics for each visit based on the child's age and history. This can allow time for meaningful discussions with patients.
- Slow down when you talk, and slow the whole visit down so the patient and family can talk.

Focus Your Messages: Keep Information Simple and Relevant, and Repeat It

- Limit the amount of information provided at each visit, and focus on the few most significant things the parent and patient need to remember. For example, when you initially diagnose a child with asthma, first tell the family the most basic information on the condition and how it can be managed. On subsequent visits, you can introduce additional—and increasingly more detailed and complex—information about the condition.
- If you add only a few messages at a time, the family is more likely to remember all of them.
- Use the Ask Me tool to assist with this; it can be found at http://practice.aap.org/content. aspx?aid=2816.

Learn From Patients and Families

- Get to know your patients.
- Address their concerns before giving advice. This can alleviate any anxiety that may block their receptiveness to information.
- Ask about their perceptions of any illnesses, their causes, and their treatments that you discussed during the visit, but do so with sensitivity and respect.
- By broadening your cultural knowledge base, you can better treat other patients who share the same condition, background, or even neighborhood.
- Try to incorporate the family's treatment beliefs (eg, herbal medicines and teas for some Latino and Asian patients) into your treatment plan, as long as doing so won't cause harm to the child.

Be Sensitive to Culture

- Use terms that your audience is comfortable or at least familiar with.
- When identifying a group of people by race or ethnicity, use a term preferred by that group, and tailor messages to each cultural or ethnic group or subgroup.

Check Your Work

- Check to make sure patients and families have understood your important messages.
- One effective method is the teach-back. In this method, the doctor, nurse, or other member of the health care team delivers a key message, then asks the patient (or caregiver) a question that causes the patient to respond by putting the message in his or her own words.

Written Techniques to Improve Patient-Doctor Communication

- Write materials using logical organization with the reader in mind; "you" and other pronouns; active voice; short sentences; common, everyday words; and easy-to-read design features.

Addressing Special Populations

- It is essential to identify special patient populations within your practice who may require additional assistance for doctor-patient communication to be successful.

Limited English Proficiency

- Consider hiring bilingual staff and doctors to help interpret and translate complex information. They can also alert you to cultural sensitivities and instill in patients a sense of trust in your practice.
- Do not use nonclinical bilingual staff members for complex health information.

- Use only trained interpreters and do not use family members, especially children.

Hearing Impaired

- Providers must first evaluate whether the preference is to use sign or spoken language. If sign language is preferred, use an interpreter and pay particular attention to the type of sign language used by the patient. If spoken language is preferred, pay particular attention to the environment.
- Do not obscure your face with a mask, your hand, or anything else.
- Keep the room well lit and quiet.
- Don't stand in front of a bright window or light.
- Use appropriate plain language written information.
- Use teach-back, pictographs, signs, videos with closed captioning, and phone reminders.

Visit the AAP Online Bookstore (www.aap.org/bookstore) to purchase *Plain Language Pediatrics: Health Literacy Strategies and Communication Resources for Common Pediatric Topics.*

Plain language handouts are available at *Patient Education Online* at http://patiented.aap.org/categoryBrowse.aspx?catID=32

Health Literacy PediaLink module is also available at http://www.pedialink.org/cmefinder/search-detail.cfm/key/6588D972-F7F4-4D37-8512-B923591A7921/type/course/grp/4/task/details.

Responding to 7 Common Parental Concerns About Vaccines & Vaccine Safety

Over the years, studies have identified 7 common parental concerns about vaccines and immunization. The following information is designed to help pediatricians and other child health professionals address these concerns in the practice setting. Additional resources, including books, articles, and Web links to patient education materials, are provided.

1. Use of Thimerosal as an Additive in Vaccines

Some parents have expressed concerns about a potential link between health problems, particularly autism, and vaccines containing thimerosal. Thimerosal is a preservative that contains a form of mercury (organomercurial). Beginning in the 1930s, thimerosal was used in very small amounts as a preservative in vaccines. Thimerosal is effective in preventing bacterial and fungal contamination, particularly in opened multi-dose vaccine containers. In 1999 the Public Health Service agencies and the American Academy of Pediatrics (AAP) recommended that thimerosal be taken out of vaccines as a precautionary measure. By the end of 2001, all routine pediatric vaccines contained no thimerosal or only trace amounts (some influenza and Td vaccines). There is no convincing evidence of harm caused by the small amounts of thimerosal in vaccines, except for minor effects like swelling and redness at the injection site due to sensitivity to thimerosal.

Prior to the recent initiative to reduce or eliminate thimerosal from childhood vaccines, the maximum cumulative exposure to mercury via routine childhood vaccinations during the first 6 months of life was 187.5 micrograms. With the newly formulated vaccines, the maximum cumulative exposure during the first 6 months of life will now be less than 3 micrograms of mercury; this represents a greater than 98% reduction in the amount of mercury a child would receive from vaccines in the first 6 months of life. (Influenza [flu] vaccine is not given until 6 months or older.)

Resources
- Offit PA, Jew RK. Addressing parents' concerns: do vaccines contain harmful preservatives, adjuvants, additives, or residuals? *Pediatrics.*

2003;112:1394–1397
- AAP. What Parents Should Know About Thimerosal: http://www.aap.org/immunization/families/ingredients.html#thimerosal
- CDC. Mercury and Vaccines (Thimerosal): http://www.cdc.gov/vaccinesafety/updates/thimerosal.htm
- CDC. Vaccine Safety Datalink (VSD) Study, Safety of Thimerosal-Containing Vaccines: A Two-Phased Study of Computerized Health Maintenance Organization (HMO) Databases: http://www.cdc.gov/nip/vacsafe/concerns/thimerosal/researchQAs.htm#vsdres
- CDC. Mercury and Vaccines (Thimerosal): http://www.cdc.gov/nip/vacsafe/concerns/thimerosal/default.htm

2. MMR Vaccine and Autism

Autism is a common developmental disability, affecting an estimated 1 in 500 children. Because the measles, mumps, rubella (MMR) vaccine is first given at age 12 to 15 months, and the first signs of autism (ie, poor social interaction and speech, repetitive behaviors, etc) often appear at 15 to 18 months of age, concerns have been raised about a possible link between the vaccine and the development of autism.

Studies conducted in the United States and Europe have found no association between the MMR vaccine and autism. Over the years, the Institute of Medicine and the AAP have organized several panels of independent scientists to study MMR and autism—again, all concluded no association between MMR and autism. Research on this topic continues in an effort to ensure the safety of vaccines.

Although the cause of autism is unknown in most instances, the theory favored by many experts is that it is a genetically based disorder that occurs before birth. Evidence that genetics is an important, but not exclusive, cause of autism includes a 3% to 8% risk of recurrence in families with one affected child. Research on the cause of autism is ongoing.

Resources
- Halsey NA, Hyman SL, Conference Writing Panel. Measles-mumps-rubella vaccine and autism spectrum disorder: a report from the New Challenges

in Childhood Immunizations. *Pediatrics.*
2001;107:84
- AAP. MMR Vaccine and Autism: What Parents
  Need to Know: http://www.aap.org/immunization/
  families/autismfacts.html
- IAC. Does MMR Cause Autism? Examine the
  Evidence: http://www.immunize.org/catg.d/
  p4026.pdf
- CDC. Vaccines and Autism Theory: http://www.
  cdc.gov/vaccinesafety/concerns/mmr_autism_
  factsheet.htm

3. Importance of Hepatitis B Vaccine in Infancy

Some parents believe that the hepatitis B vaccine
should not be given to infants and children since it
is associated with high-risk behavior including intravenous drug use and sexual activity.

The hepatitis B vaccine is the best protection a child
can have against a dangerous and lifelong disease.
Before the vaccine was introduced, 20,000 children
younger than 10 years became infected each year.
Vaccinating early against hepatitis B ensures children's immunity when they are the most vulnerable
to the worst complications of the disease and before
they enter the high-risk adolescent years. Because of
common scrapes, falls, and lack of personal hygiene,
children (particularly in child care settings) are more
exposed to bodily fluids than some adults. Infants
who catch hepatitis B from their mothers at birth
are at a greater risk of suffering a premature death
from liver cancer or liver failure later in life.

Resources
- AAP. Summary—AAP Preference for Birth Dose
  of Hepatitis B: http://www.aap.org/immunization/
  illnesses/hepb/HepBguidance.doc
- IAC. Give the Birth Dose: Hepatitis B Vaccine
  at Birth Saves Lives: http://www.immunize.org/
  catg.d/p2125.pdf
- CDC. Hepatitis B: http://www.cdc.gov/nip/vacsafe/
  concerns/hepB/default.htm

4. Importance of Pneuomococcal Conjugate Vaccine

Prior to the pneumococcal vaccine, pneumococcus
bacteria was the leading cause of bacterial meningitis
infection in children younger than 5 years. Meningitis
symptoms in children are less obvious than in adults

and often go undetected and untreated. It is important to vaccinate children to protect them from this
uncertainty. Meningitis, an inflammation of the brain
and spinal cord, can lead to brain damage, mental
retardation, and even death. Pneumococcal conjugate
vaccine provides superior protection against this
serious and deadly infection.

Resources
- Overturf GD, Committee on Infectious Diseases.
  Technical report: prevention of pneumococcal
  infections, including the use of pneumococcal conjugate and polysaccharide vaccines and antibiotic
  prophylaxis. *Pediatrics.* 2000;106:367–376
- IAC. Pneumococcal Disease in Children: http://
  www.vaccineinformation.org/pneumchild/index.
  asp
- CDC. PCV7 Vaccine Q&A: http://www.cdc.gov/
  nip/vaccine/pneumo/pneumo-vacfaqs.htm

5. Importance of Meningococcal Conjugate Vaccine

Meningococcal disease is caused by bacteria that
infect the bloodstream, lining of the brain, and spinal
cord, often causing serious illness. Every year in the
US 1,400 to 2,800 people get meningococcal disease.
Ten percent to 14% of people with meningococcal disease die, and 11% to 19% of survivors have permanent
disabilities (such as mental retardation, hearing loss,
and loss of limbs).

In 2005 a new quadrivalent conjugate vaccine to
protect against invasive meningococcal disease was
licensed and recommended for children 11 to 12
years and teens entering high school, as well as
college freshmen living in dormitories. The vaccine
is licensed for use in adolescents and adults aged 11
to 55 years. A quadrivalent polysaccharide vaccine
has been available in the United States for many
years; however, it has not been recommended for
routine use.

Resources
- CDC. Meningococcal Vaccines Vaccine
  Information Statement: http://www.cdc.gov/
  nip/publications/VIS/vis-mening.pdf
- AAP. Policy Statement on Meningococcal
  Vaccine: http://aappolicy.aappublications.org/
  cgi/content/full/pediatrics;116/2/496

6. Relative Danger of Influenza (Need for Yearly Vaccination)

Some parents question the need for a yearly dose of the flu vaccine. They believe that influenza is a relatively mild disease (one that they have had and have survived) and that the risk of vaccination outweighs the risk of the disease. Parents also may have concerns about thimerosal in the flu vaccine (see above).

Influenza is a serious disease, and people of any age can get it. In an average year, the flu causes 36,000 deaths and 200,000 hospitalizations in the United States. The "flu season" is usually from November–April each year. An annual flu vaccine (either the flu shot or the nasal spray flu vaccine [in recommended age groups]) is the best way to reduce circulation of the flu. Annual shots are necessary because flu viruses change from year to year. This means that a person can get the flu more than once during their lifetime. The immunity that is built up from having the flu caused by one virus strain doesn't always provide protection when a new strain is circulating. In other words, a vaccine made against flu viruses circulating last year may not protect against the newer viruses. Further, immunity to the disease declines over time and may be too low to provide protection after 1 year.

Resources

- CDC. Questions & Answers: Thimerosal-Containing Influenza Vaccine: http://www.cdc.gov/flu/about/qa/thimerosal.htm
- CDC. Influenza Web site: http://www.cdc.gov/flu
- AAP Childhood Immunization Support Program. Influenza Guidance Web site: http://www.aap.org/immunization/illnesses/flu/influenza.html

7. Relative Danger of Varicella Vaccine

Some parents question the need for the varicella vaccine. Like influenza, they believe that chickenpox is a harmless illness and that the risk of vaccination outweighs the risk of the disease.

In 1999 an average of 1 child a week died in the United States from complications of chickenpox. These complications include encephalitis, a brain infection; severe staph and strep secondary infections (flesh-eating strep and toxic shock syndrome); hepatitis; and pneumonia.

Before the vaccine, there were 4 million cases of chickenpox, 11,000 hospitalizations, and 100 deaths per year in the United States. The varicella vaccine prevents chickenpox in about 70% to 90% of people who get the shot and prevents severe chickenpox in over 95%.

Resources

- CDC. Varicella Vaccine Web site: http://www.cdc.gov/nip/vaccine/varicella/default.htm
- AAP Committee on Infectious Diseases. Prevention of varicella: recommendations for use of varicella vaccines in children, including a recommendation for a routine 2-dose varicella immunization schedule. *Pediatrics.* 2007;120:221–231. Available at: http://aappolicy.aappublications.org/cgi/content/full/pediatrics;120/1/221

Additional Resources

- AAP Childhood Immunization Support Program. Why Immunize?: http://www.aap.org/immunization/families/whyimmunize.html
- Immunization Action Coalition (IAC). Responding to Concerns About Vaccines: www.immunize.org/concerns/index.htm
- CDC. Six Common Misconceptions About Vaccinations and How to Respond to Them: www.cdc.gov/nip/publications/6mishome.htm

E-mail us with questions about how to respond to other parental concerns at cispimmunize@aap.org.

What Is Telephone Care?

Excerpt from Payment for Telephone Care: A Toolkit

In pediatric practice telephone care is used to a much greater extent than in other medical specialties. Pediatricians use telephone care for triage and advice, disease and case management, clarification or alteration of previous instructions, medication adjustments, acute illness care, coordination of care, test result interpretation, integration of new information into the medical treatment plan, counseling, and education.

Pediatric telephone care requires medical decision-making, incurs practice expense, and involves medical liability risk. Telephone care is often a substitute for more costly face-to-face care. Many parents find telephone care more convenient for managing certain types of medical problems. Although third-party payers have been reluctant to pay physicians for medical services provided by telephone, some are beginning to see the value of this and other non–face-to-face services.

The American Academy of Pediatrics (AAP) policy statement "Payment for Telephone Care" provides a rationale for compensation for telephone care in a complex and changing health care environment. The toolkit offers a suggested procedure and sample tools should you decide to implement charging for telephone care in your practice.

This toolkit is intended to provide the background information and tangible materials necessary for pediatricians to begin charging for telephone care in their practices. The enclosed content was developed using the collective experience of members of the AAP Section on Telephone Care (SOTC) and material submitted by the Children's Physician Network of Minnesota. Certainly there is no single set of policies and procedures that will work for every pediatric office. The content serves as sample material and should be reviewed and tailored appropriately with legal advisement to meet the needs of each practice. This toolkit will provide a summary of

- The types of telephone calls that may be eligible for compensation
- Definitions of "allowable" and "non-covered" services under insurance plans
- Ideas for notifying parents about implementing charges for telephone care

- Suggestions for notifying payers of your plans to submit charges for telephone care and a template for an appeal letter if your charges are denied
- Telephone care documentation guidelines

Pediatricians choosing to bill families directly for telephone care should be certain to undertake this practice only after
- Reviewing existing payer contracts
- Developing a clear communication plan with families and involved parties
- Establishing standard practices for *Current Procedural Terminology (CPT®)* coding and billing
- Ensuring that patients who choose not to access care by telephone have the choice to access care in a face-to face setting

This toolkit will walk you through these steps
- Deciding whether charging for telephone care is right for your practice
- Identifying the *CPT* coding guidelines for telephone care services
- Notifying patients and payers of the change in operations and the benefits of telephone care
- Documenting telephone care services appropriately
- Integrating the billing and collection staff in your transition plan
- Managing insurance denial and patient payment

Other variations and options will be discussed including the use of waivers and insurance appeals for denials of payment. A timeline and checklist for implementing charging for telephone care in your office is provided.

Pediatricians are encouraged to continue to share experiences, both clinical and business, in making this transition with the SOTC, who will collate and disseminate this material. The best way to do this is by joining the SOTC. Visit our Web site at http://www.aap.org/sections/telecare/membership.htm.

Using Web Sites to Market Your Pediatric Practice

Many pediatricians use Web sites as a way to market their practice. Not only are Web sites good marketing tools, they can also be used to educate parents about common childhood illnesses and symptoms, and developmental milestones. In addition, Web sites can help your office promote the medical home by including Web site resources that are available at all times, even when your offices are closed.

Web sites also can be used to educate families about the office including policies, forms, and more.

Following are some tips to consider when building or enhancing your practice's Web site.

Be Creative With the Design

- Consider hiring a design team.
- Include pictures and biographies of physicians and staff.
- Include pictures of children and the office building.
- Do not overcrowd your Web site. White space on the Web site is appealing.
- Use language that your audience will understand.

Incorporate Interactive Components

- Consider creating an option for parents to log on to your Web site. This can allow additional interactive components to be made available. For example, some practices that use this type of system allow parents to e-mail the physicians securely through the Web site. Others may allow patients to schedule appointments and request prescription refills online.
- Another option to consider is a patient portal where patients can view their history, previous checkups, immunization records, and more. Visit www.msimonianmd.com/ops_login.aspx for an example.
- Post monthly or quarterly newsletters.
- Consider creating a database that includes your patients' e-mails. This can allow you to send mass e-mails to your patients with recent updates, including responding to current events in the news. For example, if a retail-based clinic is opening in your county, you can use this opportunity to send all of your patients an e-mail including information about the importance of a medical home.

This might also be a good opportunity to use the following *Practice Management Online* resources: Template Letter: Retail-based Clinics Letter to Patients (http://practice.aap.org/content. aspx?aID=1943) that can be customized to fit your practice as well as a Retail-based Clinic Office Flyer (http://practice.aap.org/content.aspx?aID=1945).

Educate Your Patients

- Use this opportunity to educate your patients about your office policies by posting your practice's mission, hospital affiliations, insurance carriers, and any office forms that the parents will be asked to complete. When patients call to schedule an appointment, ask them to visit your Web site (if they have access to a computer and the Internet) to complete the forms prior to their arrival for the scheduled appointment.
- Provide instructions for parents on what to do for various common illnesses (eg, fever, vomiting) and newborn care. Include instructions on when to call the office and which number to call during various times of the day.
- If you offer classes or support groups, be sure to promote them on the Web site.

Other Tips

- Be sure that your Web site is one of the first Web sites listed when a search is conducted by entering "pediatrician" and your zip code. Be sure that your Web site contains key words that users are likely to search for.
- Keep your Web site up to date. During flu season, offer tips on preventing the flu, information about any flu clinics, and the importance of the flu vaccine. If there is a common community concern (outbreak of measles), post relevant information and resources to your Web site. The American Academy of Pediatrics (AAP) Childhood Immunization Support Program has a Web site with many valuable resources available at www.aap.org/ immunization/pediatricians.html.
- The AAP has many resources available to educate parents on specific illnesses and developmental issues. Consider providing a link to the AAP Web site, or using the AAP *Patient Education Online* service (http://patiented.aap.org), which can be incorporated right into practice Web sites.

Building Patient Loyalty and Trust: The Role of Patient Satisfaction

Maxwell Drain, MA, and Dennis O. Kaldenberg, PhD

Health care has changed dramatically in the past decade. Many physicians have found that they must participate in managed care plans not only to retain their existing patients but also to attract new ones. In the near future, the National Committee for Quality Assurance and the American Medical Association will join the Joint Commission on Accreditation of Healthcare Organizations in accrediting group practices and individual physicians.

One thing, however, has remained constant: the importance of patients' perceptions of care and service. According to The Commonwealth Fund,[1] employers rate patient satisfaction as very important in selecting plans, second only to the number and quality of physicians. Likewise, health plan members and physicians perceive members' interactions with providers (not NCQA accreditation and HEDIS information) to be the most important aspect of medical care shaping perceptions of quality.[2] The importance of patient perceptions of quality is underscored in a study done by the Kaiser Family Foundation that found that the information provided by family and friends was the most believable source of information about the quality of medical care.[3]

Financial Impact of Dissatisfaction

The long-term growth and financial health of a physician's practice is related to the satisfaction of its patients. Satisfied patients return for care, and the positive word of mouth from satisfied patients will bring new patients into the practice. The corporate customers who choose practices to be included in medical plans will select practices that satisfy patients. Clearly, health plans and primary care physicians must keep their corporate customers and patients satisfied to retain their customer base and remain competitive.

For example, consider a practice that has 6,000 patients, 5 percent of whom are dissatisfied with the service they received on their last visit. This dissatisfaction may cause not only those patients to leave but everyone in their households. Assuming that the average household has 3.5 members and each makes 2.5 visits per year, the average annual number of visits

per household is 8.75. If each of these encounters (visits plus ancillary tests) averages $57 in payments (85 percent of a $68 charge), the cost of dissatisfaction is $149,625 [(6,000 patients x .05 leaving to dissatisfaction) x ($57 payment per visit x 8.75 visits per year)]. This figure does not include the loss of existing or potential patients that results from the negative word of mouth generated by the dissatisfied patients. If each dissatisfied patient causes your practice to lose just one additional household, the financial impact doubles.

Although simplistic, this example does highlight the potential effects that patient satisfaction has on your bottom line. Furthermore, if you consider that it costs more to recruit new patients than to keep the ones you have (some estimates suggest up to six times as much) you save money every time you prevent a patient from walking out your door unhappy. Above and beyond the direct dollar benefit from satisfying patients is the leverage that the practice gains in dealing with health plans and the ability to avert frozen enrollments. Obviously, it is in the interests of both physicians and HMOs to understand the determinants of dissatisfaction and to build patient loyalty.

The Patient as Consumer

Patients may be becoming better informed and harder to please, especially those raised in a culture of immediate and predictable results (eg, ATMs and fast food). Aging baby boomers in particular demand convenience and excellent service. They ask for evidence of quality and refuse to accept advice at face value.[4] Medical groups, like other service industries, will have to deliver measurable customer service if they are to survive and flourish in today's changing marketplace.

Focusing on patient satisfaction is a smart investment. Physicians realize the return on their investment through the behavior of satisfied and loyal patients. However, what makes a patient satisfied? Better yet, how do you build long-term patient loyalty and trust?

Empowered Patients Are More Satisfied With Their Care

In drafting the Patient Bill of Rights, the American Hospital Association tried to address these questions. These rights are based on the premise that a personal relationship between the physician and the patient is essential for quality medical care. Patient rights were expected to contribute to more effective patient care and increased satisfaction for both the patient and physician. These rights are still being debated over a quarter of a century later.

In most states, the Patient Bill of Rights is voluntary. However, successful organizations understand that the consumer movement is becoming a dominant driver of change in health care and they have taken the initiative to inform patients about their rights. Today's educated and empowered patients are no longer content simply to believe, "The doctor knows best."[5] Instead, patients want to know their rights, their options, and what to expect from their health care.

Data from a quarter of a million patients in 476 hospitals from around the country confirmed the relationship between empowering patients and their satisfaction with the delivery of care. The results of a recent study conducted by Press, Ganey Associates clearly show that patients are more satisfied when health care organizations place emphasis on helping them to understand their rights as patients. Using a scale of 0 to 100 where 100 is a perfect score, the average satisfaction score of patients who reported they received information on their rights was 84.9. The average score of patients who didn't receive this information was 81.2, representing a statistically significant difference between the two groups. Providing patients with information and encouraging their participation in care decisions enhances the collaboration between patients and health care professionals; improvements in patient satisfaction and the overall quality of health care delivery follow.

Some health care professionals believe that patients don't want to think about negative outcomes and that by addressing issues such as organ donation or end of life decisions, they will see their patients become less satisfied with their overall care. When Press, Ganey looked at the satisfaction of patients who received this sort of information, it is clear that their assessment of the health care experience did not diminish. Instead, patients who received information about their decision-making options were significantly more satisfied than those who had not.

A Matter of Trust

Recently, much attention has been given to patient education. However, this is only part of the larger picture of patient-provider communication. Patients tend to be more committed to their primary care providers when both their medical and interpersonal needs have been met. Press, Ganey conducted a recent survey to determine the current needs of patients in primary care settings. Patients' perceptions of care and service were measured by asking patients to rate 31 aspects of their care and treatment. A Likert-type response scale was used with the following categories: very poor, poor, fair, good, and very good. Questions for the Press, Ganey Medical Practice Survey were developed by conducting patient focus groups, reviewing surveys from health care facilities across the country, soliciting feedback from physicians and administrators, and reviewing current professional and scientific publications on health care delivery.

Eighty-five physician offices with two-hundred-seventy care providers across five states mailed the questionnaire to randomly selected office patients within two to three days of their visit. Both single and multispecialty practices were included, serving both urban and rural patients. When the results were analyzed, interpersonal care and communication issues were highly associated with patients' overall satisfaction. Moreover, the top 10 issues associated with patients' confidence or trust in their care provider and their likelihood to recommend the care provider to others dealt with interpersonal issues, not technical or medical skill (see Table 1 and Table 2).

Building Trust

If patient-provider encounters are to be therapeutic, they must be based on respect and genuineness.[6] Trust encompasses respect; it also is the expectation that a person will act honestly and reliably. One outcome of trust is open communication, not "20 questions" asked rapidly by the physician. Communication breakdowns are among the most common causes of patient dissatisfaction and malpractice claims. Particularly in the face of adverse outcomes, patients may be more likely to equate poor communication and interpersonal care with substandard medical care.[7]

Table 1. Top 10 Issues Correlated With Patients' Confidence in Their Care Providers

Correlation Item	Coefficient
Likelihood of recommending care providers to others	0.87
Concern care providers showed for patients' questions or worries	0.76
Explanations care providers gave patients about problems or conditions	0.74
Likelihood of recommending practices to others	0.71
Amount of time care providers spent with patients	0.71
Instructions care providers gave patients about follow-up care	0.71
Care providers' efforts to include patients in treatment decisions	0.70
Overall rating of care received during office visits	0.70
Information care providers gave patients about medications	0.70
Degree to which care providers spoke using words patients could understand	0.70

Table 2. Top 10 Issues Correlated With Patients' Likelihood to Recommend Their Care Providers

Correlation Item	Coefficient
Patients' confidence in their care providers	0.87
Likelihood of recommending practices to others	0.82
Concern care providers showed for patients' questions or worries	0.75
Overall rating of care received during office visits	0.72
Explanations care providers gave patients about problems or conditions	0.72
Amount of time care providers spent with patients	0.70
Instructions care providers gave patients about follow-up care	0.70
Degree to which care providers spoke using words patients could understand	0.69
Friendliness/courtesy of care providers	0.69
Information care providers gave patients about medications	0.67

Building trust between primary care provider and patient often is the first step in caring for patients before more traditional health care begins. There is little doubt that patients want to control their own lives. By visiting a doctor, however, patients give up some of that control, adding to their anxieties about their health. Based on Press, Ganey research, the good news is that discussing life and death issues or treatment options does not diminish the patients' satisfaction. Instead, frank discussion creates an environment that contributes to patient satisfaction and trust. By addressing patient questions and discussing their options with them, care providers communicate that patients ultimately control their own care.

Hospital health systems have recognized the importance of improving patient experiences in physician offices and the role that open communication plays.[8] Many provide assistance and training to physicians who are interested in developing better therapeutic relationships with patients. These training sessions educate physicians on how to view patients as valued customers and often encourage collaboration between physicians, practice managers, and office staff in hospital department meetings and policy changes. The intent is to provide better information and explanations to patients and to help create a "seamless" care delivery experience for them.

Building patient trust and satisfaction can begin more simply however. Give patients a sense of control over their own health care as well as a perceived ability to make choices. Facilitate patients' involvement by being honest and forthright about treatment options. By bringing patients into the reality of health care, you are satisfying their needs, not intimidating them. People respond positively to being empowered. The care of patients involves not only dealing with their illness and condition but also embracing patients as individuals and recognizing their authority. Patients can handle the truth. Moreover, patients trust the physicians they perceive as honest. Honesty creates a collaborative atmosphere that empowers the patients and enables them to feel involved in their care, even when the care is ultimately placed in the hands of others.

Physician Applications

Some physicians behave in ways that distance themselves from their patients. Behaviors such as poor eye contact and lack of expression create feelings of distrust among patients.[9] In addition to non-verbal respect, physicians must ensure that verbal communication is respectful. Remember, as a physician, you must listen attentively to your patients and wait until they have expressed their concerns before fully discussing diagnoses or treatment. When you respond, you may even want to paraphrase what a patient said not only to clarify but also to demonstrate your understanding of the patient's concerns. Further, as the data presented in the tables illustrate, explaining diagnoses, medications, and prognoses in words that your patients can understand is strongly related to patient confidence and satisfaction.

Ask your patients what you could do to make their visits more comfortable. Ask them what you could do to improve the care and service you provide. Finally, check to make sure that all of your patients' questions have been answered before they leave the exam room. You may even want to encourage patients to bring a list with their questions and concerns with them to their next appointment. These practices may require some modification in the amount of time you schedule with your patients, but remember, last impressions are just as important as first ones. Success can be achieved if you constantly measure, monitor, and share patient survey feedback, and never accept excuses for poor satisfaction ratings.[10]

Conclusion

Patients are more satisfied when they are empowered through knowledge. They want to be informed, they want to have choices, and they want to be protected. Successful health care organizations respect the role that patients play in decision making.

Communication, discussion of rights, and engendering trust will create an environment in which patients feel protected and empowered. Patients are more committed to their care providers when both their medical and interpersonal needs have been met.

In this age of consumer empowerment, the more satisfied patients become, the more loyal they'll tend to be. Satisfying patients at the point of service is more cost-effective than responding to complaints after the fact. Moreover, the more loyal your patients are, the greater the likelihood they'll recommend and return to your care in the future. Ultimately, building patient loyalty and trust begins with building and sustaining effective relationships with your patients.

References

1. J.R. Gabel, K.A. Hunt, and K. Hurst. 1998. When Employers Choose Health Plans: Do NCQA Accreditation and HEDIS Data Count? New York: The Commonwealth Fund.
2. N. Goldfield, et al. 1999. The Content of Report Cards: Do Primary Care Physicians and Managed Care Medical Directors Know What Health Plan Members Think Is Important? The Joint Commission Journal on Quality Improvement, 25: 422-432.
3. The Kaiser Family Foundation/Agency for Health Care Policy Research/ Princeton Survey Associates. 1996. Americans as Health Care Consumers: The Role of Quality Information. October 28, #1203. Menlo Park, California.
4. B.A. Regrut, 1997. The Satisfaction Report, Vol. 1. South Bend, Indiana: Press, Ganey Associates.
5. M. Malone, 1998. What Do Patients Want to Know and When Do They Want to Know It? The Satisfaction Monitor, May/June, 12.
6. G. van Servellen. 1997. Communication Skills for the Health Care Professional: Concepts and Techniques. Gaithersburg, Maryland: Aspen.
7. J.W. Pichert, et al. 1998. What Health Professionals Can Do to Identify and Resolve Patient Dissatisfaction. The Joint Commission Journal on Quality Improvement, 24, 303-312.
8. M. Malone. 1999. Involving Physicians in Patient Satisfaction Initiatives. The Satisfaction Monitor, July/August, 5-8.
9. M. Malone, 1998. What Do Patients Want to Know and When Do They Want to Know It? The Satisfaction Monitor, May/June, 12.
10. S.G. Sherman and V.C. Sherman. 1999. Total Customer Satisfaction: A Comprehensive Approach for Health Care Providers. San Francisco: Jossey-Bass.

Maxwell Drain, M.A., is senior research associate and Dennis O. Kaldenberg, Ph.D., is director, research and development at Press, Ganey Associates in South Bend, Indiana.

Reprinted with permission of Group Practice Journal.

Colocation of Pediatricians and Mental Health Professionals: A Win-Win Situation

Francis Rushton, MD, FAAP

Changing morbidities and changing times cause us as pediatricians to rethink the way we provide services to our patients. Over the past quarter century, there has been a real shift in the types of problems we see. New morbidities are often psychosocial in nature and require new ways of and resources for caring for children.

One popular change in many pediatric offices is the colocation of a mental health professional with the pediatricians. We've had a mental health counselor on site for a number of years and feel that his presence is a tremendous asset for our practice. Although there are community mental health resources elsewhere, they are difficult for many of our patients to access and communicate poorly with our office.

Having a mental health professional on site has been well received by staff and patients alike. Patients like it because the pediatric office is a familiar place. Teens and preteens feel more comfortable coming to our office for counseling rather than going to a mental health center. The mental health counselor likes working with us because he has access to our records and immediate availability of a pediatrician if there are medication issues that need to be discussed. The pediatricians like the presence of the mental health counselor because of access to "hallway" mental health consultations, increased availability of mental health counseling slots in the community, and access to the mental health notes in the common chart we use.

Colocation of a mental health professional in a practice is not without difficulties, and these difficulties will vary from site to site. Payment issues are a major obstacle. In our office, which is primarily Medicaid, we provide free office space and billing services for our mental health counselor because the rates he receives for his services are insufficient to cover the total costs. But the pediatric staff feel that the effect on the office financially is minimal and worth the significant benefit the counselor brings to the practice. Mental health counselors in a busy pediatric practice also have to be flexible. We work diligently to minimize the no-show rate, but the sociodemographic factors that affect mental health conditions often also affect the propensity of families to keep their appointments.

Our colocation of a mental health professional has been so successful that we are now expanding into other areas. We colocate a public health social worker in our office and link with local providers of home-based parenting support and physical, speech, and occupational therapies. Our office is transiting toward a system of services, especially for those children with special health care needs, that can meet many of the health and developmental needs of the children we care for. We think this is community pediatrics at its best, reaching out with other providers in the community to enhance the well-being of all the children we serve.

For more information and assistance, the Mentorship and Technical Assistance Program (http://www.aap.org/sections/socp/mtap.html) of the American Academy of Pediatrics (AAP) Council on Community Pediatrics is available to help AAP members further develop their own community-specific approaches to collaboration and colocation.

Cost-effective Ways to Reduce No-shows: A Practice Management FAQ

Richard Oken, MD, FAAP
Member, Section on Administration and Practice Management

What Are Some Cost-effective Ways to Reduce No-shows?

1. Call all patients the day before an appointment, if they have an appointment that will be at least 20 minutes. This includes visits for newborns or new patients, well-visits for children 4 years and older, and conferences.

2. Devise a system for all physicians to follow. For example, on the first no-show, a phone call is placed to notify the family of the no-show and to obtain explanation. On the second no-show, a postcard reminds the family that another no-show will generate a charge for the missed appointment. On the third no-show, charge for the visit. On the fourth no-show, consider dismissing the family with a 30-day notice explaining why.

3. Identify families with late, no-show, and other compliance issues in the computer and be certain that they receive a reminder call on the day before the visit.

Additional Resources

See these sample letters for the first/second (http://practice.aap.org/content.aspx?aID=2093) and third (http://practice.aap.org/content.aspx?aID=2095) missed appointments.

Missed Appointments in Pediatric Practice, *Practice Management Online* at http://practice.aap.org/content.aspx?aID=1991 or page 166.

Missed Appointments in Pediatric Practice: A Section on Administration and Practice Management E-Mail List Summary

A discussion was posted on the American Academy of Pediatrics (AAP) Section on Administration and Practice Management e-mail list about handling missed appointments. Following is a brief summary of the responses received during this discussion:

Comments From Those Who Charge a No-show Fee

- Create a policy to charge for patient no-shows and post the policy at the check-in window.
- Once the policy was implemented, the number of missed appointments dropped from 4.7% (2002) to 3.2% (2006).
- While the written policy makes no exceptions for missed appointments, no-show fees are usually forgiven if the parent calls ahead of time to cancel the appointment.
- Teenagers old enough to drive themselves had a no-show rate of 50%. A $75 no-show fee has reduced this significantly. Parents are told of this charge when they book their teenager's appointment. It has drastically cut down on wasted office time.
- Call every family the night before an appointment as a reminder.

Comments From Those Who No Longer Charge a No-show Fee

- Charging no-show fees for missed acute care appointments became a difficult, tension-provoking exercise. Staff felt the policy was burdensome because they often had to deal with the angry parents. Therefore, the policy no longer exists.

Consequences for Not Paying

- For the first missed appointment, a warning letter is sent. Every missed appointment thereafter is charged a missed-appointment fee. The amount of the fee may vary depending on, for example, the doctor or type of visit.
- The patient is billed but is not sent to collections for the no-show fee.
- For those who do not pay, the fee is added to a bad-debt status.
- Families are sent a form letter if they are no-shows for an appointment. The letters ramp up with each subsequent infraction. After 3 no-shows, the relationship is generally terminated (unless there are extenuating circumstances, such as divorce).
- Multiple abusers are asked to leave the practice.

Tips on Charging a Fee

- If you do not charge no-show fees, you are telling patients that your time means nothing to you and they will have no problem standing you up again.
- It is absolutely essential to collect no-show and other fees (except for unusual circumstances).
- It is important to follow up and collect the fee. Otherwise, it would be better to get rid of the entire policy unless the fee is applied equally and fully.

For more information, contact the AAP Division of Pediatric Practice at dopp@aap.org.

Note: The comments in this article are the views and opinions of those who stated them and may not represent American Academy of Pediatrics policy.

Documenting Parental Refusal to Have Their Children Vaccinated

Despite our best efforts to educate parents about the effectiveness of vaccines and the realistic chances of vaccine-associated adverse events, some will decline to have their children vaccinated. Within a 12-month period, 85% of pediatricians report encountering a parent who refused or delayed one or more vaccines and 54% report encountering a parent who refused all vaccines. Even though scientific data solidly support the fact that vaccines are safe and effective, concern over harmful side effects, often taken out of context in the media and on unmonitored and biased Web sites, cause substantial and often unrealistic fears.

All parents and patients should be informed about the risks and benefits of preventive and therapeutic procedures, including vaccination. In the case of vaccination, federal law mandates this discussion. Despite doctors' and nurses' best efforts to explain the importance of vaccines and to address parental concerns about vaccine safety, some families will refuse vaccination for their children. Others will ultimately accept some or all vaccinations after repeated discussions during which the provider has listened to the parents concerns and addressed them in a non-condescending manner. The use of this or a similar form demonstrates the importance you place on appropriate immunizations, focuses the parents' attention on the unnecessary risk for which they are accepting responsibility, and may in some instances induce a wavering parent to accept your recommendations.

Providing parents (or guardians) with an opportunity to ask questions about their concerns regarding recommended childhood immunizations, attempting to understand the parent's reason for refusing one or more vaccines, and maintaining a supportive relationship with the family are all part of a good risk management strategy. The American Academy of Pediatrics (AAP) encourages documentation of the health care provider's discussion with a parent about the serious risks of what could happen to their unimmunized or under-immunized child. Provide the parents the appropriate Vaccine Information Statement (VIS) for each vaccine and answer their questions. For parents who refuse one or more recommended immunizations, document your conversation, the provision of the VIS(s), and have the parent sign the vaccine refusal form and keep the form in the patient's medical record. Revisit the immunization discussion at each subsequent appointment and carefully document the discussion, including the benefits to each immunization and the risk of not being age-appropriately immunized. For unimmunized or partially immunized children, some physicians may want to flag the chart to be reminded to revisit the immunization discussion, as well as to alert the provider about missed immunizations when considering the evaluation of future illness, especially young children with fever of unknown origin.

The AAP Refusal to Vaccinate form (see page 239) may be used as a template for such documentation but should not be considered a legal document and should not substitute for legal advice from a qualified attorney.

This form may be duplicated **or changed** to suit your needs and your patients' needs.

The AAP Section on Infectious Diseases and other contributing sections and committees hope this form will be helpful to you as you deal with parents who refuse immunizations. It will be available on the AAP Web site (www.aap.org/bookstore), the Section on Infectious Diseases Web site (http://www.aap.org/sections/infectdis/index.cfm), and the Web site for the AAP Childhood Immunization Support Program (www.aap.org/immunization).

Sincerely,

Meg Fisher, MD, FAAP
Chairperson
AAP Section on Infectious Diseases

Ed Rothstein, MD, FAAP
AAP Section on Infectious Diseases

See related form on page 239.

Parental Refusal to Accept Vaccination: Resources for Pediatricians

The following are some of the resources available to help pediatricians develop a productive dialogue with vaccine-hesitant parents and answer questions about vaccine risks and benefits:

Web sites

1. **AAP Childhood Immunization Support Program (CISP)**
   Information for providers and parents.
   www.aap.org/immunization

2. **The Immunization Education Program (IEP) of the Pennsylvania Chapter of the American Academy of Pediatrics**
   Includes answers to common vaccine questions and topics, such as addressing vaccine safety concerns, evaluating antivaccine claims, sources of accurate immunization information on the Web, and talking with parents about vaccine safety.
   http://www.paiep.org/

3. **The Immunization Action Coalition (IAC)**
   The IAC works to increase immunization rates by creating and distributing educational materials for health professionals and the public that enhance the delivery of safe and effective immunization services. Their "Unprotected People Reports" are case reports, personal testimonies, and newspaper and journal articles about people who have suffered or died from vaccine-preventable diseases.
   http://www.immunize.org/reports/

4. **Centers for Disease Control and Prevention (CDC) National Immunization Program**
   Information about vaccine safety, including Parents' Guide to Childhood Immunizations.
   http://www.cdc.gov/vaccines/hcp.htm

5. **National Network of Immunization Information (NNii)**
   Includes the NNii Resource Kit—Communicating with Patients about Immunizations. A guide to help answer patients' questions and provide the facts about immunizations.
   www.immunizationinfo.org

6. **Vaccine Education Center at Children's Hospital of Philadelphia**
   Information for parents includes Common Concerns About Vaccines, Are Vaccines Safe, and A Look at Each Vaccine.
   www.vaccine.chop.edu

7. **Institute for Vaccine Safety, Johns Hopkins University**
   Provides an independent assessment of vaccines and vaccine safety to help guide decision-makers and educate physicians, the public, and the media about key issues surrounding the safety of vaccines.
   www.vaccinesafety.edu

8. **The Canadian Coalition for Immunization Awareness and Promotion (CCIAP)**
   CCIAP aims to meet the goal of eliminating vaccine-preventable disease through education, promotion, advocacy, and media relations. It includes resources for parents and providers, including "How to advise parents unsure about immunization" by Scott A. Halperin, MD.
   http://immunize.cpha.ca/en/default.aspx

Journal Articles

1. Ball LK, Evans G, Bostrom A. Risky business: challenges in vaccine risk communication. *Pediatrics.* 1998;101:453–458. Available at: http://www.pediatrics.org/cgi/content/full/101/3/453

2. Dias M, Marcuse EK. When parents resist immunizations. *Contemp Pediatr.* 2000;17:75–86

3. Offit PA, Jew RK. Addressing parents' concerns: do vaccines contain harmful preservatives, adjuvants, additives, or residuals? *Pediatrics.* 2003;112:1394–1397

4. Offit PA, Quarles J, Gerber MA, et al. Addressing parents' concerns: do multiple vaccines overwhelm or weaken the infant's immune system? *Pediatrics.* 2002;109:124–129

5. Diekema DS, American Academy of Pediatrics Committee on Bioethics. Responding to parental refusals of immunization of children. *Pediatrics.* 2005;115:1428–1431

Books

1. Offit PA, Bell LM. *Vaccines: What Every Parent Should Know.* New York, NY: IDG Books; 1999

2. Humiston SG, Good C. *Vaccinating Your Child: Questions and Answers for the Concerned Parent.* Atlanta, GA: Peachtree Publishers; 2000

3. Fisher MC. *Immunizations and Infectious Diseases: An Informed Parent's Guide.* Elk Grove Village, IL: American Academy of Pediatrics; 2005

4. Marshall GS. *The Vaccine Handbook: A Practical Guide for Clinicians.* 2nd ed. West Islip, NY: Professional Communications, Inc.; 2008.

5. Myers MG, Pineda D. *Do Vaccines Cause That? A Guide for Evaluating Vaccine Safety Concerns.* Galveston, TX: Immunizations for Public Health; 2008

Reliable Immunization Resources for Parents

Web sites

1. **AAP Childhood Immunization Support Program (CISP)**
   Information for providers and parents.
   www.aap.org/immunization

2. **Why Should I Immunize My Child?**
   A description of the individual diseases and the benefits expected from vaccination.
   www.aap.org/immunization/families/faq/whyimmunize.pdf

3. **The Immunization Education Program (IEP) of the Pennsylvania Chapter of the American Academy of Pediatrics**
   Includes answers to common vaccine questions and topics, such as addressing vaccine safety concerns, evaluating anti-vaccine claims, sources of accurate immunization information on the Web, and talking with parents about vaccine safety.
   http://www.paiep.org/

4. **Centers for Disease Control and Prevention National Immunization Program**
   Information about vaccine safety, including Parents' Guide to Childhood Immunizations
   http://www.cdc.gov/vaccines/spec-grps/parents.htm

5. **National Network of Immunization Information (NNii)**
   Includes the NNii Resource Kit—Communicating with Patients about Immunizations. A guide to help answer patients' questions and provide the facts about immunizations.
   www.immunizationinfo.org

6. **Vaccine Education Center at Children's Hospital of Philadelphia**
   Information for parents includes Common Concerns About Vaccines, Are Vaccines Safe, and A Look at Each Vaccine.
   www.vaccine.chop.edu

7. **Institute for Vaccine Safety, Johns Hopkins University**
   Provides an independent assessment of vaccines and vaccine safety to help guide decision-makers and educate physicians, the public, and the media about key issues surrounding the safety of vaccines.
   www.vaccinesafety.edu

8. **The Canadian Coalition for Immunization Awareness and Promotion (CCIAP)**
   CCIAP aims to meet the goal of eliminating vaccine-preventable disease through education, promotion, advocacy, and media relations. It includes resources for parents and providers, including "How to advise parents unsure about immunization" by Scott A. Halperin, MD.
   http://immunize.cpha.ca/en/default.aspx

9. **Vaccinate Your Baby**
   The Every Child by Two site serves as a central resource of vaccine information for parents. The site links to the latest research and studies about vaccines, an interactive timeline on the benefits of vaccines, information about vaccine safety and ingredients, and the importance of adhering to the recommended schedule.
   www.vaccinateyourbaby.org

Books

1. Offit PA, Bell LM. *Vaccines: What Every Parent Should Know.* New York, NY: IDG Books; 1999

2. Humiston SG, Good C. *Vaccinating Your Child: Questions and Answers for the Concerned Parent.* Atlanta, GA: Peachtree Publishers; 2000

3. Fisher MC. *Immunizations and Infectious Diseases: An Informed Parent's Guide.* Elk Grove Village, IL: American Academy of Pediatrics; 2005

4. Myers MG, Pineda D. *Do Vaccines Cause That? A Guide for Evaluating Vaccine Safety Concerns.* Galveston, TX: Immunizations for Public Health; 2008

Waivers: The Basics for the Pediatric Office

Waivers should be considered as a financial policy component for pediatric practices. A waiver is a statement that the responsible party (patient/parent/guardian) signs accepting financial responsibility for a requested medical service that is or may not be covered by health insurance. To assist pediatric practices, the American Academy of Pediatrics Department of Practice has gathered information on waivers (which may also be referred to as advance beneficiary notices or advanced beneficiary notice [ABN]).

The following information (or questions and answers) have been prepared to inform pediatricians and other health care practitioners of certain basic practice principles. These materials are not a substitute for legal advice and should not be relied on or used without the advice and assistance of your legal counsel. Among other things, the contract with the insurance provider or other third-party payer and/or state law may preclude you from using these materials or may have an impact on how these materials may be used in given circumstances. These issues are beyond the scope of this information (or questions and answers).

What Is a Waiver?

A waiver is a statement that a patient/parent/guardian signs acknowledging that the requested service is or may not be covered by health insurance and accepting responsibility for payment for the service. The waiver may be accompanied by a request for payment for the service at the time of the service.

When Should You Use a Waiver?

A waiver may be used when the requested service is or may not be covered by health insurance, but only if permitted by the terms of your contract with the third-party payer and state law. It should be presented to the patient before any such service is provided. Keep in mind that a waiver may not be sufficient under certain circumstances, such as in an emergency, to shift liability for the charges to the patient/parent/guardian. You should seek the advice of legal counsel before incorporating the use of waivers into your practice.

Can I Bill for a Non-covered Service After the Service Is Provided If I Have Not Obtained a Waiver?

As a general practice it is always preferable to obtain a waiver prior to providing the service in question as a patient/parent/guardian may claim that they did not understand that they would be responsible for payment. Some third-party payer contracts may require a signed waiver be obtained prior to providing a non-covered service. A general waiver signed by the patient/parent/guardian or a notice of financial responsibility posted in a prominent place in your office may also be considered to cover these situations. It is advisable to check the terms of your contract with the third-party payer and state law regarding conditions for using a waiver. A form of general waiver follows this Q & A.

Must the Patient Be Informed Before the Service Is Provided That Insurance Will Not Cover It or Is This More of a Courtesy?

From a matter of general contract law, it is always better to clarify the terms of the payment arrangement with the patient in advance. However, it would also be reasonable to advise the patient/parent/guardian that they are responsible for knowing the terms of their insurance coverage and for following the procedures set forth in their plan for obtaining coverage, including those relating to pre-certification. Under the US Department of Labor Claims Procedure Regulations applicable to group health plans, a plan must respond to an urgent pre-certification inquiry within 72 hours after the request is made. A plan must respond to a nonurgent inquiry within 15 days. That being said, it is appropriate for the pediatrician or other health care provider to notify a patient/parent/guardian of any coverage issues that come to the pediatrician/health care provider's attention in the course of providing services.

Can I Use a Waiver When the Insurance Company Covers Only a Portion of the Charge for a Service?

Whether you can use a waiver for services only partially covered by insurance depends on your contract with the third-party payer and may also be impacted by state law and/or the circumstances under which the services are being provided. Most contracts do not allow for "balance billing" for services that are covered under the service agreement. In special circumstances, an insurance company may waive this requirement. Consult your attorney for further guidance.

How Can I Keep Providing Services With Payment Below My Cost?

You need to review carefully the contracts that you have signed with the insurance carriers and other third-party payers before implementing procedures to address this issue. Some pediatricians have elected not to provide below-cost services to ANY of their patients and refer them elsewhere because most provider contracts stipulate that you cannot discriminate based on health plan participation. Therefore, if you provide a particular service in your office, you may need to provide that service to all patients. Laboratory tests may be an exception to this rule, although certain third-party payer contracts may require that you use the contracted laboratory. Thus, if a patient/parent/guardian wants a laboratory test done in the office and is willing to pay for it even though their insurance will cover the cost of the test at an outside lab, or if a patient/parent/guardian wants Flumist™ but the health plan will only cover injectable flu vaccine, a waiver and consent to be responsible for the non-covered service may be appropriate, unless prohibited by the terms of your contract with the third-party payer or state law.

What Use of Waivers to Charge Patients Directly for Services Would Put Me in Legal Difficulty?

Care must be taken to determine that the use of waivers to charge patients directly for services does not violate the terms of your contract with the third-party payer or state law. For example, the use of a waiver to obtain full payment would likely be a breach of that agreement in the event that the provider agreement prohibited balanced billing of the patient. As a general rule, you should not seek to charge Medicaid patients for non-covered services or any shortfall in payment for the services rendered. In addition, you must exercise caution to be certain that the person signing the waiver, who should be the person responsible for payment, understands the terms of the waiver and that they will incur charges as a result of signing the waiver.

See Sample Waiver or ABN on page 243. It is essential that you consult your legal counsel before using any waivers in your practice.

Section 8

Quality Improvement

Quality Improvement Tools for Physicians

Ramesh Sachdeva, MD, PhD, JD, FAAP
American Academy of Pediatrics, Medical Director of Quality Initiatives

Physicians are being increasingly expected to participate in quality improvement endeavors. However, physicians may not have been exposed to quality improvement tools and methodologies as part of the traditional curriculum in medical schools and residencies. Quality improvement is a unique science. Although there are similarities to traditional scientific research methods, quality improvement science is distinct. The information that follows provides a framework of models for quality improvement that can be used by physicians.

What is quality? The Institute of Medicine has identified 6 dimensions of quality, which include care that is effective, efficient, equitable, timely, patient-centered, and safe. As physicians, we typically view quality synonymous with outcomes or effective care. However, this is only 1 of the 6 dimensions of quality. In addition to this clinical dimension of quality, there are other operational dimensions, which include efficiency of care. Also, of note is that safe care, representing patient safety, is 1 of the 6 dimensions of quality. Therefore, quality can be viewed from both a clinical and operational perspective. Clinical quality improvement focuses on the scope of improvement of clinical outcomes. Operational quality further expands this scope to include the business operational aspects of health care delivery in practices. Other dimensions such as equitable care, patient access, and patient-centered care further expand the scope of quality.

There are typically 4 models for improving clinical and operational quality. The Model for Improvement, the Plan Do Study Act (PDSA) model, is extensively utilized by the Institute for Healthcare Improvement. The PDSA model has been successfully applied in several inpatient and outpatient health care settings to improve clinical quality and patient outcomes. However, in addition to clinical improvement using the PDSA model, there are other business models for

quality that can significantly impact operational quality in health care. This includes the LEAN methodology used successfully by the Toyota Production System, which aims at eliminating waste in processes to enhance efficiency. In contrast to methodologies that aim to improve existing health care processes, Management Sciences offers a proactive approach of using operations research to improve flow, revenue, and safety in hospital and clinic office settings.

The following describes some basic improvement tools for physicians that are integral to implementing any quality improvement initiatives. Run charts are commonly used to monitor improvement. We could ask the question, why do we need a run chart when we can use traditional statistical methods? To answer this question, let us consider the following hypothetical situation. A practice is interested in adopting an intervention to impact obesity in children. As illustrated in Figure 1, measurements performed in 2004 showed that on average the body mass index (BMI) within a group of children in a practice was at the 97th percentile. The intervention was started in 2006. A follow-up measurement was performed in 2008, which showed that the BMI in the same patient group was at the 80th percentile. A statistical test comparing this difference was highly significant at $P<0.0001$. This would imply that there has been a statistically significant decrease in 2008 as compared to 2004 suggesting that the intervention was successful.

However, from a quality improvement standpoint it is crucial to plot a run chart to further evaluate this improvement. As illustrated in the run chart in Figure 2, there was already an ongoing improvement between 2004 and 2006. In fact, after the start of the intervention in 2006, there was an increase in the BMI to the final level of 80th percentile in 2008. This run chart illustrates that the intervention may not have been as successful as originally thought. As illustrated in Figure 2, a run chart is a plot of any process using any type of data. By providing text comments on the timeline to highlight various events, annotated run charts can be created to provide greater insights into the improvement process.

Run charts provide us insights into identifying common cause and special cause variations. Common cause variation represents the "noise" in a system. In contrast, special cause variation relates to something that is not inherent within a stable system. It

Figure 1

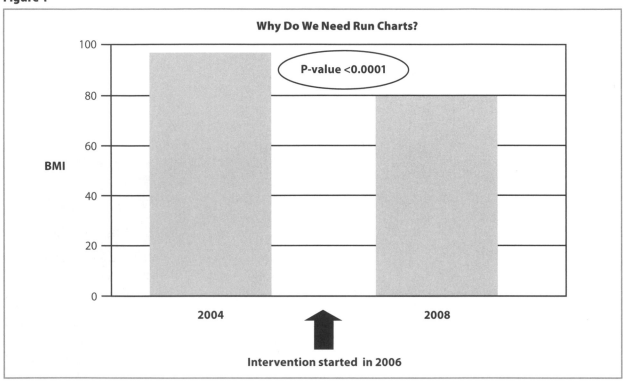

Figure 2

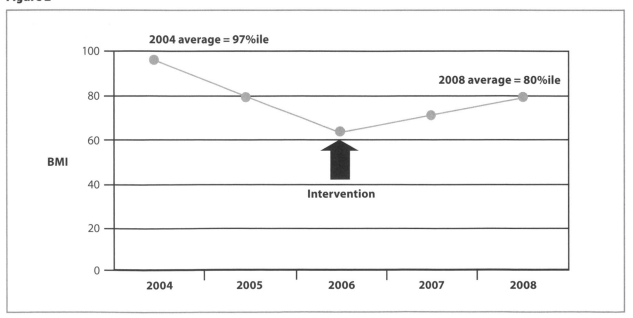

is important to highlight that a system that is stable and has common cause variations lends itself to implementation of the PDSA approach for process improvement. In contrast, a process that has special cause variations needs these variations to be investigated and addressed before implementing a change in the process itself. To illustrate this further, let us consider another hypothetical clinical situation. As illustrated in Figure 3, a run chart is created for tracking HbA_1C in a group of patients in a clinic over time. The median value is plotted on the run chart and then data points are evaluated on either side of the median (the median is the value that represents the middle point of the dataset). Figure 3 illustrates common cause variation. If special cause variation was present it would be identified by data runs of more than 7 points on either side of the median line or a trend of more than 7 points that are increasing or decreasing in any direction. The consecutive decreasing 6 data points in Figure 3 may be suggestive of a trend representing an underlying special cause variation.

Run charts are relatively easy to develop and do not need any special computer or software. Control charts, which also aim at identifying common and special cause variations are more sensitive than run charts, but typically will require software for development. In contrast to a run chart, a control chart provides an upper control limit (UCL) and a lower control limit (LCL) as illustrated in Figure 4. Furthermore, a control chart plots the mean value (average), in contrast to a run chart, which plots the median value. Using the same hypothetical example as before, HbA_1C data points that are above or below the UCL or LCL are likely to be special cause variations. As illustrated in Figure 4, the highlighted data points represent special cause variation. Data points with a trend of 6 points or data points with 8 or more consecutive values below or above the mean may signify a special cause variation. It is important to note that the UCL and LCL require special formulae for complication and are not the same as standard deviations within a statistical distribution.

As highlighted earlier, it is important to identify and distinguish between common cause and special cause variations as part of the improvement strategy. A common cause variation that needs improvement can be addressed by implementing the PDSA cycle. However, special cause variations need to be investigated and addressed and may not require a change in the process itself.

Figure 3

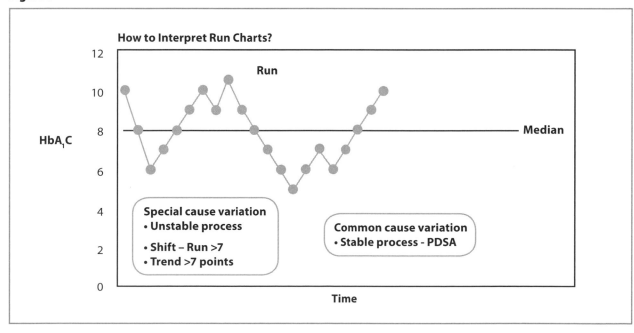

Figure 4

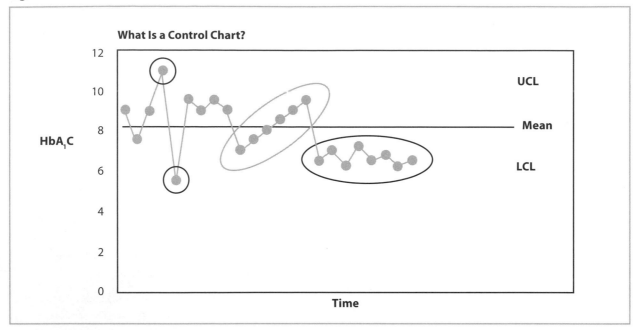

The reader is encouraged to review the selected resources below, which will provide a greater in-depth discussion of statistical process control and the use of control charts for improvement.

Resources

1. Carey RG. *Improving Healthcare with Control Charts: Basic and Advanced SPC Methods and Case Studies.* Milwaukee, WI: ASQ Quality Press; 2003

2. Lee K, McGreevey C. Using control charts to assess performance measurement data. *J Qual Improv.* 2002a;28 (2):90–101

3. Langley GJ, et al. *The Improvement Guide: A Practical Approach to Enhancing Organizational Performance.* San Francisco, CA: Jossey-Bass; 1996

4. Black K. *Business Statistics: Contemporary Decision Making.* Minneapolis, MN: West Publishing Company; 1994

Principles for the Development and Use of Quality Measures: A Summary of American Academy of Pediatrics Policy for Your Practice

The American Academy of Pediatrics (AAP) and its members are committed to providing the best and safest health care for infants, children, adolescents, and young adults. Toward that end, in February 2008, the AAP published the policy statement, "Principles for the Development and Use of Quality Measures" (http://aappolicy.aappublications.org/cgi/content/full/pediatrics;121/2/411) developed by the Steering Committee on Quality Improvement and Management and Committee on Practice and Ambulatory Medicine. The AAP strongly supports health care quality improvement endeavors and believes that measures are an important component of improving quality. The AAP believes that the primary purpose of quality measurement should be to identify opportunities to improve patient care and outcomes, including health status and satisfaction.

Following is an overview of the statement recommendations:

- **Measures should address important issues for children.** Measures should address topics of substantial impact, whether defined by prevalence, severity, or functional status, and should be chosen for their potential influence on children's health by addressing a significant gap between current and ideal practice. Additionally, measures should enable an assessment of systematic disparities in the quality of care for vulnerable groups.
- **Measures should be appropriate for children's health.** Any effort to measure quality should take into account the unique features of children's health and health care and recognize the importance of development, dependency, demographics, and disparities. Measures must reflect the differential epidemiology in children as compared with adults and include patient and family participation.
- **Measures should be scientifically valid.** Measures should be based on best evidence available and linked to evidence-based practice. Additionally, measures should be reliable and field-tested to demonstrate the potential for improvements in quality. When appropriate, measures should include risk adjustment or stratification to take into account factors beyond a practice's or health system's control, such as socioeconomic status, health insurance, and comorbid conditions.

- **Measures should be feasible.** Collection of data to support the measures should not cause undue burden on the clinician or patients and families. Issues to be considered include the number of required measures, the time interval of collection, and the resources required for collection. Ideally, data automatically collected in patient care and other health care processes should be used for measurement. Measures must have clear definitions and specific instructions for collection. Data collection must include adequate sampling. Measures also should be appropriate for the use and setting proposed and tailored to various practice settings as appropriate and must ensure patient privacy.
- **Measures should address what can be improved.** Quality measures should focus on improvable issues that clinicians and health systems can influence.

In addition to these recommendations, the AAP also supports the pay-for-performance principles (http://www.aafp.org/online/en/home/policy/policies/p/payforperformance.html) outlined by the American Academy of Family Physicians, which include involving practicing physicians in program design and providing positive physician incentives. The AAP is taking the lead in assessing quality measures proposed for children's health and health care by developing pediatric measures in collaboration with national health care quality organizations, monitoring the validity of measures developed by other organizations, and advocating for the appropriate use of measures to support improvement in the health care of children. The AAP will advocate for the use of pediatric measurement data, including use in public reporting, when data are based on validated pediatric measures that are appropriately constructed for quality improvement in children's health care and pediatric practices. The AAP is also a key partner in the Alliance for Pediatric Quality. The alliance was formed by the AAP, American Board of Pediatrics, National Association of Children's Hospitals and

Related Institutions, and Child Health Corporation of America to serve as a unified voice for children on quality improvement and health technology initiatives. Its current major initiative, Improve First, focuses on 3 clinical areas—patient safety, neonatology, and chronic care for asthma and cystic fibrosis. The role of the alliance is to spread evidence-based and proven quality improvement initiatives on the 3 areas to hospitals and medical homes. Each targeted initiative also must have an improvement measure(s) associated with it. Further information on this initiative can be found at www.kidsquality.org.

EQIPP

Helping You Improve Care for Children

- *How can practicing pediatricians ensure that they provide quality care for their patients?*
- *How can pediatricians be certain that they are consistently improving this care?*

The American Academy of Pediatrics (AAP) is committed to educating and assisting pediatricians in achieving these goals. One tool developed by the AAP to assist physicians in achieving these goals is EQIPP, a unique online learning program that teaches the principles and concepts of quality improvement in health care. EQIPP allows physicians to evaluate their practice online, using tools that can be easily implemented to enhance patient care. The goal of EQIPP is to help physicians collect and analyze practice data over time to document improved quality of care. Simulated patient data are also available for nonpracticing providers. Physicians will learn what steps are necessary to improve their quality of care on a continuous basis and be able to transfer their skills to multiple pediatric-specific clinical and practice management topics. By providing pediatricians with tools and strategies to make small cycles of change, clinicians can improve practice efficiency and patient care.

EQIPP has redesigned courses to provide user-friendly navigation in a format that encourages pediatric health care professionals to build multidisciplinary teams. EQIPP provides methods of monitoring and improving clinical care on specific topics such as pediatric nutrition, asthma, immunizations, gastroesophageal reflux disease, Bright Futures, and medical home.

Pediatricians can use this Web-based innovation to earn valuable *AMA PRA Category 1 Credit*™, meet the American Board of Pediatrics Maintenance of Certification Performance in Practice requirements, link their lifelong learning and professional development, and track all of it with PediaLink. For more information about EQIPP or PediaLink, visit www.pedialink.org.

Current EQIPP Topics

- *Nutritional Assessment for the Healthy and Chronically Ill Child:* http://www.pedialink.org/cmefinder/search-detail.cfm/key/b8c78413-6d9e-4b0f-8f4d-1eb4345b0794/type/course/grp/2/task/details
- *Diagnosing and Managing Asthma in Pediatrics:* http://www.pedialink.org/cmefinder/search-detail.cfm?key=6e04151b-fa5c-4f25-bad2-9a84255bb896&type=course&grp=2&task=details

Future EQIPP Topics

- *Give Your Immunization Rates a Shot in the Arm*
- *Differentiate and Manage: GER and GERD*
- *Bright Futures*
- *Medical Home*

Quality Improvement Innovation Network (QuIIN)

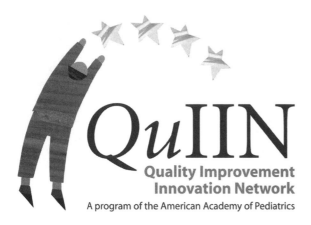

What is QuIIN?

A network of pediatricians and their staff teams that use quality improvement methods to test tools, interventions, and strategies in order to improve health care and outcomes for children and their families. QuIIN serves as a practical working lab for pediatricians to test how improvements can be implemented in practice, the child's medical home.

QuIIN Member Opportunities

- Participate in Improvement Activities
- Get Feedback on Innovations
- Talk With Fellow Innovators and Adopters
- Calls on Quality Topics for CME Credit

Who Is a QuIIN Member?

A pediatrician who likes being on the cutting-edge of practice innovations. He or she is an American Academy of Pediatrics member and clinician in practice who likes to get change started.

Benefits to QuIIN Members

- Participate in improvement activities with like-minded colleagues.
- Positively impact the pediatric profession while improving care for children and families.
- Share tools and ideas with other QuIIN members for feedback through the QuIINovation Exchange Discussion Board.

- Participate in learning opportunities such as conference calls and email lists that highlight innovative practice strategies and improvement methods.
- Have access to tools as they are developed by the network.

Variety of Project Opportunities

Opportunities vary from individual involvement in reviewing tools for a single project to participating with a staff team in an improvement learning collaborative.

Activities include
- Expert review of tools for use in practice
- Review, feedback, and testing of tools appropriate for pediatric practice
- Participation in workshops and learning collaboratives to test and evaluate tools, measures, and strategies for improving care
- Testing the use of measures on the processes and outcomes of office practice

A listing and description of QuIIN projects is available on the QuIIN Web site.

More Information

For additional information visit the QuIIN Web site at http://quiin.aap.org.

To apply to be part of QuIIN, complete the QuIIN Online Membership Application (http://www.aap.org/moc/quiin/quiin-app.cfm). It is free to join!

Questions? Contact QuIIN staff at quiin@aap.org.

Chapter Alliance for Quality Improvement (CAQI)

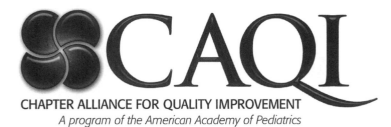

CHAPTER ALLIANCE FOR QUALITY IMPROVEMENT
A program of the American Academy of Pediatrics

This Web site for chapter leaders provides various resources and tools to support the advancement of QI initiatives within member practices. The following information and tools can be accessed on the Web site:

- Definition of chapter QI and strategies on how to get started
- Improvement Speakers Bureau
- A listing of QI activities being conducted by chapters
- *A Resource Guide for Chapters: Building Local Capacity for Improvement*
- CAQI e-mail list
- *Chapter QI Needs Assessment 2007*

For more information, visit www.aap.org/moc/chapters/caqi/index.html.

Section 9
Medical Home

Helping You Implement the Medical Home Into Your Practice

The American Academy of Pediatrics (AAP) is committed to the medical home model as a best practice model of medical care for infants, children, and adolescents. The medical home model provides accessible, family-centered, comprehensive, continuous, coordinated, compassionate, and culturally effective care for which the pediatrician and the family share responsibility. The AAP policy statement on the medical home (http://aappolicy.aappublications.org/cgi/content/full/pediatrics;110/1/184) describes this approach in more detail.

Pediatricians implementing the medical home model may require resources to assist them in this process. The AAP has created tools such as care coordination forms, educational materials for families, depositories for state-specific resources, and more. These resources are intended to support pediatricians who are seeking to implement the medical home model in their own practice and to help educate families who may not understand the importance of having a medical home for their children.

The National Center for Medical Home Implementation, a cooperative agreement between the Maternal and Child Health Bureau (MCHB) and the AAP, has pulled all of these resources together in one Web site. To access these resources, go to www. medicalhomeinfo.org.

Medical Home Implementation Educational Series

The National Center for Medical Home Implementation conducted a series of teleconferences and webinars to provide child health professionals with practical strategies for implementing the medical home in practice. These sessions provided information about the value of the family-centered primary care medical home for all children and youth and the availability of practical tools and resources, and

provided strategies for improving care and increasing patient/family satisfaction. The sessions have been archived and are available at http://www.medicalhomeinfo.org/training/archives.html.

Building Your Medical Home Toolkit (www.pediatricmedhome.org)

Brought to you by the AAP/MCHB/National Center for Medical Home Implementation, the *Building Your Medical Home* toolkit supports the primary care pediatrician's development and improvement of a pediatric medical home. It also prepares a pediatric office to apply for and potentially meet the National Committee for Quality Assurance (NCQA) Physician Practice Connections Patient Centered Medical Home Recognition program requirements. The toolkit can help a practice assess and improve its medical home capacity with resources and downloadable tools organized into 6 building blocks that provide guidance for implementation.

- **Care Partnership Support** addresses family access and communication
- **Clinical Care Organization** addresses standards for practice organization and use of clinical information
- **Care Delivery Management** addresses the promotion of clinical care that is consistent with scientific evidence, as well as patient and family preference
- **Resources and Linkages** addresses successfully linking patient and families with community resources to help meet their needs
- **Practice Performance Measurement** addresses the organization and promotion of safe and high-quality care
- **Payment and Finance** addresses the need to match quality care and NCQA recognition with payment and value

The National Center for Medical Home Implementation is a cooperative agreement between the MCHB/Health Resources and Services Administration and the AAP. The National Center works to ensure that all children and youth, including those with special health care needs, have the services and support necessary for full community inclusion through medical homes.

Building Your Medical Home toolkit content was developed by Jeanne McAllister, Director of the Center for Medical Home Improvement, Crotched Mountain Foundation in New Hampshire, with guidance from AAP leadership and the National Center's Project Advisory Committee members. For more information about the National Center, please visit www.medicalhomeinfo.org or contact Angela Tobin, manager of technical assistance, at atobin@aap.org.

The Medical Home Index: Measuring the Organization and Delivery of Primary Care for Children With Special Health Care Needs

The Medical Home Index (MHI) is a validated self-assessment and classification tool designed to translate the broad indicators defining the medical home (accessible, family-centered, comprehensive, coordinated, etc) into observable, tangible behaviors and processes of care within any office setting. It is a way of measuring and quantifying the "medical homeness" of a primary care practice. The MHI is based on the premise that "medical home" is an evolutionary process rather than a fully realized status for most practice settings. The MHI measures a practice's progress in this process. This tool can be found on *Practice Management Online* at http://practice.aap.org/content.aspx?aid=2048. A shorter version of this tool can be found on page 186.

A companion survey, the Medical Home Family Index (MHFI) is intended for use with a cohort of families whose children have special health care needs. These are families who have received care from the practice for at least a year. The MHFI provides a medical home with a valuable consumer perspective. The survey can be found on *Practice Management Online* at http://practice.aap.org/content.aspx?aid=2050 and on page 194.

Additional medical home information can be found at http://www.medicalhomeimprovement.org/knowledge/practices.html#measurement.

The Medical Home Index—Short Version

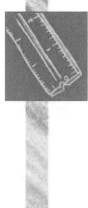

Center for Medical Home Improvement

The Medical Home Index - Short Version:

Measuring the Organization and Delivery of Primary Care for Children with Special Health Care Needs

The Medical Home Index – Short Version (MHI–SV) represents ten indicators which have been derived from the Center for Medical Home Improvement's (CMHI) original Medical Home Index (MHI). This short version can be used as an interval measurement in conjunction with the original MHI **or** it can be used as a quick "report card" or snapshot of practice quality. CMHI recommends the use of the full MHI for practice improvement purposes but offers this short version for interval or periodic measurement and/or when it is not feasible to use the full MHI.

The Medical Home Index is a nationally validated self-assessment tool designed to quantify the "medical homeness" of a primary care practice. The MHI contains twenty-five indicators which detail excellent, pro-active, comprehensive pediatric primary care. It functions both as a quality improvement tool and as a self education medium relevant to the medical home.

The Medical Home Index: Short Version (MHI-SV) is a brief representation of the more complete measurement tool. It scores a practice on a continuum of care across three levels:

- Level 1 is good, responsive pediatric primary care.
- Level 2 is pro-active pediatric primary care (in addition to Level 1)
- Level 3 illustrates pediatric primary care at the most comprehensive levels (it is in addition to Levels 1 and 2).

As the reporter for your entire practice and in response to each of the ten indicators – please score your medical home at: Level 1, Level 2 "partial", Level 2 "complete", Level 3 "partial", or Level 3 "complete".

Both the full 25-item Medical Home Index and this 10-item Medical Home Index – Short Version can be downloaded from the CMHI website at www.medicalhomeimprovement.org.

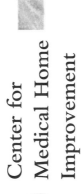
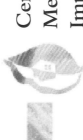

Center for Medical Home Improvement

Medical Home Index – Short Version (MHI-SV)

	Level 1	Level 2 (in addition to level 1)	Level 3 (in addition to level 2)
#1 Family Feedback *Requires both MD & key non-MD staff person's perspective.* (# 1.5 MHI-Full Version)	Pediatric primary care without the elements detailed in levels 2 and 3. ☐ Level 1	Feedback from families of *CSHCN* regarding their perception of care is gathered through systematic methods (e.g. surveys, focus groups, or interviews); there is a process for staff to review this feedback and to begin problem solving. ☐ PARTIAL ☐ COMPLETE	An advisory process is in place with families of *CSHCN* which helps to identify needs and implement creative solutions; there are tangible supports to enable families to participate in these activities (e.g. childcare or parent stipends). ☐ PARTIAL ☐ COMPLETE
#2 Cultural Competence (# 1.6 MHI-FV)	Pediatric primary care without the elements detailed in levels 2 and 3. ☐ Level 1	Materials are available and appropriate for non-English speaking families, those with limited literacy; these materials are appropriate to the developmental level of the child/young adult. ☐ PARTIAL ☐ COMPLETE	Family assessments include pertinent cultural information, particularly about health beliefs; this information is incorporated into care plans; the *practice* uses these encounters to assess patient &community cultural needs. ☐ PARTIAL ☐ COMPLETE
#3 Identification of Children in the Practice with Special Health Care Needs (# 2.1 MHI-FV)	Pediatric primary care without the elements detailed in levels 2 and 3. ☐ Level 1	A *CSHCN* list is generated by applying a definition (see pg. 6; the list is used to enhance care for define *practice* activities (e.g. to flag charts and computer databases for special attention or identify the population and its subgroups). ☐ PARTIAL ☐ COMPLETE	Diagnostic codes for *CSHCN* are documented, problem lists are current, and complexity levels are assigned to each child; this information creates an accessible *practice* database. ☐ PARTIAL ☐ COMPLETE

(The Medical Home Index – SV – Page 2)

Center for Medical Home Improvement

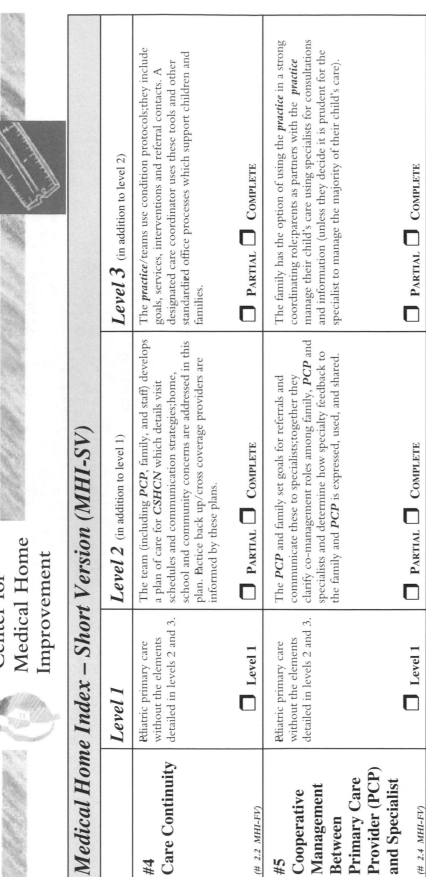

Medical Home Index – Short Version (MHI-SV)

	Level 1	*Level 2* (in addition to level 1)	*Level 3* (in addition to level 2)
#4 Care Continuity (# 2.2 *MHI-FV*)	Pediatric primary care without the elements detailed in levels 2 and 3. ☐ Level 1	The team (including *PCP*, family, and staff) develops a plan of care for *CSHCN* which details visit schedules and communication strategies: home, school and community concerns are addressed in this plan. Pactice back up/cross coverage providers are informed by these plans. ☐ PARTIAL ☐ COMPLETE	The *practice*/teams use condition protocols: they include goals, services, interventions and referral contacts. A designated care coordinator uses these tools and other standardied office processes which support children and families. ☐ PARTIAL ☐ COMPLETE
#5 Cooperative Management Between Primary Care Provider (PCP) and Specialist (# 2.4 *MHI-FV*)	Pediatric primary care without the elements detailed in levels 2 and 3. ☐ Level 1	The *PCP* and family set goals for referrals and communicate these to specialists: together they clarify co-management roles among family, *PCP* and specialists and determine how specialty feedback to the family and *PCP* is expressed, used, and shared. ☐ PARTIAL ☐ COMPLETE	The family has the option of using the *practice* in a strong coordinating role: parents as partners with the *practice* manage their child's care using specialists for consultations and information (unless they decide it is prudent for the specialist to manage the majority of their child's care). ☐ PARTIAL ☐ COMPLETE

(The Medical Home Index – SV – Page 3)

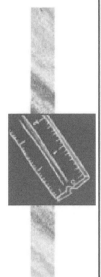

Center for Medical Home Improvement

Medical Home Index – Short Version (MHI-SV)

	Level 1	Level 2 (in addition to level 1)	Level 3 (in addition to level 2)
#6 Supporting the Transition to Adulthood	Pediatric primary care without the elements detailed in levels 2 and 3.	Pediatric and adolescent PCP support youth & family to manage their health using a transition timeline & developmental approach; they assess needs & offer culturally effective guidance related to: • health & wellness • education & vocational planning • guardianship and legal & financial issues • community supports & recreation When youth transition from pediatrician to adult provider: **Pediatricians** help to identify an adult PCP and sub-specialists and offer ongoing consultation to youth, family and providers during the transition process. **Adult Providers** offer an initial "welcome" visit and a review of transition goals.	Progressively from age 12, youth, family and PCP develop a written transition plan within the care plan; it is made available to families and all involved providers. Youth and families receive coordination support to link their health and transition plans with other relevant adolescent and adult providers/services/agencies (e.g. sub-specialists, educational, financial, insurance, housing, recreation employment and legal assistance).
(# 2.5.1 MHI-FV)	☐ Level 1	☐ PARTIAL ☐ COMPLETE	☐ PARTIAL ☐ COMPLETE
#7 Care Coordination /Role Definition	Pediatric primary care without the elements detailed in levels 2 and 3.	Care coordination activities are based upon ongoing assessments of child and family needs; the *practice* partners with the family (and older child) to accomplish care coordination goals.	Practice staff offer a set of care coordination activities, their level of involvement fluctuates according to family needs/wishes. A designated care coordinator ensures the availability of these activities including written care plans with ongoing monitoring.
(# 3.1 MHI-FV)	☐ Level 1	☐ PARTIAL ☐ COMPLETE	☐ PARTIAL ☐ COMPLETE

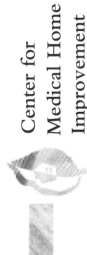

Center for Medical Home Improvement

Medical Home Index – Short Version (MHI-SV)

	Level 1	Level 2 (in addition to level 1)	Level 3 (in addition to level 2)
#8 **Assessment of Needs/ Plans of Care**	Pdiatric primary care without the elements detailed in levels 2 and 3.	The child with special needs, family, and *PCP* review current child health status and anticipated problems or needs;they create/revise action plans and allocate responsibilities at least 2 times per year or at individualized intervals.	The *PCP*/staff and families create a written plan of care that is monitored at every visit;the office care coordinator is available to the child and family to implement, update and evaluate the care plan.
(# 3.4 MHI-FV)	☐ Level 1	☐ PARTIAL ☐ COMPLETE	☐ PARTIAL ☐ COMPLETE
#9 **Community Assessment of Needs for CSHCN**	Pdiatric primary care without the elements detailed in levels 2 and 3.	Providers raise their own questions regarding the population of *CSHCN* in their practice community(ies);they seek pertinent data and information from families and local/state sources and use data to inform practice care activities.	At least one clinical practice provider participates in a community-based public health need assessment about *CSHCN*, integrates results into practice policies, and shares conclusions about population needs with community &state agencies.
(# 4.1 MHI-FV)	☐ Level 1	☐ PARTIAL ☐ COMPLETE	☐ PARTIAL ☐ COMPLETE
#10 **Quality Standards (structures)**	Pdiatric primary care without the elements detailed in levels 2 and 3.	The *practice* has its own systematic quality improvement mechanism for *CSHCN*;regular provider and staff meetings are used for input and discussions on how to improve care and treatment for this population.	The *practice* actively utilies quality improvement (Q) processes;staff and parents of *CSHCN* are supported to participate in these Qactivities;resulting quality standards are integrated into the operations of the *practice*.
(# 6.1 MHI-FV)	☐ Level 1	☐ PARTIAL ☐ COMPLETE	☐ PARTIAL ☐ COMPLETE

(The Medical Home Index – SV – Page 5)

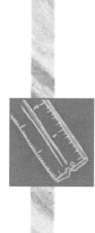

Center for Medical
Home
Improvement

The Medical Home Index – Short Version:

Measuring the Organization and Delivery of Primary Care for Children with Special Health Care Needs

<u>DEFINITIONS OF CORE CONCEPTS</u> (Words in italics throughout the document are defined below.)

Children with Special Health Care Needs (CSHCN):

Children with special health care needs are defined by the *US Maternal and Child Health Bureau* as those who have, or are at increased risk for chronic physical, developmental, behavioral, or emotional conditions and who require health and related services of a type or amount beyond that required by children generally (USDHHS, MCHB, 1997).

Medical Home:

A medical home is a community-based primary care setting which provides and coordinates high quality, planned, family-centered health promotion and chronic condition management. According to the American Academy of Pediatrics (AAP "medical home" is accessible, family-centered, continuous, comprehensive, coordinated, compassionate, and culturally competent.

Family-Centered Care (US Maternal and Child Health Bureau, 2004):

Family-Centered Care assures the health and well-being of children and their families through a respectful family-professional partnership. It honors the strengths, cultures, traditions and expertise that everyone brings to this relationship. Family-Centered Care is the standard of practice which results in high quality services.

(The Medical Home Index – SV – Page 6)

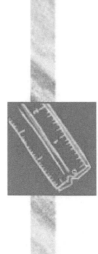

Center for
Medical Home
Improvement

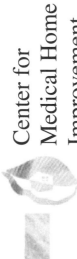

The Medical Home Index – Short Version:

Measuring the Organization and Delivery of Primary Care for Children with Special Health Care Needs

GLOSSARY OF TERMS (continued)

Care Coordination Activities:

Care and services performed in partnership with the family and providers by health professionals to:

1) Establish family-centered community-based **"Medical Homes"** for *CSHCN* and their families.
   - Make assessments and monitor child and family needs
   - Participate in parent/professional practice improvement activities

2) Facilitate timely access to the *Primary Care Provider (PCP)*, services and resources
   - Offer supportive services including counseling, education and listening
   - Facilitate communication among PCP, family and others

3) Build bridges among families and health, education and social services; promotes continuity of care
   - Develop, monitor, update and follow-up with care planning and care plans
   - Organize wrap around teams with families; support meeting recommendations and follow-up

4) Supply/provide access to referrals, information and education for families across systems.
   - Coordinate inter-organizationally
   - Advocate with and for the family (e.g. to school, daycare, or health care settings)

5) Maximize effective, efficient, and innovative use of existing resources
   - Find, coordinate and promote effective and efficient use of current resources
   - Monitor outcomes for child, family and practice

Chronic Condition Management (CCM):

CCM acknowledges that children and their families may require more than the usual well child, preventive care, and acute illness interventions. CCM involves explicit changes in the roles of providers and office staff aimed at improving:

1) Access to needed services
2) Communication with specialists, schools, and other resources, and
3) Outcomes for children and families.

(The Medical Home Index – SV – Page 7)

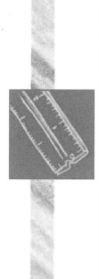
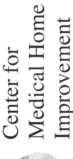

Center for
Medical Home
Improvement

The Medical Home Index – Short Version:

Measuring the Organization and Delivery of Primary Care for Children with Special Health Care Needs

GLOSSARY OF TERMS* (continued)

Quality:
Quality is best determined or judged by those who need or who use the services being offered. Quality in the medical home is best achieved when one learns what children with special health care needs and their families require for care and what they need for support. Health care teams in partnership with families then work together in ways which enhance the capacity of the family and the practice to meet these needs. Responsive care is designed in ways which incorporate family needs and suggestions. Those making practice improvements must hold a commitment to doing what needs to be done and agree to accomplish these goals in essential partnerships with families.

Office Policies
Definite courses of action adopted for expediency; "the way we do things"; these are clearly articulated to and understood by all who work in the office environment.

Practice:
The place, providers, and staff where the PCP offers pediatric care

Primary Care Provider - (PCP):
Physician or pediatric nurse practitioner who is considered the main provider of health care for the child

United States Maternal and Child Health Bureau - (USMCHB):
A division of Health Resources Services Administration

Requires both MD and key non-MD staff person's perspective - you will see this declaration before select themes; the project has found that these questions require the input of both MD and non MD staff to best capture practice activity.

(The Medical Home Index – SV – Page 8)

The Medical Home Family Index and Survey

The Medical Home Family Index and Survey

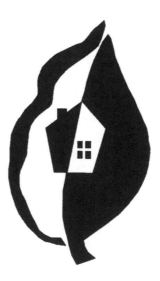

Beyond The Medical Home: Cultivating Communities of Support for
Children with Special Health Care Needs (CSHCN)
Center for Medical Home Improvement
Crotched Mountain Foundation
1 Verney Drive
Greenfield, NH 03047

Funded by: United States Maternal and Child Health Bureau Grant # H02MC02613-01-00

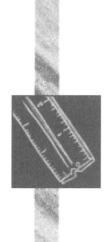

Center for
Medical Home
Improvement

THE MEDICAL HOME *FAMILY* INDEX:

Measuring the Organization and Delivery of Primary Care For Children with Special Health Care Needs

The following questions refer to the care that your child receives from his/her pediatrician or primary care provider (PCP) and the staff who work in their office. Next to each question circle the response that best describes your experience of care for your child.

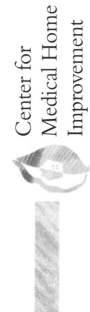

1. Through this practice/office I can get the health care that my child needs when we need it (including after office hours, on weekends and holidays).	Never	Sometimes	Often	Always
2. When I call the office: (please answer for a, b, c, and d):				
a) Staff know who we are	Never	Sometimes	Often	Always
b) Staff respect our needs and requests	Never	Sometimes	Often	Always
c) Staff remember any special needs or supports that we have asked for	Never	Sometimes	Often	Always
d) We are asked if there are any new needs requiring attention	Never	Sometimes	Often	Always
3. My primary care provider (PCP) uses helpful ways to communicate (e.g. explaining terms clearly, helping us prepare for visits, e-mail, or encouraging our questions):				
a) With me	Never	Sometimes	Often	Always
b) With my child (If (b) does not apply to your child ✔here ____)	Never	Sometimes	Often	Always
4. My PCP asks me to share with him/her my knowledge and expertise as the parent or caregiver of a child with special health care needs (CSHCN).	Never	Sometimes	Often	Always
5. I am asked by our PCP how my child's condition affects our family (e.g. the impact on siblings, the time my child's care takes, lost sleep, extra expenses, etc.).	Never	Sometimes	Often	Always
6. My PCP listens to my concerns and questions?	Never	Sometimes	Often	Always
7. Planning of care for my child includes: (please answer for a, b, c and d):				
a) The writing down of key information (e.g. recommendations, treatments, phone #)	Never	Sometimes	Often	Always
b) Setting short team goals (e.g. for the next three months)	Never	Sometimes	Often	Always
c) Setting long term goals (e.g. for the next year or more)	Never	Sometimes	Often	Always
d) Thorough follow-up with plans created	Never	Sometimes	Often	Always
8. My primary care provider and staff work with our family to create a written care plan for my child. (If your answer is "never", then skip to Question # 11)	Never	Sometimes	Often	Always

(The Medical Home *Family* Index – Page 1)

Center for Medical Home Improvement

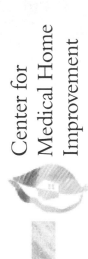

	Never	Sometimes	Often	Always
9. I receive a copy of my child's care plan with all updates and changes.	Never	Sometimes	Often	Always
10. My primary care provider (PCP) and his/her office staff (please answer a, b and c):				
a) Use and follow through with care plans they have created	Never	Sometimes	Often	Always
b) Use a care plan to help follow my child's progress	Never	Sometimes	Often	Always
c) Review and update the care plan with me regularly	Never	Sometimes	Often	Always
11. My PCP has a staff person(s) or a "care coordinator" who will:				
a) Help me with difficult referrals, payment issues, and follow-up activities	Never	Sometimes	Often	Always
b) Help to find needed services (e.g. transportation, durable equipment or home care)	Never	Sometimes	Often	Always
c) Make sure that the planning of care meets my child and my families needs	Never	Sometimes	Often	Always
d) Help each person involved in my child's care to communicate with each other (with my consent).	Never	Sometimes	Often	Always
12. When or if I ask for it, our PCP or office staff help me to:				
a) Explain my child's needs to other health professionals	Never	Sometimes	Often	Always
b) Get my child's school, early care providers or others to understand his/her condition (If (b) does not apply to your child ✔ here ___)	Never	Sometimes	Often	Always
13. Someone at the office is available to review my child's medical record with me when or if I ask to see it.		Yes	No	
14. Office providers or staff who are involved with my child's care know about their condition, history, and our concerns and priorities.		Yes	No	
15. My PCP or his/her office staff sponsor activities to support my family (e.g. support groups, parent skill building or how to support other parents).		Yes	No	
16. Office staff help me to connect with family support organizations and informational resources in our community and state.		Yes	No	
17. My PCP is a strong advocate for the rights and services important to children with special health care needs and their families.		Yes	No	
18. My PCP assists me in finding adult health care services for my child. (Check here if due to your child's age this does not apply ___).		Yes	No	

(The Medical Home *Family* Index – Page 2)

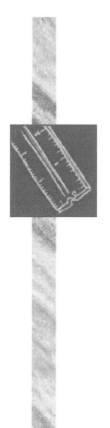

Center for Medical Home Improvement

	Yes	No
19. My primary care provider (PCP) and office staff organize and attend team meetings about my child's plan of care that include us and outside providers (when needed).	Yes	No
20. My PCP and office staff organize and attend events to talk about concerns and needs common to all children with special health care needs (CSHCN) and their families.	Yes	No
21. I have seen changes made at the office as a result of my suggestions or those made by other families.	Yes	No
22. I know the practice has conducted surveys, focus groups, or discussions with families (in the last two years) to determine if they are satisfied with their children's care.	Yes	No
23. From my experience, I believe that my PCP and the staff at his/her office have a commitment to provide the quality care and family supports that we need.	Yes	No
24. The behavior which best demonstrates the needed care and compassion I need from my child's PCP is _____ (write in here).	Comments:	

	Never	Sometimes	Often	Always
25. The frequency that I observe and experience this behavior (in #24) is?				

Would you please go back over this Family Index to check for unanswered questions; try to answer them to the best of your ability.

Please write down:

The name of the practice where you go for your child's care: _____

The name of your child's primary care provider: _____

The length of time your child has been cared for by this practice? _____   Your child's age: _____

(Optional) What is the racial/ethnic background with which you most closely identify?

❏White, Non-Hispanic   ❏ African American   ❏ Hispanic   ❏ Native American/American Indian/Alaskan Native   ❏ Asian   ❏ Other (specify)

May we have your permission to contact you further about this project? ❏ Yes ❏ No

Other comments you would like to make? (Feel free to use the other side) _____   *Thank You for Sharing Your Experiences*

(The Medical Home *Family* Index – Page 3)

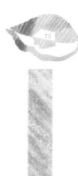

Center for Medical Home Improvement
Family/Caregiver Survey

Today's date: __/__/__

My child is a (1) ____ Boy   (2) ____ Girl

Child's date of birth (or age in total months):_____

Each of the following questions (unless otherwise stated) refers to <u>right now</u> or in the past 12 months. When questions do not apply to your family or child, circle or write NA (not applicable).

In your opinion what is your child's **(most)** primary medical condition? (**Circle only one**)

1) Arthritis	10) Deafness/trouble hearing	22) Muscular dystrophy
2) Asthma	11) Depression	23) Obesity
3) Attention deficit/hyperactivity	12) Diabetes	24) Recurrent urinary tract infection
4) Autism/pervasive development disorder	13) Down syndrome	25) Seizure disorder
5) Blindness/trouble seeing	14) Eating disorder	26) Severe allergies
6) Cerebral palsy	15) Heart disease or heart defect	27) Severe scoliosis
7) Chronic ear infection	16) Hemophilia	28) Sickle cell disease
8) Cleft lip/palate	17) HIV/AIDS	29) Spina bifida
9) Cystic fibrosis	18) Permanent deformity of arms/legs	30) Other (specify below)
	19) Kidney disease	_____
	20) Leukemia/Cancer	_____
	21) Mental retardation	_____

Select from the list above (1-29) any additional conditions that your child has, write the num ber of the condition (s) on the lines be low. If your c hild's additional condition(s) are not on the list, please also write it/them on the lines below.

a._____   d._____

b._____   e._____

c._____   f._____

Caring for Your Child

The next five questions ask about your child's health needs and whether your child has a health condition. A **health condition** can be physical, mental or behavioral. **Health conditions** may affect a child's development, daily function or need for services.

1. Does your child currently need or use **medicine prescribed by a doctor** (other than vitamins)?
    ❑ Yes → Go to Question 1a
    ❑ No → Go to Question 2

    1a. Is this because of ANY medical, behavioral or other health condition?
        ❑ Yes → Go to Question 1b
        ❑ No → Go to Question 2

    1b. Is this a condition that has lasted or is expected to last for *at least* 12 months?
        ❑ Yes
        ❑ No

2. Does your child need or use more **medical care, mental health or educational services** than is usual for most children of the same age?
    ❑ Yes → Go to Question 2a
    ❑ No → Go to Question 3

    2a. Is this because of ANY medical, behavioral or other health condition?
        ❑ Yes → Go to Question 2b
        ❑ No → Go to Question 3

    2b. Is this a condition that has lasted or is expected to last for *at least* 12 months?
        ❑ Yes
        ❑ No

3. Is your child **limited or prevented** in any way in his or her ability to do the things most children of the same age can do?
    ❑ Yes → Go to Question 3a
    ❑ No → Go to Question 4

    3a. Is this because of ANY medical, behavioral or other health condition?
        ❑ Yes → Go to Question 3b
        ❑ No → Go to Question 4

    3b. Is this a condition that has lasted or is expected to last for *at least* 12 months?
        ❑ Yes
        ❑ No

4. Does your child need or get **special therapy**, such as physical, occupational or speech therapy?
    - ☐ Yes → Go to Question 4a
    - ☐ No → Go to Question 5

    4a. Is this because of ANY medical, behavioral or other health condition?
    - ☐ Yes → Go to Question 4b
    - ☐ No → Go to Question 5

    4b. Is this a condition that has lasted or is expected to last for *at least* 12 months?
    - ☐ Yes
    - ☐ No

5. Does your child have any kind of emotional, developmental or behavioral problem for which he or she needs or gets **treatment or counseling**?
    - ☐ Yes → Go to Question 5a
    - ☐ No

    5a. Has this problem lasted or is it expected to last for *at least* 12 months?
    - ☐ Yes
    - ☐ No

6. In general, would you say your child's **health** is: (Circle one)

    (1) Excellent   (2) Good   (3) Fair   (4) Poor

7. Is there a place that your child usually goes to when he/she is sick or you need advice about his/her health?

    1) Yes   2) No   3) There is more than one place

8. A personal doctor or nurse is the health provider who knows your child best. Do you have one person that you think of as your child's personal doctor or nurse?

    1) Yes   2) No   3) Don't know

9. How **difficult** is it to take care of your child's chronic health condition(s) or disability?
    - (1) Not at all difficult   (3) Some what difficult
    - (2) A little difficult   (4) Very difficult

10. During the last 3 months, how often have you worried about your child's **health**? (Circle One)
    - (1) None of the time   (4) Most of the time
    - (2) A little of the time   (5) All of the time
    - (3) Some of the time

11. During the <u>last 3 months</u>, how often have you worried about the impact of your child's chronic health condition or disability **upon his or her siblings**?

    (1) None of the time   (4) Most of the time
    (2) A little of the time   (5) All of the time
    (3) Some of the time   (6) Does not apply to your family

12. Overall, how would you rank the <u>**severity**</u> of your child's condition or problem?
Please pick a number from "0" to "10" where "0" is the mildest severity, "10" is the most severe.

0   1   2   3   4   5   6   7   8   9   10
Mildest severity   **Most severe**

13. Which of the following statements best describes your child's health care needs?

    1) Child's health care needs change all the time
    2) Child's health care needs change only once in awhile
    3) Child's health care needs are usually stable
    4) None of the above
    5) Don't know

14. How would you measure the level of stress experienced over the last year as a result of caring for your child?
Please pick a number from "0" to "10" where "0" represents very low stress and "10" is for extremely high stress.

0   1   2   3   4   5   6   7   8   9   10
Very low stress   **Extremely high stress**

15. Does your child's doctor or office staff help to alleviate this stress (e.g. with services, supports, or referrals to other resources)?
        1) Always   3) Sometimes
        2) Often   4) Never

16. During the last month, how often have your emotions (such as feeling depressed or anxious) interfered with your work, social activities, or daily routine?

        1) None of the time   4) Most of the time
        2) A little of the time   5) All of the time
        3) Some of the time

17. During the past 12 months (1 year ago today) how many days did your child miss school because of their chronic health condition or disability?

    Write in the number of days _____ (a typical school year has ~185)

17a. Also indicate:
        (1) None (no days absent)   (3) Home schooled
        (2) Did not go to school   (4) Don't know

18. Do you have any of the following specific concerns for your child?
    (Circle the number under the response that best describes your concern):

	Never	Seldom	Sometimes	Often	Always	NA
18a. Growth and development	1	2	3	4	5	6
18b. Ability to learn	1	2	3	4	5	6
18c. Participation in activities of his/her age group	1	2	3	4	5	6
18d. Ability to make healthy choices (e.g. activity, rest, diet, medicines)	1	2	3	4	5	6
18e. Self esteem/emotional well being	1	2	3	4	5	6
18f The future	1	2	3	4	5	6

NA (not applicable)

19. How would you estimate the current overall **severity** of your child's special health care needs?
    (1) Minimal   (3) Moderate
    (2) Mild   (4) Severe

20. Are things the same from day to day with your child, or is it hard to know what to expect?
    (1) Pretty much the same day to day   (3) Lots of unexpected changes
    (2) Occasional surprises   (4) Very unpredictable one day to the next

Using the Health Care System

21. How satisfied are you with the care coordination provided outside of the family that you receive for your child?
        (1) Very satisfied   (4) Very dissatisfied
        (2) Somewhat satisfied   (5) NA (not applicable)
        (3) Dissatisfied

22. During the past year, how many times was your child seen by your child's primary care provider?
        (1) None at all   (4) More than 10 times
        (2) 1 - 3 times   (5) NA (not applicable)
        (3) 4 - 10 times

23. During the past year, how many times was your child seen by a specialist/specialty clinic?
        (1) None   (3) 4 - 10 times
        (2) 1 - 3 times   (4) More than 10 times

24. During the past year, how many times did your child require care in the emergency room?
        (1) None   (3) 4 - 10 times
        (2) 1 - 3 times   (4) More than 10 times

25. During the past year, how many <u>separate times</u> did your child have to stay in the hospital overnight?

    (1) None at all   (4) 8 - 10 times

    (2) 1 - 3 times   (5) More than 10 times

    (3) 4 - 7 times

26. In the past 3 months, how many days have you or anyone in your family had to **stay home from work** because of your child's chronic health condition(s) or disability?

    (1) None

    (2) 1 – 5 work days   (4) 16 or more work days

    (3) 6 - 16 work days   (5) No one is employed

Family Care Coordination

Parents of children with chronic health conditions often do a variety of activities to coordinate care for their child. Some parents are new at this, others have been coordinating their child's care for years. Listed below are some of the care activities parents often do. Please read each activity and **<u>circle</u>** the response that best describes <u>you and your family.</u>

	Always	Often	Some-Times	Rarely	Never	NA
27. Involving my child in regular recreational activities in the community.	1	2	3	4	5	6
28. Finding the help I need to coordinate services for my child.	1	2	3	4	5	6
29. Finding other parents to talk to who have children with similar conditions.	1	2	3	4	5	6
30. Describing how this medical condition affects my child's growth and development.	1	2	3	4	5	6
31. Taking action to correct poor care and services my child receives.	1	2	3	4	5	6
32. (*If school age or older*) Getting my child to take an active role as possible in health discussions and in decision making.	1	2	3	4	5	6
33. Communicating my concerns about my child's health needs to most professionals.	1	2	3	4	5	6
34. Getting medical professionals to give us information that we can understand.	1	2	3	4	5	6

Practice Satisfaction: How would you rate the practice for each of the following qualities?

Please circle one number on each line.	Excellent	Very Good	Good	Fair	Poor	NA
35. The length of time waiting at the office.	1	2	3	4	5	6
36. Clear directions for who to contact or where to go for aspects of your child's condition when they are not ill.	1	2	3	4	5	6
37. Provider(s) and staff have regular contact with your child's school staff.	1	2	3	4	5	6

38. How many **additional** children live in your home?
    1) none   2) one   3) two   4) three   5) four   6) five   7) six or more

39. Has anyone in your family been **unable to work** outside the home due to your child's health condition or disability?
        1) yes   2) no

40. What do you or your child currently need that you are *not* receiving?

_____

_____

Family Information	Yes	No	Don't Know
41. Do you have health insurance for yourself?	1	2	DK
42. Do you have health insurance for your child?	1	2	DK
43. Do you have Medicaid for your child?	1	2	DK
44. Do you have supplemental security income (SSI)?	1	2	DK
45. Do you receive any other assistance from the state (e.g. special medical services, children with special needs)?	1	2	DK
46. Do you have regular out of pocket health expenses (over $50/month or over $600/year) to care for your child's health condition or disability (not including insurance deductibles or co-payments)?	1	2	DK

47. Are out of pocket expenses related mostly to (circle all that apply):
1. Equipment   4) Family support
2. Supplies   5) Counseling
3. Medications   6) Respite care
                  7) Other _____ (write in)

Please use the space below to express your thoughts about this survey or any of the areas it has caused you to think about.

_____

_____

_____

_____

_____

_____

_____

_____

_____

_____

_____

_____

_____

_____

_____

_____

_____

_____

_____

Thank you for your help and time in completing this survey

The Center for Medical Home Improvement (CMHI)
Crotched Mountain Foundation & Rehabilitation Center
One Verney Drive, Greenfield, NH 03047-5000
603-547-3311 Ext 272   (Fax)--603 547-3467
www.medicalhomeimprovement.org

(Questions 1-5 are from the FACCT – Foundation for Accountability CAMHI/ Chronic Condition Screener)

Coding for Medical Home Visits

Index of Current Procedural Terminology Codes for Medical Home

The following index was originally published in November 2003 in *Medical Home Crosswalk to Reimbursement.* The information was developed by Margaret McManus, Alan Kohrt, Joel Bradley, and Linda Walsh in collaboration with the Center for Medical Home Improvement, the American Academy of Pediatrics, and the National Institute for Children's Healthcare Quality. Funded by the Maternal and Child Health Bureau, US Department of Health and Human Services through the Maternal and Child Health Policy Research Center.

Codes	Services and Description
Physician E/M Services; Face-to-Face	
	Outpatient
99201	Office or other outpatient visit, new patient; self-limited or minor problem, 10 min
99202	low to moderate severity problem, 20 min
99203	moderate severity problem, 30 min
99204	moderate to high severity problem, 45 min
99205	high severity problem, 60 min
99211	Office or other outpatient visit, established patient; minimal problem, 5 min
99212	self-limited or minor problem, 10 min
99213	low to moderate severity problem, 15 min
99214	moderate severity problem, 25 min
99215	moderate to high severity problem, 40 min
99241	Office or other outpatient consultation, new or established patient; self-limited or minor problem, 15 min
99242	low severity problem, 30 min
99243	moderate severity problem, 45 min
99244	moderate to high severity problem, 60 min
99245	moderate to high severity problem, 80 min
99341	Home visit, new patient; low severity problem, 20 min
99342	moderate severity problem, 30 min
99343	moderate to high severity problem, 45 min
99344	high severity problem, 60 min
99345	patient unstable or significant new problem requiring immediate attention, 75 min
93347	Home visit, established patient; self-limited or minor problem, 15 min
99348	low to moderate problem, 25 min
99349	moderate to high problem, 40 min
99350	patient unstable or significant new problem requiring immediate attention, 60 min
+99354	Prolonged physician services in office or other outpatient setting, with direct patient contact; first hour *(use in conjunction with time-based codes **99201–99215, 99241–99245, 99301–99350**)*
+99355	each additional 30 min (use in conjunction with **99354**)
	Preventive Medicine Services
99381	Initial comprehensive preventive medicine, new patient; infant under 1
99382	ages 1–4

Codes	Services and Description
	Preventive Medicine Services (cont)
99383	ages 5–11
99384	ages 12–17
99385	ages 18–39
99391	Periodic comprehensive preventive medicine, established patient; infant under 1
99392	ages 1–4
99393	ages 5–11
99394	ages 12–17
99395	ages 18–39
99401	Preventive medicine counseling and/or risk factor reduction provided to an individual and should address issues such as family problems, diet and exercise, substance abuse, injury prevention, and diagnostic and lab results; 15 min. Not for reporting counseling or risk factor reduction provided to patients with symptoms or established illnesses.
99402	30 min
99403	45 min
99404	60 min
99420	Administration and interpretation of health risk assessment instrument
	Group Setting
99411	Preventive medicine counseling and/or risk factor reduction provided to individuals in a *group setting;* 30 min
99412	60 min
99078	Physician educational services rendered to patients in a *group setting* (eg, obesity or diabetic instructions)
	Disability E/M services
99450	Basic life and/or disability evaluation services that include measurement of height, weight, and blood pressure; completion of a medical history following a life insurance pro forma; collection of blood sample and/or urinalysis complying with "chain of custody" protocols; and completion of necessary documentation/certificates.
99455	Work-related or medical disability evaluation services that include completion of medical history commensurate with patient's condition; performance of examination commensurate with patient's condition; formulation of diagnosis; assessment of capabilities and stability and calculation of impairment; development of future medical treatment plan; and completion of necessary documentation/certificates and report.
	Inpatient
99238	Hospital discharge day management; 30 min
99239	more than 30 min
99231	Subsequent hospital care, per day, also used for follow-up inpatient consultation services; patient is stable, recovering or improving, 15 min
99232	patient is responding inadequately to therapy or has developed minor complication, 25 min
99233	patient is unstable or has developed a significant complication or new problem, 35 min
99251	Initial inpatient consultation, new or established patient; self-limited or minor problem, 20 min
99252	low severity problem, 40 min
99253	moderate severity problem, 55 min
99254	moderate to high severity problem, 80 min
99255	moderate to high severity problem, 110 min

Codes	Services and Description
+99356	Prolonged physician services in the *inpatient* setting; first hour *(use in conjunction with time-based codes* **99221–99233, 99251–99255)**
+99357	each additional 30 min *(use in conjunction with* **99356)**
	Physician Non–Face-to-Face Services
99339	Individual physician supervision of a patient (patient not present) in home, domiciliary or rest home (eg, assisted living facility) requiring complex and multidisciplinary care modalities involving regular physician development and/or revision of care plans, review of subsequent reports of patient status, review of related laboratory and other studies, communication (including telephone calls) for purposes of assessment or care decisions with health care professional(s), family member(s), surrogate decision maker(s) (eg, legal guardian) and/or key caregiver(s) involved in patient's care, integration of new information into the medical treatment plan and/or adjustment of medical therapy, within a calendar month; 15–29 min
99340	30 min or more
+99358	Prolonged physician services without direct patient contact; first hour *(use in conjunction with other physician services and/or inpatient or outpatient E/M service codes)*
+99359	each additional 30 min *(use in conjunction with* **99358)**
99367	Medical team conference by physician with interdisciplinary team of health care professionals, patient and/or family not present, 30 min or more
99374	Care plan oversight services requiring complex and multidisciplinary care modalities involving regular physician development and/or revision of care plans, review of subsequent reports and related lab studies, communications, integration of new information into treatment plan, and/or adjustment of medical therapy, patient under care of home health agency, 15–29 min
99375	Same, 30 min or more
99377	Care plan oversight services, patient under care of hospice, 15–29 min
99378	Same, 30 min or more
99379	Care plan oversight, patient in a nursing facility, 15–29 min
99380	Same, 30 min or more
99441	Telephone E/M to patient, parent or guardian not originating from a related E/M service within the previous 7 days nor leading to an E/M service or procedure within the next 24 hours or soonest available appointment; 5–10 min of medical discussion
99442	11–20 min of medical discussion
99443	21–30 min of medical discussion
99444	Online E/M service provided by a physician to an established patient, guardian, or health care provider not originating from a related E/M service provided within the previous 7 days, using the Internet or similar electronic communications network
	Psychiatric Diagnostic or Evaluative Interview Procedures
90801	Psychiatric diagnostic interview examination
90802	Interactive psychiatric diagnostic interview examination using play equipment, physical devices, language interpretation, or other communication mechanisms
	Psychotherapy
90804	Individual psychotherapy, 20–30 min face to face with patient
90805	with medical E/M
90806	Individual psychotherapy, 45–50 min face to face with patient;
90807	with medical E/M services
90808	Individual psychotherapy, 75–80 min face to face with patient
90809	with medical E/M services

Codes	Services and Description
	Psychotherapy (cont)
90810	Individual psychotherapy, interactive, using play equipment, or other mechanisms, 20–30 min face to face with patient;
90811	with medical E/M services
90812	Individual psychotherapy, interactive, 45–50 min face to face with patient;
90813	with medical E/M services
90814	Individual psychotherapy, interactive 75–80 min face to face with patient;
90815	with medical E/M services
90846	Family psychotherapy (without patient present)
90847	Family psychotherapy (conjoint psychotherapy) (with patient present)
90849	Multiple-family group psychotherapy
90857	Interactive group psychotherapy
	Other Psychiatric Services/Procedures
90862	Pharmacologic management, including prescription, use, and review of medication with no more than minimal medical psychotherapy
90885	Psychiatric evaluation of hospital records, other psychiatric reports, and psychometric and/or projective tests, and other accumulated data for medical diagnostic purposes
90887	Interpretation or explanation of results of psychiatric, other medical exams, or other accumulated data to family or other responsible persons, or advising them how to assist patient
90889	Preparation of reports on patient's psychiatric status, history, treatment, or progress (other than for legal or consultative purposes) for other physicians, agencies, or insurance carriers
	Special Otorhinolaryngologic Services
92506	Evaluation of speech, language, voice, communication, and/or auditory processing
92551	Audiologic screening test, pure tone, air only
92552	Pure tone audiometry (threshold); air only
92553	air and bone
96101	Psychological testing (includes psychodiagnostic assessment of emotionality, intellectual abilities, personality and psychopathology, eg, MMPI, Rorschach, WAIS), per hour of the *psychologist's or physician's* time, both face-to-face time administering tests to the patient and time interpreting these test results and preparing the report
96102	Psychological testing (includes psychodiagnostic assessment of emotionality, intellectual abilities, personality, and psychopathology, eg, MMPI, Rorschach, WAIS), with *qualified health care professional* interpretation and report, administered by technician, per hour of technician time, face to face
96103	Psychological testing (includes psychodiagnostic assessment of emotionality, intellectual abilities, personality and psychopathology, eg, MMPI, Rorschach, WAIS), administered by a computer, with *qualified health care professional* interpretation and report
96105	Assessment of aphasia (includes assessment of expressive and receptive speech and language function, language comprehension, speech production ability, reading, spelling, writing, eg, Boston Diagnostic Aphasia Examination) with interpretation and report, per hour
96110	Developmental testing, limited (eg, Developmental Screening Test II, Early Language Milestone Screen), with interpretation and report
96111	Developmental testing, extended (includes assessment of motor, language, social, adaptive, and/or cognitive functioning by standardized developmental instruments, eg, Bayley Scales of Infant Development) with interpretation and report
96116	Neurobehavioral status exam (clinical assessment of thinking, reasoning, and judgment, eg, acquired knowledge, attention, language, memory, planning and problem solving, and visual spatial abilities), per hour of the *psychologist's or physician's* time, both face to face with the patient and time interpreting test results and preparing the report

Codes	Services and Description
96118	Neuropsychological testing (eg, Halstead-Reitan, Neuropsychological Battery, Wechsler Memory Scales, and Wisconsin Card Sorting Test), per hour of the psychologist's or physician's time, both face-to-face time administering tests to the patient and time interpreting these test results and preparing the report
96119	Neuropsychological testing (eg, Halstead-Reitan, Neuropsychological Battery, Wechsler Memory Scales, and Wisconsin Card Sorting Test), with qualified health care professional interpretation and report, administered by *technician*, per hour of technician time, face to face
96120	Neuropsychological testing (eg, Halstead-Reitan, Neuropsychological Battery, Wechsler Memory Scales, and Wisconsin Card Sorting Test), administered by a computer, with qualified health care professional interpretation and report
Nonphysician Provider (NPP) Services	
99366	Medical team conference with interdisciplinary team of health care professionals, face to face with patient and/or family, 30 minutes or more, participation by a nonphysician qualified health care professional
99368	Medical team conference with interdisciplinary team of health care professionals, patient and/or family not present, 30 minutes or more, participation by a nonphysician qualified health care professional
96150	Health and behavior assessment performed by nonphysician provider (health-focused clinical interviews, behavior observations) to identify psychological, behavioral, emotional, cognitive, or social factors important to management of physical health problems, 15 min, initial assessment
96151	reassessment
96152	Health and behavior intervention performed by nonphysician provider to improve patient's health and well-being using cognitive, behavioral, social, and/or psychophysiological procedures designed to ameliorate specific disease-related problems), individual, 15 min
96153	group (2 or more patients)
96154	family (with the patient present)
96155	family (without the patient present)
97802	Medical nutrition therapy performed by nonphysician provider; initial assessment and intervention, individual, face to face with patient, each 15 min
97803	reassessment and intervention, individual, face to face, each 15 min
97804	group (2 or more individuals), each 30 min
Non–Face-to-Face Services: NPP	
98966	Telephone assessment and management service provided by a qualified nonphysician health care professional to an established patient, parent, or guardian not originating from a related assessment and management service provided within the previous 7 days nor leading to an assessment and management service or procedure within the next 24 hours or soonest available appointment; 5–10 min of medical discussion
98967	11–20 min of medical discussion
98968	21–20 min of medical discussion
98969	Online assessment and management service provided by a qualified nonphysician health care professional to an established patient, parent, guardian, or health care provider not originating from a related assessment and management service provided within the previous 7 days nor using the internet or similar electronic communications network
Other Services, Procedures, and Reports	
99050	Service(s) provided in office at times other than regularly scheduled office hours, or days when the office is normally closed (eg, holidays, Saturday, or Sunday), in addition to basic service
99051	Service(s) provided in the office during regularly scheduled evening, weekend, or holiday hours, in addition to basic service
99056	Services typically provided in the office, provided out of the office at request of patient, in addition to basic service

Codes	Services and Description
	Other Services, Procedures, and Reports (cont)
99058	Service(s) provided on an emergency basis in the office, which disrupts other scheduled office services, in addition to basic service
99060	Service(s) provided on an emergency basis, out of the office, which disrupts other scheduled office services, in addition to basic service
99071	Educational supplies, such as books, tapes, and pamphlets provided to patient at cost to physician
99078	Physician educational services rendered to patients in group setting (eg, obesity or diabetic instructions)
99080	Special reports such as insurance forms, more than conveyed in usual medical communications
99090	Analysis of clinical data stored in computers
99091	Collection and interpretation of physiologic data
99173	Screening test of visual acuity, quantitative, bilateral (must employ graduated visual acuity stimuli that allow a quantitative estimate of visual estimate of visual acuity—eg, Snellen chart). Other identifiable services unrelated to this screening test provided at the same time may be reported separately (eg, preventive services).
99174	Ocular photoscreening with interpretation and report, bilateral
	Modifiers
21	Prolonged E/M services
22	Unusual procedural services
25	Significant, separately identifiable E/M service by the same physician on the same day of the procedure or other service
32	Mandated services
59	Distinct procedural services (non-E/M services)

+ = Add-on code

Current Procedural Terminology (CPT®) 5-digit codes, nomenclature, and other data are copyright 2008 American Medical Association (AMA). All Rights Reserved.

Important note: Given the relative frequency with which code and valuation revisions occur, articles related to coding may not reflect the most current information available. Please check the online version of this article at http://practice.aap.org/content.aspx?aid=2560 and the *AAP Pediatric Coding Newsletter* at http://coding.aap.org for updated guidance.

Because the American Academy of Pediatrics (AAP) is not able to verify the accuracy of the facts relating to a patient encounter, we cannot be held responsible for any coding decisions that you make based on the guidance you receive from the AAP. It is your responsibility to only code for what you do during a patient encounter.

Section 10

Physician Health/Wellness

Personal and Family Needs

Excerpt from Launching Your Career in Pediatrics Handbook: Opening a New Practice

Family needs and wants are often at the top of the list when considering where to practice. Many pediatricians who have young children often choose to move closer to family and relatives for support. The location of where a spouse can work is an important factor when determining a location, as well. Also important is the availability of educational, cultural, and recreational activities. If you love outdoor activities, you may wish to move to regions that offer those advantages.

As more women enter the field of pediatrics, there has been an increase in demand for careers that offer a work/life balance. This demand has prompted many pediatricians to seek careers that offer job sharing and part-time and flexible work schedules. The American Academy of Pediatrics Women in Pediatrics Web site (http://www.aap.org/womenpeds/) has more information about issues facing women in pediatrics. The same dynamics hold true for those on the opposite end of the spectrum—retiring pediatricians (Shrier DK, Shrier LA, Rich M, Greenberg L. Pediatricians leading the way: integrating a career and a family/personal life over the life cycle. *Pediatrics.* 2006;117:519–522).

To make a decision about where to practice, it is important to assess your goals.

Clarify Your Career Objectives

- Do you want to practice a specific style or philosophy of pediatrics?
- Are you a team player or someone who likes to go it alone?
- What type of location would you like to be in—rural, suburban, or urban?
- What kinds of patients do you want to serve?
- What are your future goals?
- Do you enjoy working shifts?
- Do you prefer inpatient or outpatient care?

Do You Like the Idea of Hospital or Academic Practice, a Clinic Practice, or a Private Office?

- How many hours do you want to work?
- Do you mind working a lot of evenings and weekends?
- How often do you want to be on call?
- Is the practice committed to being a medical home for its families?

What Kind of Lifestyle Do You Want Outside the Office?

- Exposure to urban life opportunities
- Outside adventures

Making Time for Balance

Hanna B. Sherman, MD, FAAP

Most physicians and other professionals perpetually struggle to manage the competing responsibilities and desires of personal and professional lives. The capacity to be in balance, first and foremost, requires understanding the meaning and personal values in one's life and then matching attention and actions to what is individually discerned to be important. Another critical part of balance is managing time well so that we can use our time as effectively and meaningfully as possible. While most physicians are masterful at multitasking and managing large-volume lives, a fresh look at how we prioritize and approach our tasks can be useful.

Judy Sorum Brown's poem, "Fire," opens with

What makes a fire burn is the space between the logs, a breathing space.

How can we better manage our time to create the necessary breathing spaces that allow us to reduce our stress and better balance our lives? The following guidelines are adapted from Brian Tracy's book, *Eat That Frog! 21 Great Ways to Stop Procrastinating and Get More Done in Less Time.* Some guidelines may be more applicable than others for your personal style and particular work setting.

1. **Choose goals and objectives.** Decide what you want, both in your work and in balancing your life. Put your thoughts in writing so you can review and edit them when you need to.
2. **Plan your day.** Think on paper. Make lists of tasks and each component to accomplish them. Every minute spent in planning can save 5 to 10 minutes in execution. Some people like writing their lists at the end of the day, so they settle their next-day tasks before leaving work. It allows them to lay the work down and better transition to their personal time. Others prefer to draft their lists with a fresh look at the start of the day.
3. **Create large chunks of time.** Organize tasks that require focused attention and effort around large blocks of time where you can concentrate for extended periods. However, also remember to optimize small bits of time when they are available by attending to simple, limited tasks.

4. **Be selective.** There is never enough time to do everything, now or in the future. What are the most important things to give your attention to? Be self-reflective and get additional help from family, friends, and colleagues in discerning where to concentrate your efforts. Say "no" when necessary and be prepared to make hard choices about what to let go. Figure out what is "enough."
5. **Consider the consequences.** The most important tasks and priorities are those that have the most serious consequences, positive or negative. Focus on these first. Resist the temptation to clear up small tasks. Leave those as breaks or time fill-ins.
6. **Do what is most stressful first.** Worrying slows down efficiency. Tackle what is hardest first and get it out of the way or into a manageable state.
7. **Practice the ABCDE method continually.** Before beginning to work on a list of tasks, organize them by value and priority.
   A: Must do
   B: Should do
   C: Nice to do
   D: Can delegate to someone else
   E: Can eliminate doing
   This guideline is my personal favorite, particularly E. I have piles of papers and items on my list that, if I leave them long enough, tend to fall off completely. When I can discern proactively that a task can be eliminated, it greatly reduces my stress.
8. **Break tasks down into smaller components.** Break large, complex tasks down into smaller pieces. Work on one small part of the task to get started. Plan how long it will take to complete each part.
9. **Do it now.** Work as though you are leaving on vacation and have to get all your major tasks completed before you leave. If you get your work done, you'll end up creating free time to enjoy without leaving town.
10. **Know your best time of day.** Identify your periods of highest mental and physical energy each day and, as best you can, structure the most important and demanding tasks around those times.
11. **Know your strengths.** Have a positive attitude about your work. Know what you can accomplish.

12. **Identify your key constraints.** Determine the areas, internally or externally, that set the speed at which you achieve your most important goals and focus on alleviating them. Know your work style and needs.

13. **Single handle tasks.** Finish tasks in one sitting if possible. Make less-important decisions quickly. Touch each piece of paper once. Two-minute rule: If a task can be done in 2 minutes or less, do it now.

14. **Be intentional about interruptions.** Don't set out the candy jar unless you want company. Open your door, answer your phone, and check your e-mail on your schedule. Protect your time and energies.

15. **Guard your energy and spirit.** Treat yourself well and keep yourself healthy. Eat well, sleep well, and exercise often. Nurture your heart and spirit regularly. Have a creative outlet. Know when to trust something is good enough. Maintain a supportive and trustworthy community.

16. **Look for solutions to every problem.** Believe in yourself. Have an "I can do" attitude. Be an optimist. See the good and learn from the challenges. Create what you want to live. Develop habits for the positive and share them.

If you find managing your time to be impossible, it may be that the roles and responsibilities you have taken on are more than can be managed reasonably and in a balanced way by one person. Carefully list the major roles you play in your life, including all the different ways you contribute to your work, your family, your community, and your personal growth. As you look at the list, are you in balance in the way you would like to be? If not, is there a particular area that is over-attended to? Are there areas that are under-attended to? When you look at your life list with honesty and emotional integrity, are there hard choices that need to be made? While balance is never static and rarely achievable consistently on a day-to-day basis, through self-awareness, mindfulness, hard choices, discipline, and practice, it is possible to have overall balance. Maximizing our time management helps to loosen up the space to enjoy a fuller balance and a more whole life.

Work Smarter, Not Harder

Phillip Itkin, MD, FAAP

At the April 2004 SuperCME in Orlando, FL, I discussed some practice tips that, if incorporated into a physician's life, should enhance his or her quality of practice and the quality of life. We can be more successful by bringing balance to our lives—professionally and personally. Our patients prefer a medical home that is efficiently run by caring, happy, and satisfied practitioners.

You can divide your work and life into 5 areas: (1) family, (2) work, (3) health, (4) friends, and (5) spirituality. These are in no particular order; you can place them in the order you find best and then bring them into balance. I am summarizing my talk with bullet-pointed items.

Work

- Aim to run your office smoothly, efficiently, and profitably.
- Hire employees to expect excellence in their work. Incorporate this in office manuals, training, meetings, and discipline.
- Diversity of employees helps patients and other staff to be more at ease and sensitive of others' cultural, ethnic, and gender-driven points of view.
- Delineate a chain of command to allow the physician to spend time with patients rather than with tasks others can handle.
- Trusted, bonded employees should handle accounts under careful supervision of a managing partner.
- Regular collection procedures should be followed to ensure a regular flow of money to the practice (and by extension to the practitioners).
- Provide comfort, convenience, compassion, consistency, competence, and value for patient services.
- Schedule flexibly and appropriately—this keeps patients, staff, and family happy. It reduces hassles and still will ensure patients' needs are met and enough income generated.
- Use staff wisely. Extenders can see more patients. Have staff do what they are capable of. Do not have a nurse do what a certified medical assistant can do at half the price. Time-sharing of positions may give you a greater flexibility with personnel and hold down benefit packages.
- Invest wisely at work. Get new equipment to expedite care or obtain a new stream of revenue. Practices that invest in themselves tend to have higher net revenues.
- Allow and encourage credit card usage. This is less expensive than billing for services rendered.
- Collect all co-pays before seeing patients unless there is a true emergency.
- Charge interest on account receivables in conformity with state laws.
- Use a collection agency. The average pediatrician has $6,100 in bad debt per year. Once you have turned over a patient, quit seeing that patient in the future. Keep collections under 120 days, as collections fall drastically after this time period.
- Fund pension plans, flexible savings plans, educational savings accounts, or 529 plans for children's education. These can go a long way toward making your life less stressful.
- Avoid credit card debt.
- Don't get insurance poor. Reprice and rebid your policies routinely.
- Use professional advice from your accountant and lawyer.
- Coding properly is the easiest way to maximize revenue. Attend American Academy of Pediatrics (AAP) coding conferences when offered.
- Participate in the management of your practice. Be part of decisions concerning contracts, schedules, income splits, etc.
- Spouses, as a general rule, should not be in the office, as they can easily disrupt relationships, create jealousy, and cause hard feelings.
- Mentor or get mentored to understand the history of the practice and how things run. Sources for practice management information are available at www.aap.org or the AAP Section on Administration and Practice Management Web site. Remember, reinventing the wheel is expensive and time-consuming.

Family, Health, Friends, Spirituality

- To feel more involved in life away from the white coat and stethoscope, ensure your schedule allows time. If you have trouble finding time, schedule it! Each member of our practice takes a full day off every week and it's inviolate.

- Break up your routines to avoid burnout.
- Do regular workouts.
- Schedule an afternoon with your spouse.
- Do an activity with friends.
- Volunteer at your church, mosque, or synagogue.

Keeping a balance with work, health, family, spirituality, and friends will let you work smarter, not harder.

Physician Satisfaction: Improving Your Work Environment

Margie Andreae, MD, FAAP

For many health care providers, delivering services is more difficult and stressful than ever. Our workloads have increased, leaving little flexibility in our schedules and creating more hassles. We feel pressured to meet patient and productivity demands while at the same time, reimbursement for our services and the cost of health care threaten our job security.

How do we recapture our enthusiasm for medicine and make our practice more rewarding?

The following practical and easy-to-implement strategies are a culmination of ideas that have been gathered from the literature, seminars, and speaking to many practicing clinicians.

Time Management

- Determine your priorities then adjust your schedule to reflect your priorities.
  - If attending a monthly education session or class in the gym is important to you, then work with your partners to build your schedule around this. It may mean that you will need to be willing to accommodate their request.
- Determine what's important.
  - Review your schedule with these questions in mind
    1. Is this a high priority for me?
    2. What, if anything, will happen if I do less of this?
    3. Can I delegate this to someone else?
    4. In 3 years, will my doing this matter to anyone?
- Block your tasks.
  - Nonurgent paperwork.
  - Return phone calls.
  - Prescription refills.
- Be more efficient on the phone.
  - Delegate calls to assistants.
  - Provide effective written instructions to patients to avoid call backs.
  - Write legibly (saves calls from pharmacies).

Hassle-Free Work Environment

- Support your staff.
  - Keep good staff at all costs. Use non-monetary rewards/recognition. Buy them lunch.
  - Remember the "I CARE" of staff values.

Input	ask for their ideas
Consistency	maintain an even temper
Attention	acknowledge by name
Recognition	reward performance
Empathy	be aware of their challenges

- Model the behavior you want staff to exhibit.

Effective Communication

- Build rapport with patients.
- Stick to your schedule. Learn to say no to additional requests from patients, amid others that are not necessary or urgent.
- Find opportunities to enhance your professional challenge.
  - Mentor a resident or student.
  - Participate on committees of interest.
  - Have a hobby.

Career Transitions

Negotiating Change: Making the Switch From Practice to Administration

Peter D. Wallace, MD, MS, FAAP

Do it? Or not?

Many of our pediatric colleagues have made the switch from clinical practice to administration. Some have done it full time, while others have opted for part time. Most have made this dramatic career decision with forethought and some have done it quickly and rashly.

Making the switch from practice to administration involves 3 important stages: (1) thought, (2) preparation, and (3) implementation. The first is the most important and time-consuming and requires research and self-evaluation. It is beneficial to talk with physician executives about their jobs, what made them make the switch, and their satisfaction with it. Your family and colleagues also can provide you with ideas and insight. The American College of Physician Executives (ACPE—http://www.acpe.org) has a wealth of information, including the publications *The Physician Executive*, edited by Wesley Curry, and *Hope for the Future*, by Barbara Linney.

More important is the soul-searching that is crucial in contemplating a career change. Two distinct thoughts will occur to you—am I doing this because of a positive motivation or because of dissatisfaction with my present situation? Most physicians move into administration because of a motivation for the change. Several factors attend here; the most prominent is the challenge inherent in taking on different issues in a different venue using different skills. Many wish to take a leadership role in dealing with the ever-present changes around us. Some look at a desire for professional growth. Others genuinely feel that they can make an impact on health care at a higher level than in their offices. A smaller number choose to change because of a dissatisfaction element. Competition may be forcing practices to contract or to be unpleasant. Some may feel stale and tired of doing the same thing every day. Some may feel unable to keep up with the changes in practice and the limitations imposed by third parties. Others may be attracted to the concept of more regular hours with no call.

The second stage involves the process of preparing oneself for a transition. This stage requires a plan and may be expensive. Many of my executive colleagues and I dabbled in seminars, books, and meetings with and about physician executives. These activities were part of the first stage to contemplate and make a decision; however, they are also very helpful in educating the clinician on the necessary skills and exposing the clinician to the milieu in which they will find themselves.

Another area of preparation involves experience in management, such as participating in the American Academy of Pediatrics in chapters, committees, and sections; directing or managing your office or division; serving on hospital committees; or holding a leadership position with an independent practice association, physician hospital organization, or health maintenance organization (HMO). These experiences will help provide you with a more complete picture of the executive without making a commitment and will serve you well when you are job hunting.

Formal education also is beneficial in preparing for the career change. An MBA or similar degree was not important 15 years ago, but now most recruiters insist on it, especially for the full-time positions. Formal, degree-granting graduate business programs are available throughout the country with many specifically designed for physicians. Many of these programs are conducted extensively on the Internet and accommodate part-time on-campus attendance. I received my graduate degree at the University of Wisconsin (affiliated with the ACPE), which was fabulous training for me as a vice president of medical affairs. There are alternatives to obtaining a business degree. The ACPE offers a series of courses called "Physicians in

Management" and a number of meetings and educational experiences in print and through the Internet. Unfortunately, these and other introductory courses do not supply the depth that a graduate program provides. In addition to business education, many physician executive positions require 3 or more years of clinical practice and board eligibility or certification.

Now, you've decided to go for it. Consider several steps. The first might be to become aware of, and inquire into, a position in your area, such as a hospital, clinic system, insurance agency, or HMO. Go through the process or inquiry, resume and curriculum vitae (CV) preparation, and interview. Respond to ads in *Pediatrics, The Physician Executive,* or hospital journals your chief executive officer can feed you. If the situation doesn't appeal to you at all, withdraw your name, clarify your feelings, and learn from the experience of being interviewed (something with which few clinicians have any experience).

A key point here is that executives must be prepared to move away from their community; if not initially, then when they desire advancement or a change in duties.

Let your hospital and clinic administrators know what your wishes are. Like the clinical side, health administrators have a network and can alert their own colleagues of your interest.

The already mentioned ACPE meetings and seminars are excellent venues to meet physician executives and inquire about opportunities. Prepare a resume or a CV and begin calling some physician executive search firms. There are several—I've worked with the Physician Executive Management Center in Tampa, Witt Kiefer, and Heidrick and Struggles. They can keep your inquiry on file (and in confidence if you wish), and will ask you for preferences such as job desires and locale.

You will find that the recruiters are fond of pediatricians. We are many times more represented than our 5% share of the physician population. For reasons not elaborated, our surgical friends are very underrepresented.

In sum: think carefully, talk with people, do your research and educate yourself, and talk with physician executives locally or through meetings. Do I regret the move? No, although I was very happy with my 25 years of clinical practice. I'm challenged on a different plane, and can see my work as affecting far more people than I ever could in my private practice.

Preretirement Checklist

Michael O'Halloran, MD, FAAP; Jerold M. Aronson, MD, FAAP; and Avrum Katcher, MD, FAAP
Excerpt from the Closing a Practice Handbook

This section provides an overview of various considerations associated with retirement. Many of the organizational issues listed herein will happen automatically; they are included because this list is partly generated from the experiences of already-retired physicians who think a comprehensive list such as this would have helped them. This is not meant to substitute for discussions with your department chair, the institution medical director, or the human resources department. There can be some complexity to this process, having to do in part with personal circumstances and federal guidelines. Therefore, this overview will necessarily deal in generalities.

Also included is a template for recording information that is personal and possibly important to a person's family on one's death.

This material was prepared by Michael O'Halloran, MD, FAAP, with revisions by Jerold M. Aronson, MD, FAAP; American Academy of Pediatrics (AAP) Section for Senior Members (SFSM) webmaster; and Av Katcher, MD, FAAP, AAP SFSM chairperson.

Insurance and Retirement Funds

Department of Human Resources (Employer): If you are working where there is such a department, it is likely to be of considerable help with retirement plans and should be contacted.

Health Insurance: After retirement, clinics and organizations will sometimes continue to help pay for this. For example, premiums might be paid for you and possibly your spouse until death, subject to age and years of service rules. If you retire prior to eligibility for Medicare, ask about Consolidated Omnibus Budget Reconciliation Act (COBRA) insurance from your employer.

Dental Insurance: The same. Depending on your circumstances, if your coverage ends, you might consider COBRA depending on your circumstances.

Life Insurance: The same, but a conversion option may also be available.

Long-term Disability Insurance: The same, also with the possible availability of a conversion option.

Retirement Plans, Individual Retirement Accounts (IRAs): You will likely need to contact your pension carrier about this. Your plan may have special rules with which you will need to comply. Also, several distribution options are usually available. These areas of legal and financial planning may require consultation with specialists in elder law or estate planning. To learn more about elder law, view the information at public interest elder law groups such as the Connecticut Legal Services Elder Law Project (http://www.ctelderlaw.org/) or the Elder Law Center of the Coalition of Wisconsin Aging Groups (http://cwag.org/), or resources of the American Association of Retired Persons (AARP) http://www.aarp.org/.

Health Care Spending Account: If you have such an account, you should learn whether there are special retirement rules depending on such things as your organization's fiscal year and your actual date of retirement.

Social Security: If you are old enough to receive benefits, you'll need to check with your Social Security office. Contact the office at least 90 days prior to retirement to discuss the initiation of benefits. Consider and make arrangements via direct deposit for your bank to receive your Social Security income electronically.

Medicare: Timely application is essential. Delays in applying, if age eligible, can result in delays in benefits and higher premiums (eg, Part D—Prescription Drugs).

Malpractice Insurance: The 2 issues that must be addressed are arranging for tail coverage should a claim be brought against you after retirement and professional liability coverage in the event you choose to perform part-time or volunteer medical work. Tail coverage requirements depend, in part, on whether your current insurance is for *claims made* or *occurrence*. The former refers to when a claim is filed by the attorney. The latter refers to when the patient about whom the claim is filed was actually treated. In any event, check directly with your current malpractice insurer to assess your specific needs. When you check, also note the financial stability of your current malpractice insurer and inquire about arrangement for claims payment in the event of bankruptcy. Your state department of insurance or state medical society may also help in this area. Many arrangements may be available to you depending on your circumstances. As to the need for professional liability insurance for volunteer work, you may be eligible for free malpractice coverage. Check with your existing malpractice carrier or contact your state department of health.

For more information, see the Fidelity Preretirement Checklist (http://personal.fidelity.com/planning/retirement/content/pre-retirement_checklist.shtml) on Social Security, pension benefits, Medicare, and estate planning.

Organizational Issues

If you are part of or employed by a medical organization, there are often several steps to take for a smooth retirement (in addition to contacting your human resources department for matters mentioned previously).

1. Contact your department chair, department supervisor, and medical director. This is especially important when your retirement will require recruiting a replacement or changes in support staff. In some organizations the actual retirement date is only established after considering the needs of the department, organization, and retiree.
2. An exit interview with the leadership of your group may be an option.
3. Attend to mailing address, phone number, and e-mail address changes.
4. Contact medical staff secretaries of hospitals with which you are affiliated.
5. There may be ways to maintain some contact with your colleagues, clinics, or hospitals after retirement. Making contact with someone in your group who has already retired will usually be helpful.
6. If your group has an information systems department, you may need to contact the department director.
7. Notify your mail room.
8. Contact your financial services payroll person.

9. Determine whether there are any continuing privileges such as access to doctor's parking at the hospital or clinic, e-mail, or access to a fax machine.
10. Learn whether there are special arrangements for vacation benefits during the retirement year.

Personal Issues

In addition to the previous issues, you may want to consider taking care of some of these more personal matters.

1. Get a physical examination. Be sure that you have established a long-term relationship with a medical home that includes a personal physician of your choice, whom you respect and with whom you get along well. Be sure that this physician and the practice will continue to care for you as a Medicare recipient.
2. Execute appropriate financial and health care powers of attorney.
3. Seek financial and estate planning advice (eg, money manager, financial planner, accountant, lawyer). A financial advisor can help you learn about special opportunities available to you (eg, the place for use of Roth IRAs).
4. Learn about financial planning software (http://www.aap.org/sections/seniormembers/docs/finplancht.pdf), Web resources, and how to select a financial advisor from the AAP SFSM Web site. Visit http://estate.findlaw.com/estate-planning/estate-planning-overview/estate-planning-overview-process-checklist.html to view an estate planning checklist from the American Bar Association. Estate planning seminars are also available, but while some are excellent, others turn out to be sales pitches, so be careful.
5. Review and update your will, living will/health care proxies/advance health directives, durable powers of attorney, and estate plans. General attorneys do this, of course, but there are those who specialize in estate law and elder law.
6. Notify your academic and professional groups about your retirement and decide whether to volunteer to help, continue under a retiree status, or cancel. Remember, the AAP offers a reduced membership fee status as an AAP Retired Fellow or AAP Emeritus Fellow. Fellows who are at least 65 years of age and have been an AAP member for 30 years or more are eligible for Emeritus Fellow. Emeritus Fellows receive a discount on dues.

Fellows who are at least 55 years of age, have been an AAP member for 5 years or more, and no longer derive income from professional activities are eligible for Retired Fellow. For more information, check with the AAP at 800/433-9016, ext 5897.

7. Consider volunteering your medical expertise or child advocacy skills. Licensing and liability issues are different for each state. Check with your AAP chapter or your state department of health. Find information about volunteering in the Opportunities section of the AAP SFSM Web site (www.aap.org/sections/seniormembers/ opportunities/opportunities.htm).

8. Remain active in the AAP with the SFSM. The section mission is to "provide opportunities for our members to remain involved with the AAP in a meaningful way, to foster the growth and development of younger members through effective mentorship, and to provide experience and resources that will support our members as they make transitions in their personal and professional lives." Visit the AAP SFSM Web site to see the variety of contributions you can continue to make to children and the ways in which the AAP can continue to serve you.

9. Depending on your age, you may want get information about Social Security and Medicare. Many issues can come up relating to your situation, and application needs to be made several months ahead.

10. Web site help—there are many such sites. Among them are www.nolo.com for estate planning and www.medicare.gov for Medicare. AARP (www. aarp.org) also maintains a good Web site. Don't forget the AAP SFSM Web site at www.aap.org/ sections/seniormembers! Check out the Living Well and Health & Fitness sections to aid in planning your retirement.

11. Check out other opportunities depending on your inclination. These are all over the place and include hospital committees, state specialty organizations, local free clinic boards, health-related boards such as United Cerebral Palsy, local arts boards, hospital advisory committees, assisting in research projects, political activities, university courses, and courses from retirement organizations.

12. Compose or update a document or letter to help your heirs and personal representative on your death. Such documents include, but are not limited to, vital personal information such as Social Security, bank, trusts, and location of resources and important documents. They may also include an inventory or description of where everything is kept, bank safe deposit box, or where in the home things are located. Be certain that your heirs receive these documents in sufficient time to discuss them with you to understand your specific wishes after death, or in the event one or both of you are not competent or one or both of you are in a state such that care should be withdrawn except for relief of discomfort. Note that this may be in addition to your will but will provide your heirs with information about immediate action steps that may be required and a guide to accomplishing them in accordance with your wishes. Visit Template for Recording Important Personal Information at http://www.aap.org/sections/ seniormembers for tips.

Appendices

Supplies Needed to Start a Practice

Coker Publishing Company and modified by Somerset Pediatric Practice, PA

This checklist includes 3 sample lists of the various supplies needed to start a medical practice. Tab 1 outlines the medical office supplies, tab 2 the office supplies needed, and tab 3 the equipment.

Medical Supply Checklist (Tab 1)

Item	Qty	Cost	Item	Qty	Cost
INSTRUMENTS			**FORCEPS (cont)**		
Blades and Handles			Nail Clipper		
Cervical Biopsy Punch			Nasal Specula		
Cervical Tenaculum			Needle Holders		
Circumcision Clamp			Pelvimeter		
Cutaneous Punch			Rectal Probe and Hooks		
Ear Curettes			Rectal Specula		
Ear Piercer			Rectal Suction Tube		
Ear Spoon and Hook			Retractors		
Ear Syringe			Scalpels, Disposable		
Eye, Needle, and Spud			**SCISSORS**		
Fingernail Drill			Bandage Dissecting		
Finger Ring Cutter			Iris		
FORCEPS			Operating		
Dressing			Stitch		
Ear			Tuning Forks		
Hemostatic			Uterine Curette		
Mosquito			Uterine Sounds		
Splinter			Urethral Sound		
Sponge Holding			**STERILIZATION, DISINFECTION, AND CLEANERS**		
Tissue					
Towel			Autoclave Test Record		
Uterine			Air Deodorizers		
Hemorrhoidal Ligator			Dialdehyde Solution		
IUD Extractor			Disinfectant/Deodorant Spray		
Laryngoscopes			Foam Surface Cleaners		

This sample document is provided only as a reference for practices developing their own materials and may be adapted to local needs. This document may or may not represent official American Academy of Pediatrics (AAP) policy or guidelines and the AAP is not responsible for its use. You should consult an attorney who is knowledgeable about the laws of the jurisdiction in which you practice before creating or using any legal documents.

Medical Supply Checklist (Tab 1) (continued)

Item	Qty	Cost
STERILIZATION, DISINFECTION, AND CLEANERS (cont)		
Germicidal Solution		
Heat Sealer		
Instrument Lubricant		
Instrument Sterilization		
Sterilization Monitors, Strips/Tape/Sheets		
Sterilizer Forceps		
Sterilizing Record Systems		
Ultrasonic Cleaners		
Ultrasonic Solutions		
SYRINGES AND NEEDLES		
Allergist Packs		
Destruction Devices		
Hypodermic Needles		
Special Procedure Needles		
Syringe/Needle Combinations		
SYRINGES		
Allergy		
Control		
Insulin		
Irrigation		
Tuberculin		
Utility		
Trays, Special Procedure		
LABORATORY SUPPLIES		
Labels, Precut		
Latex Tubing		
Markers		
Media, Plated		
MICROSCOPE		
Cover Glasses		
Slides		
Mixer, Orbital Motion		
pH Paper		
PIPETTES		
Blood Diluting, Red Blood Cell/White Blood Cell		
Lambda, Disposable		
Sahli		
Transfer		
Pipetter Shaker/Washer		

Item	Qty	Cost
PIPETTES (cont)		
Plastic Laboratory Ware		
Potassium Analyzer		
Prothrombin Meter/Supplies		
Reagent Strips, Dip, & Read		
Refractometer		
Refrigerator		
Rh View Box		
Rotator		
Sedimentation Apparatus		
Serology Analyzer		
Serum Separation Tubes		
Specimen Collectors, Urine/Feces		
Stool, Laboratory		
Thyroid Function Tester		
Timers, Ty Systems, Laboratory		
TUBES		
Capillary		
Centrifuge		
Hematocrit		
Sedimentation Apparatus		
Serum Separation Tubes		
Urinalysis Reagent Strips/Tablets		
Urinometer		
Water Bath		
BIOLOGICALS, INJECTABLES		
Biologicals		
Chemicals		
Injectables		
Liquids		
Ointments and Creams		
Tablets and Capsules		
Miscellaneous		
DRESSINGS		
Adherent Wrap		
Adhesive Closures		
Adhesive Pads, Sterile		
Adhesive Strips, Patches, Spots		
Adhesive Tapes		
Adhesive Tape Remover, Pad/Spray		
Ammonia Inhalant Pads		
Benzoin Spray		

Medical Supply Checklist (Tab 1) (continued)

Item	Qty	Cost	Item	Qty	Cost
DRESSINGS			**SUNDRIES (cont)**		
Butterfly Closures			Cotton-Tipped Applicators		
Combine Dressings			Diaphragms		
Conforming Bandages			Dilators, Rectal/Vaginal		
Cotton or Rayon Balls			Diapers		
Cotton Rolls			Disinfectant/Deodorant Spray		
Elastic Tape			Dressing Jars, Stainless Steel or Glass		
Eye Pads			Ear Basin		
Finger Splints (Decorative)			Finger Cots		
First Aid Kit			Flashlights		
Flame Photometer			Forceps Jar		
Gauze Bandages			Gloves, Examination/Surgical		
Gauze Dressings			Gloves, Latex		
Gauze Packing Strips			Hand Lotion		
Gauze Sponges			Instrument Trays, Stainless Steel w/o Cover		
Glucose Tolerance Test			Intrauterine Devices		
Hematocrit Tube Reader			Labels		
Hematocrit Tube Sealer			Lubricating Jelly		
Hemolysis Applicators			Markers, Waterproof		
Incontinent Cleaners			Nebulizers		
Inoculating Loop and Holder			Organizers and Bins		
Inoculating Loop Sterilizer			Patient Bibs		
Ointment Dressings			Pillow Cases		
Lubricating Jelly			Room Deodorizers		
Merthiolate Spray			Sanitary Napkins/Belts		
Non-adherent Dressings			Sheets, Paper		
Patellar-stabilizing Knee Sleeves of Various Sizes			Sigmoidoscope Applicators		
Petrolatum Gauze			Signs and Signage		
Spray On Dressings			Silver Nitrate Applicators		
Topical Anesthetic Spray			Soap, Lotion/Bar		
Topical Skin Freeze Spray			Straws, Drinking		
Towelettes			Sundry Jars With Lids, Labeled		
Transparent Dressing			Table Paper and Holder		
Tubular Gauze			Tape Measures		
Velcro Wrist Splints			Tapewriter		
Wound Closure Strips			Thermometer Holder/Sheathes		
SUNDRIES			Thermometers, Oral and Rectal		
Alcohol Dispenser			Toilet Tissue		
Atomizer			Tubing, Latex		
Bags, Doctors, Nurses, EMT			Tongue Depressors		
Batteries, General Use					

Medical Supply Checklist (Tab 1) (continued)

Item	Qty	Cost
SUNDRIES (cont)		
Towels, Paper/Dispenser		
Wash Cloths		
Wood Applicators		
PAPER AND PLASTIC PRODUCTS		
Capes, Examination		
Cup Dispenser		
Cups, Paper and Plastic		
Drape Sheets		
Face Masks		
Facial Tissues		
Gowns, Examination		
Labels, Medical		
Laboratory Coat		
Medicine Cups		
Office Coat, Disposable		
LABORATORY SUPPLIES		
Automatic Pipettes		
Bacteria Identification System		
BLOOD COLLECTION		
Chair		
Lancets		
Needles and Holders		
Prep Applicators		
Syringe/Needle		
Tourniquet		
Vacuum Tubes		
Blood Glucose Monitor/Strips		
Blood Grouping/Typing Strips		
Blood Grouping Slides		
Cervical Scraper		
Coagulating Cups/Tips		
Cytological Fixative		
Detergent, Laboratory		
DIAGNOSTIC SCREENING TESTS		
Gonorrhea		
Meningitis		
Mononucleosis		
Occult Blood		

Item	Qty	Cost
DIAGNOSTIC SCREENING TESTS (cont)		
Pregnancy		
Rheumatoid Factor		
Rubella		
Sickle Cell		
Streptococcus		
Syphilis		
ORTHOPEDIC		
Ankle Supports		
Ankle Wrap		
Arm Slings		
CAST		
Boots		
Padding		
Walking Heels		
Cervical Collar		
Clavicle Strap		
Colles Splint		
Elastic Bandages		
Felt		
Fiberglass Casts		
Finger Splints, Assorted		
Head Halter		
Knee Immobilizers		
Lumbosacral Support		
PLASTER		
Apron		
Bandages		
Knife		
Shears		
Splints		
Rib Belts		
Shoulder Immobilizer		
Casting System		
Traction Kit		
Tubular Bandages/Stockinette		
Wrist Supports		

This sample office supply list was reprinted with permission from Coker Publishing Company and modified by Somerset Pediatric Practice, PA. This checklist is meant to serve as a guide and only contains suggestions, as some of these items may not be needed in your practice.

Office Supply Checklist (Tab 2)

Item	Qty	Cost	Item	Qty	Cost
Health Care Financing Administration 1500 Claim Forms			Scissors		
Copier/Fax Paper			Desk Calendars		
Printed Billing Statements			Letter Trays		
Pens and Pencils			Door Pockets		
Patient Chart Folders			Electric Pencil Sharpener		
Post-it Notes			Coil Pen (for Reception Desk)		
Cellophane Tape			Light Bulbs		
Stapler			Petty Cash Box		
Staples			Bulletin Board		
Staple Remover			Thumb Tacks		
Paper Clips (Assorted Sizes)			Rubber Bands (Assorted)		
Manila Envelopes			Stamp Pads		
Memo Pads			Wall Clock		
Wite-Out			Letter Openers		
Tape Dispensers			Expandable Paper Sorter		
Clip Boards			Lined Pads		
Manila File Folders			Index Card File		
File Folder Index Sheets			Pen and Pencil Holders		
Hanging Folders			CDs or Memory Sticks		
Year Labels			Liquid Glue Stick		
Alpha Tabs (for Chart Folders)			Money Box With Lock		
2-Hole Punch			Step Stool		
3-Hole Punch			Mop/Broom		
Paper Clip Holders			Message Holder		
Binder Clips (Assorted Sizes)			Highlighters		
Prescription Pads			Rulers		
Envelopes			Stamps		

This sample office supply list was reprinted with permission from Coker Publishing Company and modified by Somerset Pediatric Practice, PA. This checklist is meant to serve as a guide and only contains suggestions, as some of these items may not be needed in your practice.

Equipment Checklist (Tab 3)						
Item	**Qty**	**Cost**		**Item**	**Qty**	**Cost**
Examination Tables				Toolbox With Assorted Tools		
Procedure Table				Extension Cords		
Handheld Pulse Oximeter				ENT Wall Unit		
Autoclave				Ophthalmoscope		
Microscope				Otoscope		
EKG Machine				Wall Unit Sphygmomanometer		
Executive Desks (Physicians and Managers)				Outpatient Examination Light		
Credenza				MidMark Spin Stool		
Refrigerator (Vaccinations)				Two Section X-ray Viewbox		
Refrigerator (Staff)				Tycos Stethoscope		
Fax Machine				Mayo Stands		
High-Volume Copy Machine				Infant Scale		
File Cabinet				Adult Scale		
Front Office Chairs				Eye Chart		
Back Office Chairs				Double Lock Narcotics Cabinet		
Bookcases				Handheld Cobalt Blue Light		
Reception Chairs				Pelvic Light		
End Tables				Digital Thermometers		
Break Table				Pulmonary Function Unit		
Parson Table				Biohazard Trash Hampers		
Step Stool With Handle				Wheelchair		
Coffee Maker				EKG Stand/Utility Cart		

This sample office supply list was reprinted with permission from Coker Publishing Company and modified by Somerset Pediatric Practice, PA. This checklist is meant to serve as a guide and only contains suggestions, as some of these items may not be needed in your practice.

Sample Employee Handbook Outline

Note: a full sample employee handbook can be found on Practice Management Online at http://practice.aap.org/content.aspx?aID=2091

Table of Contents

Table of Contents (cont)

This sample document was created by Catawba Pediatric Associates, P.A. It is provided only as a reference for practices developing their own materials and may be adapted to local needs. This document does not represent official American Academy of Pediatrics (AAP) policy or guidelines and the AAP is not responsible for its use. You should consult an attorney who is knowledgeable about the laws of the jurisdiction in which you practice before creating or using any legal documents.

Staff Evaluations: Guidelines and Instructions

Performance Appraisal: _____

Evaluation Period: From _____ to _____

Evaluators: _____

1. Performance appraisals are an important and effective tool. They are an opportunity for a manager and employee to discuss an individual's performance over the past 6 to 12 months, offer positive recognition where appropriate, as well as identify areas that require improvement.

2. The coordinator with direct supervision of the administrator will be responsible for completing the evaluation with input from the physician staff.

3. Comments should be made on all assigned ratings that are greater than 3.5 and less than 2.00.

4. The rating guide we are using is

   4.00 Frequently Exceeds Requirements: Performance frequently exceeds the expectations of the job requirements and the individual demonstrates self-motivation and initiative in accomplishing tasks. This category is to be used for strong performances.

   3.00 Meets All Requirements: Performance meets the reasonable requirements of and usual expectations for assigned responsibilities. Generally evidences self-motivation and accomplishes tasks within scope of responsibility.

   2.00 Meets Most Requirements: Performance meets most requirements for the position. This category is to be used for employees who are learning their jobs or have assumed new responsibilities or where a plan of action is in place to correct any performance deficiencies.

   1.00 Meets Minimal Requirements: Performance meets just the minimal requirement for the position. The employee should know the duties but elects to meet them only minimally.

   0.00 Does Not Meet Requirements: Performance does not meet minimum requirements and is unacceptable. Requires a greater degree of supervision and follow-up than can be expected. Substantial improvement and corrective action is required.

5. An employee with an overall rating of less than 2.00 must be reevaluated in 3 months. If the employee fails to achieve the minimum standard within the 3-month time frame, termination of employment may occur.

Staff Evaluations: Template

Name: _____

Front Office

Criteria	Evaluator #1	Evaluator #2	Evaluator #3	Average
Answer phones and retrieve voice mail in a timely manner.				
Schedule appointments in appropriate time slots.				
Register new patients into computer in timely manner.				
Verify demographics and insurance information regularly.				
Check in patients within 5 to 7 minutes of sign-in time.				
Collect co-payment and print receipt for patients as needed.				
Post all charges and payments before end of shift.				
Prove out money at end of shift.				
Communicate with business office when needed.				
Confirm appointment schedule and document results.				
Scan all paperwork on a regular basis.				
Handle patient complaints and concerns.				
Get information requested by doctors in a timely manner.				
Maintain waiting room for a tidy appearance.				
Communicate professionally with coordinator in office and other staff members.				
Use downtime appropriately and professionally (eg, filing).				
Accept change in a positive and cooperative manner.				
Work well with colleagues; enhance teamwork in the office.				
Attendance/Reliability				
OVERALL AVERAGE				

Employee Comments:

SIGNATURE

This sample document was created by Somerset Pediatric Group. It is provided only as a reference for practices developing their own materials and may be adapted to local needs. This document does not represent official American Academy of Pediatrics (AAP) policy or guidelines and the AAP is not responsible for its use. You should consult an attorney who is knowledgeable about the laws of the jurisdiction in which you practice before creating or using any legal documents.

Sample Financial Policy

OFFICE FINANCIAL POLICY

Our goal is to provide and maintain a good physician-patient relationship. Letting you know in advance of our office policy allows for a good flow of communication and enables us to achieve our goal. Please read this carefully and if you have any questions, please do not hesitate to ask a member of our staff.

1. On arrival, please sign in at the front desk and present your current insurance card at every visit. You will be asked to sign and date the file copy of the card. This is your verification of the correct insurance and consent to bill them on your child's behalf. IF THE INSURANCE COMPANY THAT YOU DESIGNATE IS INCORRECT, YOU WILL BE RESPONSIBLE FOR PAYMENT OF THE VISIT AND TO SUBMIT THE CHARGES TO THE CORRECT PLAN.
2. If we are your primary care physician, make sure our name or phone number appears on your card. If your insurance company has not been informed that we are your primary care physicians as of this date, you may be financially responsible for the visit.
3. According to your insurance plan, you are responsible for any and all co-payments, deductibles, and coinsurances.
4. We do not submit to secondary insurance plans. If you have secondary insurance, we will provide you with a receipt to submit for reimbursement. Your secondary insurance will send the reimbursement check directly to you. YOU ARE RESPONSIBLE FOR ANY BALANCE ON YOUR ACCOUNT.
5. It is your responsibility to understand your benefit plan. It is your responsibility to know if a written referral or authorization is required to see specialists, if preauthorization is required prior to a procedure, and what services are covered.
6. If our physicians do not participate in your insurance plan, payment in full is expected from you at the time of your office visit. For scheduled appointments, prior balances must be paid prior to the visit.
7. If you have no insurance, payment for an office visit is to be paid at the time of the visit.
8. Co-payments are due at time of service. A **$XX processing fee (or service fee)** will be charged in addition to your co-payment if the co-payment is not paid at time of service or by the end of the next business day.
9. Patient balances are billed immediately on receipt of your insurance plan's explanation of benefits. Your remittance is due *within* 10 business days of your receipt of your bill.
10. If previous arrangements have not been made with our finance office, any account balance outstanding greater than 28 days will be charged a $X re-bill fee. Any balance over 60 days will be forwarded to a collection agency.
11. If you participate with a high-deductible health plan, we require a copy of the health savings account debit/ credit card or a personal credit card remain on file. There are addenda to this financial policy, which are signed separately.
12. We require 24-hour notice for canceling any appointments. There is a **$XX** charge for weekday appointments and **$XX** charge for Saturday appointments if they are not canceled OR if 24-hour notice is not given.
13. A **$XX** fee will be charged for any checks returned for insufficient funds, plus any bank fees incurred.
14. We charge **$XX** per child to copy or transfer medical records.
15. If your child has school, camp, or sport forms to be completed, there is a **$XX** charge per form. Payment is due when the forms are dropped off. We have a 3- to 5-day turnaround time for forms. If a form is needed sooner than 3 days, there is an additional **$XX** *rush* fee.
16. Advance notice is needed for all non-emergent referrals, typically 3 to 5 business days. It is your responsibility to know if a selected specialist participates in your plan. Remember your primary care physician must approve referrals before being issued.

17. Before making an annual physical appointment, check with your insurance company whether the visit will be covered as a healthy visit. Not all plans cover annual healthy physicals or hearing and vision screenings. It is your responsibility to know your insurance plan benefits. If it is not covered, you will be responsible for payment at the time of visit.

18. Not all services provided by our office are covered by every plan. Any service determined to not be covered by your plan will be your responsibility.

I have read and understand this office financial policy and agree to comply and accept the responsibility for any payment that becomes due as outlined previously.

Patient Name(s)

Responsible party member's name _____

Relationship _____

Responsible party member's signature _____

Date _____

This sample document was created by Watchung Pediatrics. It is provided only as a reference for practices developing their own materials and may be adapted to local needs. This document does not represent official American Academy of Pediatrics (AAP) policy or guidelines and the AAP is not responsible for its use. You should consult an attorney who is knowledgeable about the laws of the jurisdiction in which you practice before creating or using any legal documents.

Patient Survey

Thank you for taking the time to complete this questionnaire. Our goal is to provide you with the best pediatric care possible. We appreciate you letting us know how we are doing. Your feedback helps us measure our performance so we may meet the high standards we set for ourselves.

Please Rate Our Scheduling.	Excellent	Good	Fair	Poor
For a sick-child visit: Able to get an appointment within a reasonable amount of time.				
For a well visit: Able to get an appointment within a reasonable amount of time.				
The convenience of our hours and available appointment times				
The ability to see the doctor of your choice				
The wait time to see your doctor or nurse was reasonable.				
	15–30 min	30–45 min	45–60 min	60+ min
Please estimate your wait time to see the physician.				
Please estimate the wait time to see a nurse.				
Comments:				

Please Rate Our Facilities.	Excellent	Good	Fair	Poor
The cleanliness and comfort of the office itself				
Our parking facilities				
Availability of adult reading materials and children's books or toys				
Comments:				

Please Rate the Courtesy, Helpfulness, and Knowledge of Our Staff.	Excellent	Good	Fair	Poor
Billing				
Receptionist				
Schedulers				
Nurse Treats you and your child in a caring, respectful manner				
Knowledge and ability				
Comments:				

Please Rate Our Communication.	Excellent	Good	Fair	Poor
Your ease in reaching our office by phone				
If your call required a return call from a nurse, the call was returned in a reasonable amount of time.				
If your call required a return call from a doctor, the call was returned in a reasonable amount of time.				
Quality of information or medical advice provided by phone				
Description of tests and procedures prior to performing them				
Timely reporting of your test and procedure results				
Our timeliness in completing any form or paperwork requests				
Keeping you informed of any delays with your appointment				
Comments:				

Please Rate Your Visit With the Doctor.	Excellent	Good	Fair	Poor
Courtesy of the doctor				
Doctor's patience and interest in your or your child's problem				
Explanations of diagnosis and treatment options				
The thoroughness of the examination				
Your overall satisfaction with the medical care you received				
Comments:				

Please Rate Your Overall Satisfaction With Our Practice.	Excellent	Good	Fair	Poor

Would you recommend this practice to a family member or friend?   ☐ Yes   ☐ No

How many years have you been a patient in our practice? _____

Have you visited our Web site?   ☐ Yes   ☐ No

Comments and suggestions: _____

_____

_____

_____

Optional Information	Date of Appointment	Appointment Time	Dr Seen

Name _____ Phone _____

This sample document was created by a pediatric practice. It is provided only as a reference for practices developing their own materials and may be adapted to local needs. This document does not represent official American Academy of Pediatrics (AAP) policy or guidelines and the AAP is not responsible for its use. You should consult an attorney who is knowledgeable about the laws of the jurisdiction in which you practice before creating or using any legal documents.

Parental Refusal to Vaccinate Form

Refusal to Vaccinate

Child's Name _____ Child's ID# _____

Parent's/Guardian's Name _____

My child's doctor/nurse, _____, has advised me that my child (named above) should receive the following vaccines:

Recommended		Declined
☐	Hepatitis B vaccine	☐
☐	Diphtheria, tetanus, acellular pertussis (DTaP or Tdap) vaccine	☐
☐	Diphtheria tetanus (DT or Td) vaccine	☐
☐	*Haemophilus influenzae* type b (Hib) vaccine	☐
☐	Pneumococcal conjugate or polysaccharide vaccine	☐
☐	Inactivated poliovirus (IPV) vaccine	☐
☐	Measles-mumps-rubella (MMR) vaccine	☐
☐	Varicella (chickenpox) vaccine	☐
☐	Influenza (flu) vaccine	☐
☐	Meningococcal conjugate or polysaccharide vaccine	☐
☐	Hepatitis A vaccine	☐
☐	Rotavirus vaccine	☐
☐	Human papillomavirus vaccine	☐
☐	Other _____	☐

I have read the Vaccine Information Statement from the Centers for Disease Control and Prevention explaining the vaccine(s) and the disease(s) it prevents. I have had the opportunity to discuss this with my child's doctor or nurse, who has answered all of my questions regarding the recommended vaccine(s). I understand the following:

- The **purpose** of and the need for the recommended vaccine(s).
- The **risks and benefits** of the recommended vaccine(s).
- If my child does not receive the vaccine(s) according to the medically accepted schedule, **the consequences** may include
  - Contracting the illness the vaccine should prevent (The outcomes of these illnesses may include one or more of the following: certain types of cancer, pneumonia, illness requiring hospitalization, death, brain damage, paralysis, meningitis, seizures, and deafness. Other severe and permanent effects from these vaccine-preventable diseases are possible as well.)
  - Transmitting the disease to others
  - Requiring my child to stay out of child care or school during disease outbreaks
- My child's doctor or nurse, the American Academy of Pediatrics, the American Academy of Family Physicians, and the Centers for Disease Control and Prevention all strongly recommend that the vaccine(s) be given according to recommendations.

Nevertheless, I have decided at this time to decline or defer the vaccine(s) recommended for my child, as indicated above, by checking the appropriate box under the column titled "Declined."

I know that failure to follow the recommendations about vaccination may endanger the health or life of my child and others with whom my child might come into contact.

I know that I may readdress this issue with my child's doctor or nurse at any time and that I may change my mind and accept vaccination for my child anytime in the future.

I acknowledge that I have read this document in its entirety and fully understand it.

Parent/Guardian Signature _____ Date _____

Witness _____ Date _____

I have had the opportunity to rediscuss my decision not to vaccinate my child and still decline the recommended immunizations.

Parent's initials _____ Date _____ Parent's initials _____ Date _____

Parent's initials _____ Date _____ Parent's initials _____ Date _____

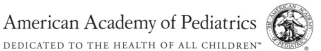

American Academy of Pediatrics

DEDICATED TO THE HEALTH OF ALL CHILDREN™

Parental Refusal to Accept Vaccination: Resources for Pediatricians

The following are some of the resources available to help pediatricians develop a productive dialogue with vaccine-hesitant parents and answer questions about vaccine risks and benefits:

Web Sites

1. **AAP Childhood Immunization Support Program (CISP)**
   Information for providers and parents.
   http://www.aap.org/immunization
2. **The Immunization Education Program (IEP) of the Pennsylvania Chapter of the American Academy of Pediatrics**
   Includes answers to common vaccine questions and topics, such as addressing vaccine safety concerns, evaluating anti-vaccine claims, sources of accurate immunization information on the Web, and talking with parents about vaccine safety.
   http://www.paiep.org
3. **The Immunization Action Coalition (IAC)**
   The IAC works to increase immunization rates by creating and distributing educational materials for health professionals and the public that enhance the delivery of safe and effective immunization services. Their "Unprotected People Reports" are case reports, personal testimonies, and newspaper and journal articles about people who have suffered or died from vaccine-preventable diseases.
   http://www.immunize.org/reports
4. **Centers for Disease Control and Prevention (CDC) National Immunization Program**
   Information about vaccine safety, including Parents' Guide to Childhood Immunizations.
   http://www.cdc.gov/vaccines/hcp.htm
5. **National Network of Immunization Information (NNii)**
   Includes the NNii Resource Kit—Communicating with Patients about Immunizations, a guide to help answer patients' questions and provide the facts about immunizations.
   www.immunizationinfo.org
6. **Vaccine Education Center at Children's Hospital of Philadelphia**
   Information for parents includes Common Concerns About Vaccines, Are Vaccines Safe, and A Look at Each Vaccine.
   www.vaccine.chop.edu
7. **Institute for Vaccine Safety, Johns Hopkins University**
   Provides an independent assessment of vaccines and vaccine safety to help guide decision-makers and educate physicians, the public, and the media about key issues surrounding the safety of vaccines.
   www.vaccinesafety.edu
8. **The Canadian Coalition for Immunization Awareness and Promotion (CCIAP)**
   CCIAP aims to meet the goal of eliminating vaccine-preventable disease through education, promotion, advocacy, and media relations. It includes resources for parents and providers, including "How to Advise Parents Unsure About Immunization" by Scott A. Halperin, MD.
   http://immunize.cpha.ca/en/default.aspx

Journal Articles

1. Ball LK, Evans G, Bostrom A. Risky business: challenges in vaccine risk communication. *Pediatrics*. 1998;101:453–458. Available at: http://www.pediatrics.org/cgi/content/full/101/3/453 (subscription needed)
2. Dias M, Marcuse EK. When parents resist immunizations. *Contemp Pediatr*. 2000;17:75–86
3. Offit PA, Jew RK. Addressing parents' concerns: do vaccines contain harmful preservatives, adjuvants, additives, or residuals? *Pediatrics*. 2003;112:1394–1397
4. Offit PA, Quarles J, Gerber MA, et al. Addressing parents' concerns: do multiple vaccines overwhelm or weaken the infant's immune system? *Pediatrics*. 2002;109:124–129
5. Diekema DS, American Academy of Pediatrics Committee on Bioethics. Responding to parental refusals of immunization of children. *Pediatrics*. 2005;115:1428–1431

Books

1. Offit PA, Bell LM. *Vaccines: What Every Parent Should Know*. New York, NY: IDG Books; 1999
2. Humiston SG, Good C. *Vaccinating Your Child: Questions and Answers for the Concerned Parent*. Atlanta, GA: Peachtree Publishers; 2000
3. Fisher MC. *Immunizations and Infectious Diseases: An Informed Parent's Guide*. Elk Grove Village, IL: American Academy of Pediatrics; 2005
4. Marshall GS. *The Vaccine Handbook: A Practical Guide for Clinicians*. 2nd ed. West Islip, NY: Professional Communications, Inc.; 2008

Reliable Immunization Resources for Parents

Web Sites

1. **AAP Childhood Immunization Support Program (CISP)**
   Information for providers and parents.
   http://www.aap.org/immunization
2. **Why Should I Immunize My Child?**
   A description of the individual diseases and the benefits expected from vaccination.
   http://www.aap.org/immunization/families/faq/whyimmunize.pdf
3. **The Immunization Education Program (IEP) of the Pennsylvania Chapter of the American Academy of Pediatrics**
   Includes answers to common vaccine questions and topics, such as addressing vaccine safety concerns, evaluating anti-vaccine claims, sources of accurate immunization information on the Web, and talking with parents about vaccine safety.
   http://www.paiep.org
4. **Centers for Disease Control and Prevention National Immunization Program**
   Information about vaccine safety, including Parents' Guide to Childhood Immunizations
   http://www.cdc.gov/vaccines/spec-grps/parents.htm
5. **National Network of Immunization Information (NNii)**
   Includes the NNii Resource Kit—Communicating with Patients about Immunizations, a guide to help answer patients' questions and provide the facts about immunizations.
   www.immunizationinfo.org
6. **Vaccine Education Center at Children's Hospital of Philadelphia**
   Information for parents includes Common Concerns About Vaccines, Are Vaccines Safe, and A Look at Each Vaccine.
   www.vaccine.chop.edu
7. **Institute for Vaccine Safety, Johns Hopkins University**
   Provides an independent assessment of vaccines and vaccine safety to help guide decision-makers and educate physicians, the public, and the media about key issues surrounding the safety of vaccines.
   www.vaccinesafety.edu
8. **The Canadian Coalition for Immunization Awareness and Promotion (CCIAP)**
   CCIAP aims to meet the goal of eliminating vaccine-preventable disease through education, promotion, advocacy, and media relations. It includes resources for parents and providers, including "How to Advise Parents Unsure About Immunization" by Scott A. Halperin, MD.
   http://immunize.cpha.ca/en/default.aspx
9. **Vaccinate Your Baby**
   The Every Child by Two site serves as a central resource of vaccine information for parents. The site links to the latest research and studies about vaccines, an interactive timeline on the benefits of vaccines, information about vaccine safety and ingredients, and the importance of adhering to the recommended schedule.
   www.vaccinateyourbaby.org

Books

1. Offit PA, Bell LM. *Vaccines: What Every Parent Should Know*. New York, NY: IDG Books; 1999
2. Humiston SG, Good C. *Vaccinating Your Child: Questions and Answers for the Concerned Parent*. Atlanta, GA: Peachtree Publishers; 2000
3. Fisher MC. *Immunizations and Infectious Diseases: An Informed Parent's Guide*. Elk Grove Village, IL: American Academy of Pediatrics; 2005

Local List of Possible Community Resources for Pediatric Practices

Pediatric practices can use this form to insert the names and contact information of local referral sources and family groups so that the information is readily available when needed.

EVALUATION AND DEVELOPMENTAL SERVICES

Early Intervention (EI) Program

EI Coordinator Name:	
Telephone Number:	
Fax Number:	
Email Address:	
Address:	

Developmental Pediatricians

	Name	Telephone	Fax	Address	Email Address
1					
2					
3					

Child Psychologists

	Name	Telephone	Fax	Address	Email Address
1					
2					
3					

Child Neurologists

	Name	Telephone	Fax	Address	Email Address
1					
2					
3					

Other Evaluation/Developmental Referral Sources (OT, PT, Speech, Audiology, etc)

	Name	Telephone	Fax	Address	Email Address
1					
2					
3					
4					
5					

Local List of Possible Community Resources for Pediatric Practices

Pediatric practices can use this form to insert the names and contact information of local referral sources and family groups so that the information is readily available when needed.

FAMILY ASSISTANCE AND FAMILY SUPPORT SERVICES

Family Voices State Contact

Name:	
Telephone:	
Fax:	
Email:	
Address:	

Family Resource Centers

	Name	Telephone	Fax	Address	Email Address
1					
2					
3					

Family Support Groups

	Name	Telephone	Fax	Address	Email Address
1					
2					
3					

Other Family Support Networks:

1					
2					
3					
4					
5					

Resources and contacts in your state can be found at http://www.medicalhomeinfo.org/states/index.html

Sample Waiver or Advance Beneficiary Notice (ABN)

Patient's name: _____

Insurance Co.: _____

Advance Beneficiary Notice (ABN)

Note: You will need to make a choice about receiving these health care items or services.

Your health insurance may not pay for the items or services that are described below. Health insurers do not necessarily pay for all of your health care costs. Insurance only pays for covered items and services. The fact that insurance may not pay for a particular service does not mean that you should not receive it, if your doctor recommends that you do receive this service.

Items or Services:

The purpose of this form is to help you make an informed choice about whether or not you want to receive these items or services, knowing that you might have to pay for them yourself. By signing below you agree to take financial responsibility for the cost of the items or services, if your health insurance does not include this as a covered items or services.

Responsible party signature: _____

Date: _____

This is a sample document. It is provided only as a reference for practices developing their own materials and may be adapted to local needs. This document does not represent official American Academy of Pediatrics (AAP) policy or guidelines and the AAP is not responsible for its use. You should consult an attorney who is knowledgeable about the laws of the jurisdiction in which you practice before creating or using any legal documents.

Template Letter: Appeal to Payers for Payment

NAME
STREET ADDRESS
CITY, STATE, ZIP

Re: PATIENT NAME

DATE

To Whom It May Concern:

I am writing to appeal your refusal to make payment on NAME OF PATIENT for INSERT DATE OF SERVICE. On this date of service the child was seen for INSERT REASON FOR VISIT. HIS/HER examination was significant for INSERT DIAGNOSIS AND JUSTIFICATION FOR EXAMINATION.

The charges that were filed with your company reflect the services rendered on that date. Attached please find the office notes documenting the services performed on this date of service. The primary reason for the child's visit was INSERT REASON FOR OFFICE VISIT. The INSERT APPROPRIATE CODE code is appropriate for the services provided. The SERVICE PROVIDED was required to properly diagnose this child's condition. Many major insurance plans now recognize this code and pay appropriately.

Your reconsideration and prompt payment of these charges is appreciated. Please contact my office should you require further assistance.

Sincerely,

NAME, CREDENTIALS

Template Letter: Unable to Continue Medical Care

Denise Doctor, MD
ABC Pediatric Group
1111 First St, Suite 200
Hometown, ST 54321
444/555-6666

<Date>

<Inside address>

Dear <Patient's Name:>

I regret to inform you that I will no longer be able to provide medical care to your children. If you require medical care within the next 30 days, I will be available, but will not be available to care for your children after <month, day, year>.

Please secure the care of another pediatrician. If you do not know another pediatrician, please call your health plan or the American Academy of Pediatrics Referral Program to locate a pediatrician in your area. To assist you in continuing to receive medical care, I will make a copy of your children's medical records available to the new pediatrician you designate.

After you have chosen another pediatrician, please complete and return the enclosed Authorization to Transfer Medical Records form.

If you have any concerns about this transition or need my help, please call my office. Again, I will be available to you for the next 30 days. After that time, my office will not be in a position to serve you. I extend to you best wishes for your future health and happiness.

Sincerely,

Denise Doctor, MD

Template Letter: Outstanding Patient Account Balance

[INSERT DATE]

PARENT/GUARDIAN NAME
ADDRESS
CITY, STATE ZIP

RE: ACCT #_____

Dear _____:

It has come to my attention that we have made several attempts to contact you by phone and mail about your outstanding account balance. If there has been a problem or you are unhappy with the care that your family has received, please contact me to discuss the situation. However, our attempts have gone unanswered; therefore, according to our office policy, [INSERT OUTCOME].

[IF OUTCOME IS OPPORTUNITY TO PAY—]We are providing you with a final opportunity to pay your balance within the next [X] days. If the balance is unpaid by [INSERT DATE], your account will be sent to [INSERT] for collections.

[IF OUTCOME IS DISMISSAL—]We will continue to provide care for your child(ren) for any emergent situations that may arise over the next 30 days, from the date of this letter. However, you should make arrangements to retain another physician to care for your child(ren) after those 30 days. Once you have identified a new pediatrician, please contact our office staff to request that your medical records be forwarded. If you need assistance locating a pediatrician, we can provide you with contact information for local pediatricians.

Please contact me at [(XXX) XXX-XXXX] if you have any questions or need to arrange a payment plan.

Sincerely,

Name
Title

This sample document was created by the Practice Management Online Editorial Advisory Board. It is provided only as a reference for practices developing their own materials and may be adapted to local needs. This document does not represent official American Academy of Pediatrics (AAP) policy or guidelines and the AAP is not responsible for its use. You should consult an attorney who is knowledgeable about the laws of the jurisdiction in which you practice before creating or using any legal documents.

Template Letter: Notification of Retirement or Closing a Practice

[DATE]

[INSIDE ADDRESS]

Dear [INSERT NAME OF PATIENT/PARENT]:

I have enjoyed the opportunity of being [INSERT NAME OF CHILD's] pediatrician. As some of my patient's families already know, I have decided to retire from clinical practice on [INSERT DATE]. [INSERT NAME OF PRACTITIONER(S)] have agreed to assume care of my patients on my retirement, if you wish to continue to bring your child to our practice. If you prefer to transfer care to another group, our staff will be able to assist you in transferring medical records to your new physician, with your consent. I wish you the very best of health and good fortune in the future and will always be grateful for your allowing me, as a pediatrician, to have been part of your child's and family's lives.

Sincerely,

Name of MD

This is a sample document. It is provided only as a reference for practices developing their own materials and may be adapted to local needs. This document does not represent official American Academy of Pediatrics (AAP) policy or guidelines and the AAP is not responsible for its use. You should consult an attorney who is knowledgeable about the laws of the jurisdiction in which you practice before creating or using any legal documents.

Additional Resources

- **Practice Management Online:**
  http://practice.aap.org
  - **Practice Basics:**
    http://practice.aap.org/topicBrowse.aspx?nodeID=1000
  - **Payment and Finance:**
    http://practice.aap.org/topicBrowse.aspx?nodeID=2000
  - **Office Operations:**
    http://practice.aap.org/topicBrowse.aspx?nodeID=3000
  - **Quality Improvement and Patient Safety:**
    http://practice.aap.org/topicBrowse.aspx?nodeID=8000
  - **Office Operations:**
    http://practice.aap.org/topicBrowse.aspx?nodeID=4000
  - **Practice Toolbox:**
    http://practice.aap.org/toolbox.aspx
  - **Sample Office Documents:**
    http://practice.aap.org/sampleofficedocs.aspx
  - **Sample Personnel Documents (including job descriptions):**
    http://practice.aap.org/samplepersonneldocs.aspx
  - **Template Letters:**
    http://practice.aap.org/templateletters.aspx
  - **Sample Employee Handbook:**
    http://practice.aap.org/content.aspx?aID=2091
  - **Sample Employment Contract:**
    http://practice.aap.org/content.aspx?aID=2100
- **AAP Pediatric Coding Newsletter Online:**
  http://coding.aap.org
- **Patient Education Online:**
  http://patiented.aap.org
- **Pediatric Care Online:**
  http://pediatriccareonline.org
- **PedJobs:**
  http://www.pedjobs.org
- **Quality Improvement Innovation Network:**
  http://quiin.aap.org
- **Education in Quality Improvement in Pediatric Practice (EQIPP):**
  www.eqipp.org
- **Chapter Alliance for Quality Improvement (CAQI):**
  www.aap.org/moc/chapters/caqi/index.html
- **Safer Health Care for Kids:**
  www.aap.org/saferhealthcare

AAP Practice Publications
(www.aap.org/bookstore)

- *AAP Pediatric Coding Newsletter*
- *Coding for Pediatrics 2010*
- *2010 Pediatric ICD-9-CM Coding Pocket Guide*
- *Quick Reference Card for Pediatric Coding and Documentation,* 5th ed.
- *Quick Reference Guide to Neonatal Coding and Documentation*
- *AAP Pediatric Visit Documentation Forms*
- *Pediatric Growth Charts*
- *Pediatric Telephone Protocols, Office Version,* 12th ed.
- *Adult Telephone Protocols, Office Version,* 2nd ed.
- *The Complete Guide: Developing a Telephone Triage and Advice System for a Pediatric Office Practice: During Office Hours and/or After-Hours*
- *The Complete Guide: Providing Telephone Triage and Advice in a Family Practice*
- *AAP Textbook of Pediatric Care: Tools for Practice*
- *Coding for Pediatric Preventive Care 2010*
- *Pediatric Patient Safety in the Emergency Department*
- *Socioeconomic Survey of Pediatric Practices*
- *HIPAA: A How-To Guide for Your Medical Practice*
- *Medical Liability for Pediatricians,* 6th ed.
- *Refusal to Vaccinate Form*
- *Vaccine Administration Record*
- *Short Medical Record*

AAP Practice-Oriented Sections and Councils
(http://www.aap.org/sections/sintro.htm)

- Council on Clinical Information Technology (COCIT)
- Section on Administration and Practice Management (SOAPM)
- Section on Telehealth Care (SOTC)

For a complete list of AAP section and councils, go to http://www.aap.org/sections/shome.htm.

Index